Aortopathy

Koichiro Niwa • Harald Kaemmerer
Editors

Aortopathy

Springer

Editors
Koichiro Niwa
Cardiovascular Center
St Luke's International Hospital
Tokyo, Japan

Harald Kaemmerer
ACHD Unit
German Heart Centre Munich
Munich, Bayern
Germany

ISBN 978-4-431-56069-2   ISBN 978-4-431-56071-5 (eBook)
DOI 10.1007/978-4-431-56071-5

Library of Congress Control Number: 2016963621

Printed on acid-free paper

This Springer imprint is published by Springer Nature
The registered company is Springer Japan KK
The registered company address is: Chiyoda First Bldg. East, 3-8-1 Nishi-Kanda, Chiyoda-ku, Tokyo 101-0065, Japan

Preface

Aortic ectasia and aneurysm formation is well recognized in Marfan syndrome, bicuspid aortic valve, and coarctation of the aorta, and these disorders are consistently associated with ascending aortic and/or para-coarctation medial abnormalities. However, medial abnormalities in the ascending aorta are also prevalent in other congenital heart anomalies, such as univentricular heart, persistent truncus arteriosus, transposition of the great arteries, hypoplastic left heart syndrome, and tetralogy of Fallot. They encompass a wide age range and may predispose to dilatation, aneurysm, and rupture necessitating aortic valve and root surgery or even death.

Aortic medial abnormalities – formerly often called "cystic medial necrosis" – reach their severest form in Marfan syndrome and annuloaortic ectasia. They are prevalent and qualitatively similar but seldom quantitatively as marked in a wide variety of congenital heart diseases with a wide age range.

These congenital heart anomalies exhibit ongoing ectasia of the aortic root, reduced aortic elasticity, and increased aortic stiffness that may relate to intrinsic properties of the aortic root. Aortic dilatation and increased stiffness can induce aortic aneurysm, aortic ulcerations, intramural hematoma, rupture of the aorta, and aortic regurgitation, but also provoke left ventricular hypertrophy, reduced coronary artery flow, and left ventricular failure. Therefore, the association of aortic pathophysiological abnormalities, aortic ectasia, and aorto-left ventricular interaction is a new clinical entity: "aortopathy."

For prevention and management of this type of aortic dilatation, the usefulness of beta-blockers and angiotensin II receptor blockers is not yet established.

As "aortopathy in congenital anomalies of the heart and the great vessels" is a new entity, this textbook *Aortopathy* is written in a comprehensive and educational style by international authors. The first part of the sections is a general overview, while the second part deals with conventional as well as innovative diagnosis and management, followed by various disorders that represent aortopathy.

We are grateful to the Springer JP team, especially Ms. Makie Kambara and Kanako Honma, for their great support.

We hope this textbook is useful in clinical medicine and especially in the field of congenital heart anomalies.

Tokyo, Japan Koichiro Niwa
Munich, Germany Harald Kaemmerer

Contents

Part I
Overview

Chapter 1
History of Aortopathy

Koichiro Niwa

Abstract After Maude Abbott mentioned in 1928 in her atlas of congenital heart disease that the presence of a bicuspid aortic valve appears to indicate a tendency for spontaneous rupture, the following story started: recognized were a high incidence of aortic dissection and medial intrinsic abnormalities of the aorta in the presence of a bicuspid aortic valve, medial abnormalities (resembling Marfan aorta) in various congenital heart anomalies with dilated aorta, risk factors for this dilatation, reduced aortic elasticity influencing coronary artery, and ventricular performance, and finally, the concept of aortopathy in congenital heart diseases has been established.

Medial abnormalities in the ascending aorta were prevalent in a variety of congenital heart anomalies such as bicuspid aortic valve, coarctation of the aorta, single ventricle with pulmonary atresia or stenosis, persistent truncus arteriosus, transposition of the great arteries, hypoplastic left heart syndrome, and tetralogy of Fallot and may predispose to dilatation and aneurysmal formation. These congenital heart diseases exhibit ongoing dilatation of the aortic root and reduced aortic elasticity that may relate to intrinsic properties of the aortic root. Aortic dilatation and increased stiffness can also induce left ventricular hypertrophy, reduced coronary artery flow, and left ventricular dysfunction. This association of aortic pathophysiological abnormality, aortic dilation, and aorto-ventricular interaction could be recognized as a new clinical entity: "aortopathy."

Keywords Aortic dilatation • Cystic medial necrosis • Aortopathy • Aortic stiffness

K. Niwa, M.D., Ph.D., FACC, FAHA, FJCC (✉)
Cardiovascular Center, St Luke's International Hospital, 9-1 Akashi-cho, Tokyo 104-8560, Japan
e-mail: koniwa@luke.ac.jp; kniwa@aol.com

K. Niwa, H. Kaemmerer (eds.), *Aortopathy*, DOI 10.1007/978-4-431-56071-5_1

1.1 Introduction

The ascending aorta in congenital heart disease may dilate out of proportion to hemodynamic or morphogenetic expectations, may become aneurysmal, and may rupture [1, 2]. Aortic dilation in Marfan syndrome, Turner syndrome, bicuspid aortic valve, and coarctation of the aorta is well recognized, and these disorders are consistently associated with ascending aortic and/or paracoarctation medial abnormalities [2, 3]. Congenital heart anomalies such as single ventricle with pulmonary atresia or stenosis, persistent truncus arteriosus, transposition of the great arteries, hypoplastic left heart syndrome, or tetralogy of Fallot are also associated with aortic medial abnormalities, aortic dilatation, and aortic regurgitation [1] (Table 1.1). Aortic medial abnormalities reach their severest form in Marfan syndrome and are prevalent and qualitatively similar but seldom quantitatively as marked in a wide variety of congenital heart diseases with a wide age range [1]. Now various types of congenital heart disease are known to harbor an aortic medial abnormality that reflects a common developmental fault that weakens and attenuates the aortic wall. These congenital heart diseases with aortic dilatation are often associated with latent complications, such as decreased elasticity and increased stiffness of the aorta [4–6]. Due to increased afterload and ventricular hypertrophy, the pathophysiological aortic changes are negatively influencing systolic and diastolic systemic ventricular functions [5].

This review deals with the aortic manifestations of congenital heart disease, such as dilatation, aneurysm, and dissection, with specific consideration of the history and importance of new clinical entity "aortopathy" [7, 8].

1.2 Historical Perspective (Table 1.2)

Bicuspid aortic valve is the most common gross morphologic congenital abnormality of the heart and great vessels in adults.

The well-known artist, Leonardo da Vinci, illustrated that anomaly firstly in 1513 in his remarkable *Anatomical, Physiological, and Embryological Drawings* [9]. In 1928, Maude Abbott, Montreal [9], mentioned in her textbook of congenital heart disease that the presence of a bicuspid aortic valve appears to indicate, at least in a portion of the cases in which it occurs, a tendency for spontaneous rupture."

The association of a congenital bicuspid aortic valve with coarctation of the aorta is also well recognized. Abbott [3] found a bicuspid aortic valve in 47 of 200 cases of coarctation.

In 1930, Erdheim referred to medionecrosis aortae idiopathica cystica, and cystic medial necrosis was defined as [10]:

- Noninflammatory smooth muscle cell loss
- Fragmentation of elastic fibers

Table 1.1 Congenital heart diseases associated with aortic dilatation in adults

Marfan syndrome
Turner syndrome
Bicuspid aortic valve
Coarctation of the aorta
Tetralogy of Fallot
Single ventricle with pulmonary atresia or stenosis
Persistent truncus arteriosus
Transposition of the great arteries
Hypoplastic left heart syndrome
Post-Fontan procedure

Table 1.2 Historical overview

Year	Topics	Author	Refs.
1513	Illustration of BAV	Leonardo da Vinci	[9]
1928	"The presence of a BAV appears to indicate, at least in a portion of the cases in which it occurs, a tendency for spontaneous rupture."	Maude Abbott	[9]
1928	Medionecrosis	Gsell O	[3]
1928	Aortic rupture in BAV and coarctation of the aorta	Abbott ME	[3]
1930	Medionecrosis aortae idiopathica cystica	Erdheim J	[10]
1957	Aortic valve disease and CMN	McKusick VA	[11]
1972	BAV and Erdheim's cystic medial necrosis	McKusick VA	[3]
1978	BAV and aortic dissection	Edwards WD	[12]
1987	Coarctation of the aorta and CMS	Isner JM	[19]
2000	TGA and impaired aortic distensibility	Murakami T	[51]
2001	CMS in various CHDs	Niwa K	[1]
2002	Progressive aortic dilatation in TOF	Niwa K	[49]
2003	HLHS and neo-aortic dilatation	Cohen MS	[29]
2004	TGA and aortic dilatation, AR	Schwartz M	[28]
2005	Aortopathy and TOF	Niwa K	[24]
2008	Arterial hemodynamics influence LV	Senzaki H	[5]
2009	Fontan and dissection	Egan M	[36]

BAV bicuspid aortic valve, *CMN* cystic medial necrosis, *CHD* congenital heart disease, *TOF* tetralogy of Fallot, *TGA* complete transposition of the great arteries, *HLHS* hypoplastic left heart syndrome, *AR* aortic regurgitation, *LV* left ventricle

- Accumulation of basophilic ground substance within cell-depleted areas of the medial layer of the vessel wall

An association between aortic valve disease and cystic medial necrosis of the aorta was pointed out in 1957 [11] and often documented after that. It was suggested that the valve disease places unusual hemodynamic stress on the aortic wall, leading to structural fatigue, expressed as congenital heart disease [3] and/or "inborn" congenital weakness [3].

In 1972, maKusick (3) reported a man and his son with a bicuspid aortic valve with aortic regurgitation without phenotype of Marfan syndrome. Intraoperatively "cystic medial necrosis" in aortic media was found, and they reported that the association of bicuspid aortic valve and "cystic medial necrosis" is more than a coincidence.

In 1978, Edwards et al. [12] reported that among 119 necropsy specimens from aortic dissection, 11 had occurred in patients with bicuspid aortic valve (9 %). Roberts et al. [2] also reported that among 186 necropsy specimens with aortic dissection, 14 were from bicuspid aortic valve (7.5 %) with a mean age of 52 and severe degeneration of the elastic fiber was found in the aortic wall in 90 % of them. High incidence of bicuspid aortic valve among patients with aortic dissection is suggesting a causative relationship between bicuspid aortic valve and aortic dissecting aneurysm.

In 1990s, Harn et al. [13] and Nistri et al. [14] reported a high prevalence of aortic root enlargement in bicuspid aortic valves that occurs irrespective of altered hemodynamics, aortic valve stenosis, and regurgitation, suggesting that bicuspid aortic valve and aortic root dilatation may reflect a common developmental defect. It has been recognized that patients with aortic valve harbor cystic medial necrosis in the aortic media, and the aortic root has a tendency to dilate, sometimes followed by aortic dissection. Bicuspid aortic valve was the first non-syndromic congenital heart anomaly in which aortic dilation and dissection were reported [15].

In 2001, Niwa and Perloff et al. [1] reported for the first time that aortic medial abnormalities – so-called cystic medial necrosis – are prevalent in a wide variety of congenital heart disease with dilated aortic root, other than bicuspid aortic valve or coarctation of the aorta.

After that, progressive aortic dilatation and aortic valve regurgitation have been reported in various types of congenital heart disease, regardless of intracardiac repair [16–29].

1.3 Congenital Heart Diseases associated with Aortic Dilatation (Table 1.1)

1.3.1 Bicuspid Aortic Valve and Ross Procedure

Aortic dissection is found to be 9–18 times more prevalent in patients with bicuspid aortic valve than in those with tricuspid aortic valve [30]. Aortic dilation begins during childhood in patients with bicuspid aortic valve, regardless of the presence of aortic stenosis [31]. Histologic abnormalities in the ascending aorta in patients with bicuspid aortic valve are similar to those found in Marfan patients [3].

After Ross procedure, in 118 patients (bicuspid aortic valve in 81 %) with age of 34 years and 44 months of follow-up, the diameter of the sinuses of Valsalva increased from 31 +/− 0.4 to 33 +/− 0.5 mm [16]. In 13 (11 %) with the ascending aortic diameter ranged from 40 to 51 mm, 7 (6 %) developed moderate aortic regurgitation, and 3 (3 %) required aortic valve replacement. The predicted probability of no or trivial aortic regurgitation decreased from 63 % in the early postoperative period to 24 % after 16 years.

The most common cause for a failing Ross is pulmonary autograft dilation [18], occurring because of an intrinsic abnormality of the pulmonary root in congenital aortic valve disease.

1.3.2 Coarctation of the Aorta

Isner et al. [19] in 1987 described the light microscopic features of the coarctation segment in 33 patients aging 1 day to 15 years and found cystic medial necrosis, deletion, and disarray of elastic tissue in all 33 specimens. Remarkably, these findings are already observed in neonates, suggesting that cystic medial necrosis in the aortic wall in coarctation of the aorta is possibly intrinsic. The mentioned cystic medial necrosis may represent the pathologic basis for the aneurysm formation observed after balloon angioplasty of coarctation.

As coarctation of the aorta is often accompanied by a bicuspid aortic valve [9], this disorder harbors the risk of medial abnormalities not only at paracoarctation site but also in the ascending aorta.

1.3.3 Aortic Dilatation of Tetralogy of Fallot

Enlarged aorta is one of the specific anatomical features of tetralogy of Fallot that is observed even during fetus. Among the cyanotic congenital heart anomalies, tetralogy of Fallot was the first in which significant aortic dilation was recognized in 1960s–1970s [20, 21].

Aortic dilatation is a well-known feature of unrepaired tetralogy of Fallot and correlates well with severity of right ventricular outflow tract stenosis and is greatest in pulmonary atresia and ventricular septal defect. Aortic regurgitation in unrepaired adult tetralogy of Fallot is often observed, and it imposes volume overload on both ventricles [22].

A significant subset of adults late after repair of tetralogy of Fallot exhibits progressive aortic root dilatation that may lead to aortic regurgitation and predispose to dissection and rupture. The aortic dilatation relates medial abnormalities coupled with previous long-standing volume overload of the ascending aorta. Such a dilatation and histological abnormalities have been found from fetus life to childhood [23]. Fifteen percent of repaired tetralogy of Fallot had a dilated aortic root in adulthood [24].

Different from the Marfan syndrome, dissection is rarely reported in tetralogy of Fallot. In 2005, aortic dissection was reported from two different institutions in two patients with repaired tetralogy of Fallot with the aortic root size of 93×83 mm and 70 mm [32, 33].

1.3.4 Neo-aortic Dilation After Arterial Switch Operation in Complete Transposition of the Great Artery

In 2000s, aortic dilation and aortic regurgitation became known complications after arterial switch operation in complete transposition of the great artery [25, 26]. The freedom from aortic regurgitation was 78 % at 10 years and 69 % at 15 years, and the freedom from aortic valve replacement was 98 % at 10 years and 97 % at 15 years [25]. Severe neo-aortic valve regurgitation was present in only 3.7 %, and trivial to mild regurgitation in 81 % of patients at midterm follow-up [26]. Cystic medial necrosis is observed after arterial switch operation in both neo-aorta and pulmonary artery (20 %) in neonate. Therefore, in transposition of the great arteries, histologic aortic abnormalities are, along with the operative technique, one of the causes of this aortic dilatation after repair [27]. Progressive dilation of the neo-aortic root is out of proportion to somatic growth, and the incidence of aortic regurgitation increases with the duration of follow-up. During a long-term follow-up, aortic regurgitation will possibly increase with age. Previous pulmonary artery banding is a risk factor for aortic dilation, while older age at arterial switch operation and presence of ventricular septal defect are other risk factors for aortic regurgitation [28].

1.3.5 Hypoplastic Left Heart Syndrome

Neo-aortic root dilation and aortic regurgitation after staged reconstruction for hypoplastic left heart syndrome are known complications, progressing over time. In 2003, Cohen et al. [29] reported on a 9-year follow-up of 53 patients with hypoplastic left heart syndrome after Fontan procedure. They found the neo-aortic root progressively dilated out of proportion to body size, with 98 % having a Z-score >2 at most recent follow-up. Neo-aortic regurgitation was present in 61 %. In general, mild pulmonary regurgitation can physiologically be seen in normal subjects, while any degree of aortic regurgitation is considered abnormal [34]· Therefore, a different texture of the arterial wall may be one of the causes of regurgitation.

1.3.6 Persistent Truncus Arteriosus

A dilated aortic root is found in the majority of operated patients with truncus arteriosus, but none of them had aortic dissection or rupture [35]. Although, in this disorder, the anatomical truncal valve is commonly abnormal and regurgitant, the role of dilatation of the aorta on truncal valve regurgitation is unclear.

1.3.7 Fontan and Cyanotic Congenital Heart Disease with Pulmonary Stenosis/Atresia

The incidence of aortic dissection in congenital heart disease other than bicuspid aortic valve and coarctation of the aorta is extremely rare [8].

Aortic dissection has been seen in patients with Fontan circulation [36], and a patient with tricuspid atresia after Fontan operation experienced aortic dissection (personal communication). Also a patient with tricuspid atresia post Glenn procedure revealed an aortic aneurysm with aortic size of 50 mm (personal communication).

1.4 Cause of Aortic Dilatation in Congenital Heart Disease (Table 1.3)

Independent variables that alter the structure of the ascending aortic media include genetic abnormalities, such as Marfan syndrome, annuloaortic ectasia, or Turner syndrome. Systemic hypertension [37], aging [38], and pregnancy [39] are also accompanied with aortic root dilatation (Table 1.1). In patients with systemic hypertension, abnormalities of aortic medial elastin and collagen were reported in 1970, and these histological changes are prevalent [37]. With advancing age, the aortic diameter is gradually increasing, along with layers of parallel aortic elastic fiber fragment, and smooth muscle decreases, especially in the thoracic aorta [38]. In pregnancy, gestational changes for supplying blood for the fetus with increased cardiac output happen in accordance with elastic fiber fragmentation and hypertrophy/hyperplasia of smooth muscle cells in ascending aortic media. The resulting histological changes were recognized in 1967 [39]; however, it is not known whether these changes are reversible after delivery or not.

Marfan syndrome is characterized by a defect in the chromosome 15 gene that codes for fibrillin-1 [40], in the absence of which elastin is more readily degraded by metalloproteinase [41]. Apoptosis plays a pathogenetic role in the medial abnormalities of abdominal aortic aneurysm [42]. Deletion of TGF-β receptor has a relation with aortic dilatation [43]. The genetic fault in Marfan syndrome

Table 1.3 Cause of cystic medial necrosis in ascending aortic media

1.	Systemic hypertension
2.	Aging
3.	Pregnancy
4.	Chromosome abnormality: Marfan syndrome, Turner syndrome, Noonan syndrome
5.	Gene abnormality: fibrillin-1 defect (15q21.1)
6.	Deletion of transforming growth factor-β receptor, ALK5 signaling in neural crest cell
7.	Medial smooth muscle cell apoptosis
8.	Metalloproteinase and elastin
9.	Hemodynamic abnormality (increased aortic flow)
10.	Intrinsic abnormality of aortic wall in congenital heart diseases

apparently impairs aortic medial elastic fibers more extensively than impairment in congenital heart disease [1].

In 2008, Chowdhury et al. [44] reported comparison of patients with A-P phenotype (R-L cusp fusion) bicuspid aortic valve with R-L phenotype (R-N cusp fusion); the former is more common in male and larger and stiffer at the sinus of Valsalva and smaller at ascending aorta and aortic arch than the latter. This aortic shape difference is possibly attributed rather to inborn errors of the aortic wall than to hemodynamic effects [45, 46]. Therefore, bicuspid aortic valve phenotype can predict elastic properties of ascending aorta and has a potential impact on clinical outcomes [47].

50.9 % prevalence of fibrillin-1 gene polymorphisms or mutations is found in patients with coarctation of the aorta and a dilated aorta, and there is >8 times risk of aortic dilation in patients with these variants [44]. In patients with chromosome 22q11.2 partial deletion without conotruncal abnormality, aortic dilation is found in 10/93 (10.8 %) [48]. Therefore, it is a possibility, but aortic dilatation is a novel cardiovascular finding in patients with chromosome 22q11.2 partial deletion, and after repair of tetralogy of Fallot, chromosome 22q11.2 partial deletion is one of the risk factors of aortic dilatation [24].

1.5 Aortic Root Dilation and Aortic Elastic Properties in the Aortic Wall in CHDs

The concept of vasculopathy/aortopathy is evolving in 2000s. In 2006, Chong et al. [49] found, at 8.3 years after tetralogy of Fallot repair in 67 children, a significant increased stiffness, reduced strain, and distensibility of the aorta in patients with dilated aorta.

In 2008, Senzaki et al. [5] compared 38 repaired tetralogy of Fallot patients with 55 controls. The former had higher characteristic of impedance and pulse wave velocity, lower total peripheral arterial compliance, and higher arterial wave reflection. They also observed that the increase in aortic wall stiffness was closely associated with the increase in aortic root diameter. Therefore, central and peripheral arterial wall stiffness is characteristically increased after tetralogy of Fallot repair. Abnormal arterial elastic properties have negative impact on left ventricle and provoke aortic dilatation. This may induce left ventricular hypertrophy and systolic and diastolic dysfunction of the left ventricle. Also after tetralogy of Fallot repair, a decreased aortic elasticity and increased augmentation index are found [50].

Aortic properties in transposition were reported earlier than in tetralogy of Fallot. In patients after arterial switch operation, a decreased aortic elasticity and distensibility are confirmed by increased pulse wave velocity [51], and the stiffness index is increased [52].

These pathophysiological aortic abnormalities are observed in the other types of congenital heart disease with aortic dilatation, and these abnormalities may have a negative impact not only on aorta but also on the left ventricle (or systemic right ventricle). These characteristics induce aortic dilation and aortic regurgitation and increase pulsatile load on the left ventricle, followed by a decreased cardiac output. They also provoke a decreased coronary blood flow that may negatively influence left ventricular function [5]. Aortic regurgitation may also develop and progress due to stiffness of aortic root [52].

1.6 Age of New Clinical Entity " Aortopathy": Dilatation of Aortic Root, Abnormality in Aortic Pathophysiological Function, Low Coronary Artery Flow, and Systemic Ventricular Dysfunction in CHDs

We can recognize several pathophysiological abnormalities of the aorta and an abnormal aorto-ventricular interaction as a new clinical entity "aortopathy": aortic dilation, aortic regurgitation, and decreased coronary artery flow and left ventricular dysfunctions.

1.7 Conclusions

A subset of adult patients with congenital heart disease exhibits ongoing dilatation of the aortic root and reduced aortic elasticity that may relate to intrinsic properties of the aortic root. This new concept of aortic dilatation is shifting a paradigm of aortic dilatation from so-called post-stenotic dilatation to primary intrinsic aortopathy. These aortic dilatation and increased stiffness can induce aortic aneurysm, rupture, and aortic regurgitation but also provoke systemic ventricular hypertrophy, reduced coronary artery flow, and systemic ventricular failure. We can recognize this association of aortic pathophysiological abnormalities, aortic dilation, and aorto-ventricular interaction as a new clinical entity: "aortopathy."

References

1. Niwa K, Perloff JK, Bhuta SM et al (2001) Structural abnormalities of great arterial walls in congenital heart disease. Light and electron microscopic analyses. Circulation 103:393–400
2. Roberts CS, Roberts WC (1991) Dissection of the aorta associated with congenital malformation of the aortic valve. J Am Coll Cardiol 17:712–716
3. Mckusick VA (1972) Association of congenital bicuspid aortic valve and Erdheim's cystic medial necrosis. Lancet I 299:1026–1027
4. Seki M, Kurishima C, Kawasaki H et al (2012) Aortic stiffness and aortic dilation in infants and children with tetralogy of Fallot before corrective surgery: evidence for intrinsically abnormal aortic mechanical property. Eur J Cardiothorac Surg 41:277–282
5. Senzaki H, Iwamoto Y, Ishido H et al (2008) Arterial haemodynamics in patients after repair of tetralogy of Fallot: influence on left ventricular after load and aortic dilatation. Heart 94:70–74
6. Chong WY, Wong WH, Chiu CS et al (2006) Aortic root dilation and aortic elastic properties in children after repair of tetralogy of Fallot. Am J Cardiol 97:905–909
7. Niwa K (2005) Aortic root dilatation in tetralogy of Fallot long-term after repair–histology of the aorta in tetralogy of Fallot: evidence of intrinsic aortopathy. Int J Cardiol 103:117–119
8. Niwa K (2013) Aortopathy in congenital heart disease in adults: aortic dilatation with decreased aortic elasticity that Impacts negatively on left ventricular function. Korean Circ J 43:215–220
9. Perloff JK (2012) Congenital aortic stenosis. Congenital aortic regurgitation. In: Perloff JK, Marelli AJ (eds) Clinical recognition of congenital heart disease, 6th edn. Elsevier Saunders Company, Philadelphia, pp 74–75
10. Erdheim J (1929) Medionecrosis aortae idiopathica. Virchows Arch (Pathol Anat) 273:186
11. Mckusick VA, RB L, HT B (1957) Association of aortic valvular disease and cystic medial necrosis of the ascending aorta; report of four instances. Circulation 16:188–194
12. Edwards WD, Leaf DS, Edwards JE (1978) Dissecting aortic aneurysm associated with congenital bicuspid aortic valve. Circulation 57:1022–1025
13. Hahn RT, Roman MJ, Mogtader AH et al (1992) Association of aortic dilation with regurgitant, stenotic and functionally normal bicuspid aortic valves. J Am Coll Cardiol 19:283–288
14. Nistri S, Sorbo MD, Marin M et al (1999) Aortic root dilatation in young men with normally functioning bicuspid aortic valves. Heart 82:19–22
15. Reid RT (1952) Bicuspid aortic valve associated with aneurysmal dilatation of the ascending aorta. Med J Aust 2:628–629
16. de Sa M, Moshkovitz Y, Butany J et al (1999) Histologic abnormalities of the ascending aorta and pulmonary trunk in patients with bicuspid aortic valve disease: clinical relevance to the Ross procedure. J Thorac Cardiovasc Surg 118:588–594
17. Elkins RC, Thompson DM, Lane MM et al (2008) Ross operation: 16-year experience. J Thorac Cardiovasc Surg 136:623–630
18. David TE, Omran A, Ivanov J et al (2000) Dilation of the pulmonary autograft after the Ross procedure. J Thorac Cardiovasc Surg 119:210–220
19. Isner JM, Donaldson RF, Fulton D et al (1987) Cystic medial necrosis in coarctation of the aorta: a potential factor contributing to adverse consequences observed after percutaneous balloon angioplasty of coarctation sites. Circulation 75:689–695
20. Bahnson HT, Spencer FC, Landtman B et al (1962) Surgical treatment and follow-up of 147 cases of tetralogy of Fallot treated by correction. J Thorac Cardiovasc Surg 44:419–432

21. Rieker RP, Berman MA, Stansel HC Jr (1975) Postoperative studies in patients with tetralogy of Fallot. Ann Thorac Surg 19:17–26
22. Capelli H, Ross D, Somerville J (1982) Aortic regurgitation in tetrad of Fallot and pulmonary atresia. Am J Cardiol 49:1979–1983
23. Tan JL, Davlouros PA, McCarthy KP et al (2005) Intrinsic histological abnormalities of aortic root and ascending aorta in tetralogy of Fallot: evidence of causative mechanism for aortic dilatation and aortopathy. Circulation 112:961–968
24. Niwa K, Siu S, Webb G et al (2002) Progressive aortic root dilatation in adults late after repair of tetralogy of Fallot. Circulation 106:1374–1378
25. Losay J, Touchot A, Capderou A et al (2006) Aortic valve regurgitation after arterial switch operation for transposition of the great arteries: incidence, risk factors, and outcome. J Am Coll Cardiol 247:2057–2062
26. Marino BS, Wernovsky G, McElhinney DB et al (2006) Neo-aortic valvar function after the arterial switch. Cardiol Young 16:481–489
27. Takeuchi T, Imai Y, Takanashi Y et al (1996) Histological study of the great arteries in patients with arterial switch operation. Act Ped Cardiol Jpn 12:506–512
28. Schwartz ML, Gauvreau K, del Nido P et al (2004) Long-term predictors of aortic root dilation and aortic regurgitation after arterial switch operation. Circulation 110:128–132
29. Cohen MS, Marino BS, McElhinney DB et al (2003) Neo-aortic root dilation and valve regurgitation up to 21 years after staged reconstruction for hypoplastic left heart syndrome. J Am Coll Cardiol 42:533–540
30. Larson EW, Edwards WD (1984) Risk factors for aortic dissection: a necropsy study of 161 cases. Am J Cardiol 53:849–855
31. Gurvitz M, Chang RK, Drant S et al (2004) Frequency of aortic root dilation in children with a bicuspid aortic valve. Am J Cardiol 94:1337–1340
32. Kim WH, Seo JW, Kim SJ et al (2005) Aortic dissection late after repair of tetralogy of Fallot. Int J Cardiol 101:515–516
33. Rathi VK, Doyle M, Williams RB et al (2005) Massive aortic aneurysm and dissection in repaired tetralogy of Fallot; diagnosis by cardiovascular magnetic resonance imaging. Int J Cardiol 101:169–170
34. Yoshida K, Yoshikawa J, Shakudo M et al (1988) Color Doppler evaluation of valvular regurgitation in normal subjects. Circulation 78:840–847
35. Carlo WF, McKenzie ED, Slesnick TC (2011) Root dilation in patients with truncus arteriosus. Congenit Heart Dis 6:228–233
36. Egan M, Phillips A, Cook SC (2009) Aortic dissection in the adult Fontan with aortic root enlargement. Pediatr Cardiol 30:562–563
37. Carlson RG, Lillehei CW, Edwards JE (1970) Cystic medial necrosis of the ascending aorta in relation to age and hypertension. Am J Cardiol 25:411–415
38. Schlatmann TJ, Becker AE (1977) Histologic changes in the normal aging aorta: implications for dissecting aortic aneurysm. Am J Cardiol 39:13–20
39. Monalo-Estrell P, Barker AE (1967) Histopathologic findings in human aortic media associated with pregnancy. Arch Pathol 83:336–341
40. Dietz HC, Pyeritz RE (1995) Mutations in the human gene for fibrillin-1 (FBN1) in the Marfan syndrome and related disorders. Hum Mol Genet 4:1799–1809
41. Segura AM, Luna RE, Horiba K et al (1998) Immunohistochemistry of matrix metalloproteinases and their inhibitors in thoracic aortic aneurysms and aortic valves in patients with Marfan's syndrome. Circulation 98(Suppl II: II):331–338
42. Bonderman D, Gharehbaghi-Schnell E, Walleneck G et al (1999) Mechanisms underlying aortic dilatation in congenital aortic valve malformations. Circulation 99:2138–2143
43. Wang J, Nagy A, Larsson J et al (2006) Defective ALK5 signaling in the neural crest leads to increased postmigratory neural crest cell apoptosis and severe outflow tract defects. BMC Dev Biol 6:51–64

44. Chowdhury UK, Mishra AK, Balakrishnan P et al (2008) Role of fibrillin-1 genetic mutations and polymorphism in aortic dilatation in patients undergoing intracardiac repair of tetralogy of Fallot. J Thorac Cardiovasc Surg 136:757–766
45. Schaefer BM, Lewin MB, Stout KK et al (2008) The bicuspid aortic valve: an integrated phenotypic classification of leaflet morphology and aortic root shape. Heart 94:1634–1638
46. Jackson V, Petrini J, Caidahl K et al (2011) Bicuspid aortic valve leaflet morphology in relation to aortic root morphology: a study of 300 patients undergoing open-heart surgery. Eur J Cardiothorac Surg 40:e118–e124
47. Schaefer BM, Lewin MB, Stout KK et al (2007) Usefulness of bicuspid aortic valve phenotype to predict elastic properties of the ascending aorta. Am J Cardiol 99:686–690
48. John AS, McDonald-McGinn DM, Zackai EH et al (2009) Aortic root dilatation in patients with 22q11.2 deletion syndrome. Am J Med Genet A149A:939–942
49. Chong WY, Wong WH, Chiu CS et al (2006) Aortic root dilation and aortic elastic properties in children after repair of tetralogy of Fallot. Am J Cardiol 97:905–909
50. Cheung YF, Ou X, Wong SJ (2006) Central and peripheral arterial stiffness in patients after surgical repair of tetralogy of Fallot: implications for aortic root dilatation. Heart 92:1827–1830
51. Murakami T, Nakazawa M, Momma K et al (2000) Impaired distensibility of neoaorta after arterial switch procedure. Ann Thorac Surg 70:1907–1910
52. Sievers HH, Lange PE, Arensman FW et al (1984) Influence of two-stage anatomic correction on size and distensibility of the anatomic pulmonary/functional aortic root in patients with simple transposition of the great arteries. Circulation 70:202–208

Chapter 2
Pathological Background

Koichiro Niwa

Abstract A bicuspid aortic valve and/or coarctation of the aorta are consistently associated with ascending aortic and paracoarctation medial abnormalities. Congenital heart diseases (CHDs) such as single ventricle, truncus arteriosus, transposition of the great arteries, and tetralogy of Fallot are also associated with aortic medial abnormalities. A significant subset of adults with these CHD exhibits progressive dilatation of the aortic root even after repair owing to medial abnormalities that may lead to regurgitation and predispose to dissection and rupture that can be fatal and necessitating aortic valve and aortic root surgery.

Aortic medial abnormalities—incorrectly called "cystic medial necrosis"—reach their severest form in Marfan syndrome and are prevalent and qualitatively similar in a variety of CHDs with a wide age range. In Marfan syndrome, impairment of aortic medial elastic fibers is apparently more extensive than in CHD. Accordingly, the incidence of ascending aortic dilatation, dissection, or rupture is lower, and the degree of aortic root medial lesions is smaller in congenital heart disease patients with aortic dilatation. These aortic abnormalities in CHD with aortic dilatation. These aortic abnormalities in CHD are either from intrinsic factors or result from volume overload of the aorta due to right to left shunting.

Keywords Cystic medial necrosis • Aortic medial elastic fibers • Aortic dilatation • Congenital heart disease • Aortic medial abnormalities

2.1 Introduction

The ascending aorta in congenital heart disease (CHD) may dilate out of proportion to hemodynamic or morphogenetic expectations, may become aneurysmal, and may rapture [1, 2]. Aortic dilatation in Marfan syndrome, Turner syndrome, bicuspid aortic valve, and coarctation of the aorta is well recognized, and these disorders are consistently associated with ascending aortic and/or paracoarctation

K. Niwa, M.D., Ph.D., FACC, FAHA, FJCC (✉)
Cardiovascular Center, St Luke's International Hospital, 9-1 Akashi-cho, Tokyo 104-8560, Japan
e-mail: koniwa@luke.ac.jp; kniwa@aol.com

K. Niwa, H. Kaemmerer (eds.), *Aortopathy*, DOI 10.1007/978-4-431-56071-5_2

Fig. 2.1 Definition of so-called cystic medial necrosis

1, Non-inflammatory smooth muscle cell loss

2, Fragmentation of elastic fibers

3, Accumulation of basophilic ground substance within cell-depleted areas of the medial layer of the vessel wall

medial abnormalities [2, 3]. Congenital heart anomalies such as single ventricle, persistent truncus arteriosus, transposition of the great arteries, hypoplastic left heart syndrome, and tetralogy of Fallot are also associated with aortic medial abnormalities, aortic dilatation, and aortic regurgitation [1]. Aortic medial abnormalities—incorrectly called "cystic medial necrosis" (Fig. 2.1)—reach their severest form in Marfan syndrome and are prevalent and qualitatively similar but seldom quantitatively as marked in a variety of CHD with a wide age range [1].

In CHD with great artery dilatation (aortic or pulmonary dilatation), six morphologic variations are possibly represented:

1. Marfan syndrome (intrinsic connective tissue defect)
2. Bicuspid aortic valve and/or paracoarctation aorta
3. Cyanotic CHD with progressive aortic dilatation such as tetralogy of Fallot and pulmonary stenosis/atresia, truncus arteriosus, and single ventricle with pulmonary atresia or stenosis
4. CHD with pulmonary vascular disease
5. CHD with large left to right shunt (e.g., atrial septal defect) without pulmonary obstructive disease
6. Tricuspid aortic stenosis or pulmonary stenosis or "idiopathic pulmonary artery dilatation"

Marfan syndrome, which has a causal association with mutations of fibrillin, involves dilatation of the ascending aorta with morphological finding of the so-called cystic medial necrosis (elastic fiber fragmentation, smooth muscle cell loss) [4–6].

Dilatation of the ascending aorta and pulmonary trunk in CHD has been considered secondary to the basic anomaly. However, a dilated paracoarctation aorta and a dilated ascending aorta above a bicuspid aortic valve may harbor "cystic medial necrosis" that is indistinguishable from Marfan syndrome [7–11], and such dilatation can be observed in bicuspid aortic valve patients even without aortic stenosis or regurgitation. Therefore, this dilatation of the aorta possibly develops due to intrinsic rather than hemodynamic abnormalities. These observations have led us to hypothesize that various types of CHD harbor an aortic medial abnormality that reflects a common developmental fault weakening and attenuating the aortic wall.

2.2 Cause of Aortic Dilatation in Congenital Heart Disease and Histology of the Aortic Media

There are several independent variables that alter the structure of ascending aortic media. In pregnancy [12], gestational changes in ascending aortic and pulmonary truncal media are characterized by elastic fiber fragmentation, a decrease in ground substance, and hypertrophy/hyperplasia of smooth muscle cells. Those induce reduced peripheral arterial resistance and an increased fetal blood flow and also reduced peripheral pulmonary arterial resistance for an increased cardiac output during pregnancy. With aging, layers of parallel aortic elastic fibers fragment, smooth muscle decreases, and collagen and ground substance increase, especially in the thoracic aorta [13]. In patients with systemic hypertension and increased share stress to the aortic wall, abnormalities of aortic medial elastin and collagen are significantly more prevalent than in normotensive subjects of comparable age [14]. Deletion of transposing growth factor-β (TGF-β) receptor has a relation with aortic dilatation [15]. The genetic fault in Marfan syndrome apparently impairs the aortic medial elastic fibers more extensively than impairment in CHD, and the incidence of ascending aortic dilatation, dissection, or rupture is higher, and the degree of aortic root medial lesions is greater in former than the latter [1].

After Erdheim referred to medionecrosis aortae idiopathica cystica [16] in 1929, "cystic medial necrosis" became a part of the medical term. However, the term is misnomer, as the so-called cyst is in fact non-cystic medial structure faults, instead, accumulation of basophilic ground substance. McKusick et al. reported that the association of bicuspid aortic valve and cystic medial necrosis is more than coincidence and cystic medial necrosis was defined as [3, 8]:

1. Non-inflammatory smooth muscle cell loss
2. Fragmentation of elastic fibers
3. Accumulation of basophilic ground substance within cell-depleted areas of the medial layer of the vessel wall

2.3 Marfan Syndrome, Annulo-aortic Ectasia, and Cystic Medial Necrosis

Marfan syndrome is an autosomal dominant disorder with partial deletion of chromosome 15 and fault in making fibrillin which is the main component of elastic fibers [4, 5]. In Marfan syndrome, the morphological analysis of the arterial media in the ascending aorta and pulmonary trunk reveals fragmentation of elastic fiber and smooth muscle cell loss [4, 5, 17, 18]. Annulo-aortic ectasia has been defined as an entity comprising dilatation of the ascending aorta, dilatation of the aortic annulus, and progressive insufficiency of the aortic valve with cystic medial necrosis in the ascending aortic wall. Those without classic Marfan syndrome phenotype [19, 20] possibly have some relation with unknown responsible genes.

Marfan syndrome and annulo-aortic ectasia are the typical cases revealing cystic medial necrosis in the aortic media.

2.4 Bicuspid Aortic Valve, Paracoarctation of the Aorta, and Cystic Medial Necrosis

As mentioned before, McKusick et al. suggested that manifestations of an abnormal aortic media are too frequently observed in the paracoarctation aorta and bicuspid aortic valve as to allow postulation of a common underlying defect [8, 21]. After this report, close relations in the incidence among bicuspid aortic valve, paracoarctation aorta, aortic dilatation or dissection, and cystic medial necrosis in the ascending aorta were observed [9–11, 18–24] (Fig. 2.2). Aortic aneurysm and dissection are not rare in paracoarctation aorta, and aortic rupture is a frequently described cause of death in adults with coarctation of the aorta [25]. Arterial hypertension, accompanied by turbulent flow produced at the coarcted segment or the bicuspid aortic valve, can provide an explanation for cystic medial necrosis and aortic rupture [11]. However, aortic aneurysm and rupture may also occur years after successful repair of coarctation [26, 27]. Moreover, dissection in the distal compartment of the paracoarctation aorta is difficult to explain on the basis of hypertension alone [27, 28]. In histological study in CHD with aortic dilatation [1], 11 of 17 specimens from patients with bicuspid aortic valve and eight of nine specimens from the paracoarctation aorta (including above and below the

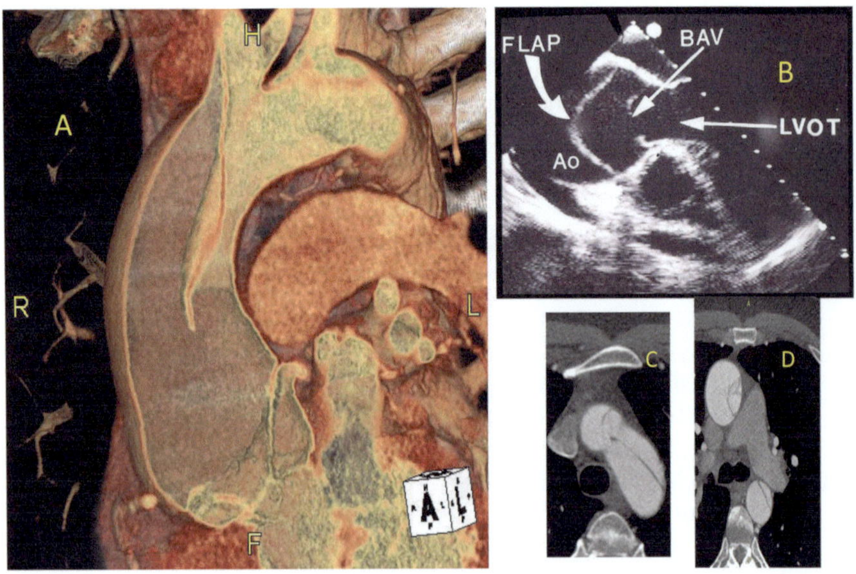

Fig. 2.2 A 51-year-old male with bicuspid aortic valve aortic dissection. (**a**), (**c**), and (**d**) CT images and (**b**) echo image. *Ao* aorta, *BA* bicuspid aortic valve, *LVOT* left ventricular outflow tract

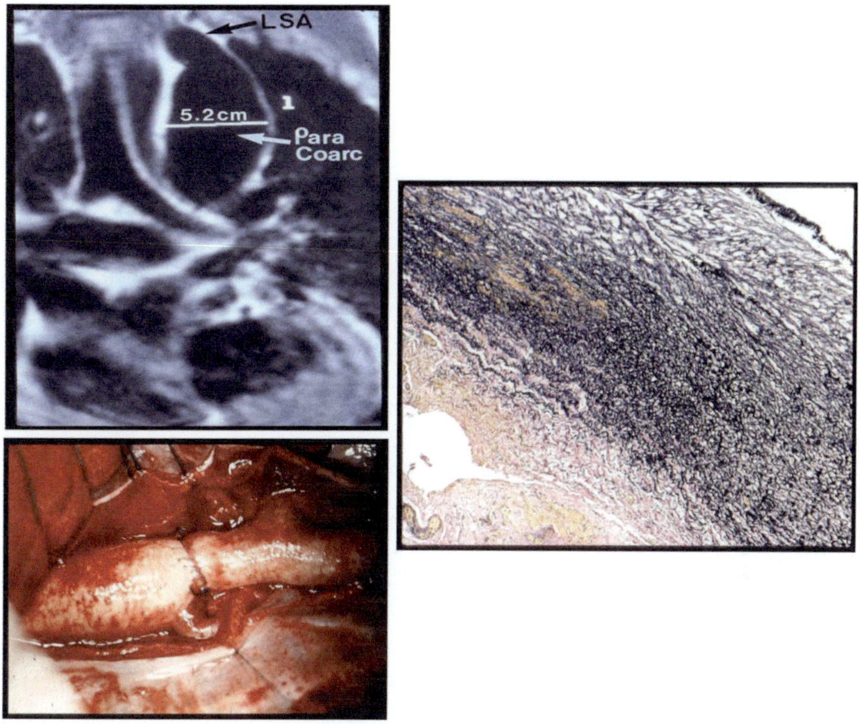

Fig. 2.3 A 20-year-old male with coarctation of the aorta (COA). *Left upper panel*: Paracoarctation aneurysm is clearly seen (5.2 cm diameter). *Left lower panel*: Postsurgical repair (end-to-end repair). *Right panel*: Severely fragmented elastic fibers (E) and smooth muscle cell (SM) are observed. Light microscopy, EVG (Courtesy by Perloff JK MD)

coarctation), specific cystic medial necrosis could be revealed (Fig. 2.3). Isner et al. [29] reported that 22 of 33 children, including five infants, with the coarctation of the aorta revealed extensive cystic medial necrosis in the paracoarctation aorta and a 3-week-old coarctation patient revealed typical cystic medial necrosis in the ascending aorta. Therefore, in bicuspid aortic valves or in the paracoarctation aorta, an inherent fragility of the aortic wall may provide an explanation for the high incidence of cystic medial necrosis in ascending aorta. The possible occurrence of an abnormal aortic media in the paracoarctation aorta might contribute to the prevalence of aneurysm formation after balloon dilatation for the coarctation of the aorta [29, 30].

2.5 Histopathological Abnormalities in Various Congenital Heart Diseases

A similar developmental fault in connective tissue possibly exists in other forms of CHD with great artery dilatation [1]. Niwa K et al.[1] reported that in 88 CHD patients with dilated aorta, aging 3 weeks to 81 years (32 ± 6 years) (48 males,

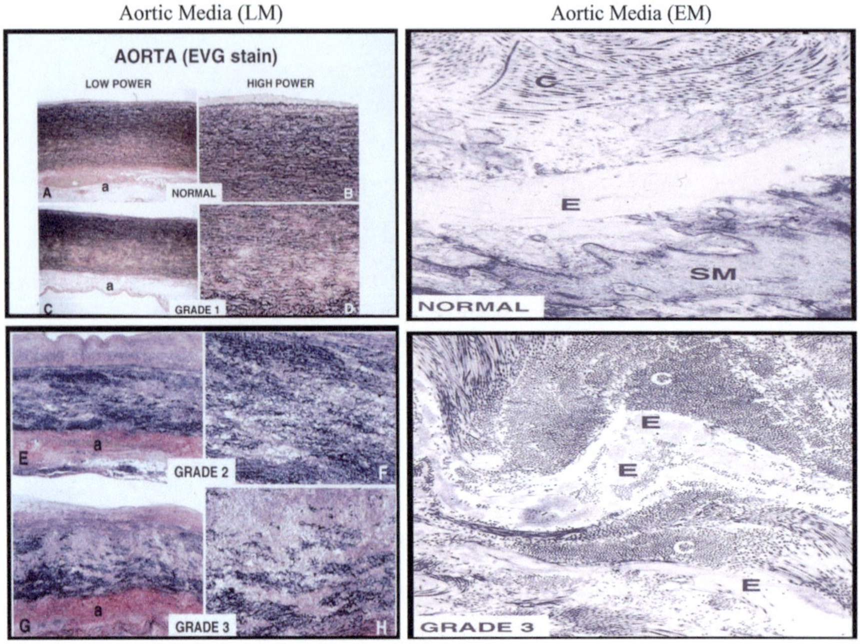

Fig. 2.4 Aortic medial histological findings: Light (*left side panel*) and electron microscopy (*right side panel*). *Left panel*: Histological severity is shown with the grading from normal to grade 3 (EVG stain). *Right panel*: Elastic fibers are severely fragmented. *SM* smooth muscle cell, *E* elastic fiber

40 females), surgical biopsy aortic specimens were obtained, and cystic medial necrosis was observed in the aortic media in all of them (Figs. 2.4 and 2.5).

2.6 Progressive Ascending Aorta Dilatation and Cystic Medial Necrosis in Cyanotic Congenital Heart Disease

There is an age-related increase in the incidence and degree of aortic regurgitation in tetralogy of Fallot, especially with pulmonary atresia. Regurgitation is related to the mechanical effects of a dilated aortic root above the aortic valve [31, 32]. Patients with a dilated aortic root in tetralogy of Fallot share similar histological changes of the aortic root, suggestive of cystic medial necrosis, indistinguishable from the aortic root in patients with Marfan syndrome [1]. Higher histologic grading scores in tetralogy of Fallot patients are found

	Normal	Grade1	Grade2	Grade3
Marfan				10
AAE				5
BAV AS		2	6	4
BAV AR		4	3	3
TOF			9	6
SV PS			2	1
TA PS			2	1
DORV			1	1
DOLV			1	
VSD				1
Do. Ao A			1	
PTA			3	2
d-TGA			6	2
Controls	21			

Fig. 2.5 Histological severity of aortic media by aortic biopsy specimens in various CHD with dilated aorta (n=88). *AAE* annulo-aortic ectasia, *BAV AS* bicuspid aortic valve with aortic stenosis, *BAV AR* bicuspid aortic valve with aortic regurgitation, *tetralogy of Fallot* tetralogy of Fallot, *SV PS* single ventricle with pulmonary stenosis, *TA PS* tricuspid atresia with pulmonary stenosis, *DORV* double outlet right ventricle, *DOLV* double outlet left ventricle, *VSD* ventricular septal defect, *Do Ao A* double aortic arch, *PTA* persistent truncus arteriosus, *d-TGA* d-transposition of the great arteries, *controls* transplant donor heart

even in infants, suggesting the intrinsic abnormality has crucial role for this dilatation [33].

Dilatation of the ascending aorta in truncus arteriosus or single ventricle with pulmonary atresia or stenosis is also thought to be progressive. In the former study [1], six of seven patients with tetralogy of Fallot with pulmonary atresia or severe pulmonary stenosis (including three younger than 10 years), a 4-year-old patient with truncus arteriosus, and a 16-month-old patient with complete transposition of the great arteries revealed specific cystic medial necrosis in the dilated ascending aorta. Complete transposition of the great arteries with a nonrestrictive ventricular septal defect was associated with grade 2 medial abnormalities in hypertensive pulmonary trunk. A patient with tetralogy of Fallot and an obstructive pulmonary vascular disease, induced by an oversized Blalock-Taussig shunt, suffered from a rupture of a hypertensive aneurysmal pulmonary trunk with grade 3 medial abnormalities that may have been acquired, although vulnerability might have been enhanced by an inherent reduction in elastic fibers. Truncus arteriosus is neither an aorta nor a pulmonary trunk, differing from a large aorta with pulmonary atresia or a large pulmonary trunk with aortic atresia, both of which have an aortopulmonary septum [34, 35]. Medial abnormalities in neonates and infants with truncus arteriosus may be inherent, albeit facilitated by systemic arterial pressure, volume overload, and a wide pulse pressure. In adults with truncus arteriosus and obstructive pulmonary vascular disease, medial abnormalities must be considered in light of abnormalities in neonates and infants.

It is reported that cystic medial necrosis was observed in 3 of 21 patients with transposition of the great arteries with the mean age of 5 months [36]. Therefore, it is

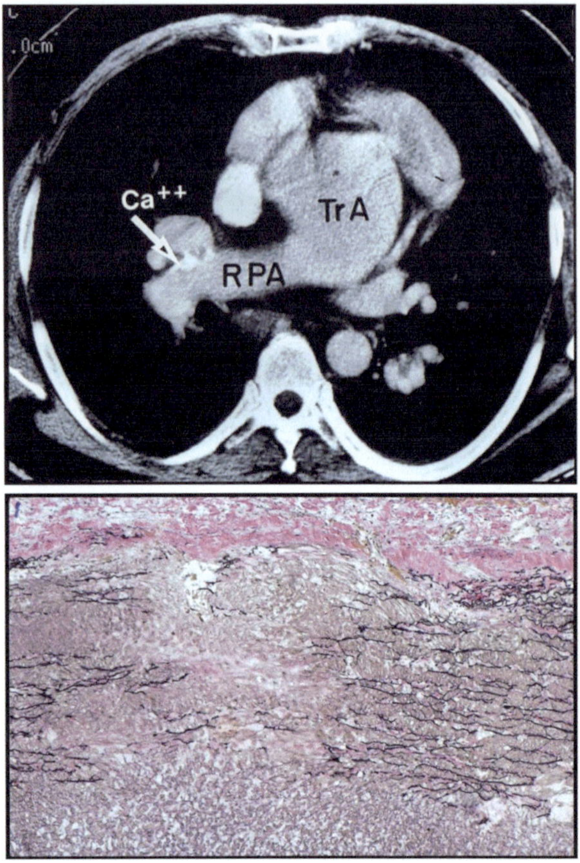

Fig. 2.6 Persistent truncus arteriosus, male 41 years old. *Upper panel*: MRI finding, the truncal artery is severely dilated. *Lower panel*: Histopathological findings of the truncus. Severely fragmented elastic fiber in the aortic media, aortic root grade 3 (polychromatic stain). *TrA* truncal artery, *RPA* right pulmonary artery, *Ca* calcium deposition

suggested that cystic medial necrosis observed in the ascending aorta in tetralogy of Fallot, truncus arteriosus (Fig. 2.6), and complete transposition of the great arteries may be related to intrinsic weakness of the aortic wall, because it is observed even in early childhood. Also, the ascending aorta in univentricular hearts with pulmonary stenosis/atresia may dilate out of proportion (Fig. 2.7). Dissection or rupture of the ascending aorta in these anomalies is very rare, but it can happen in Fontan patients [37]. Also another Fontan case with aortic dissection was experienced (personal communication). Decreased elasticity in the aortic wall in these patients can possibly induce low coronary flow and systemic ventricular dysfunction in the future. As these patients have a prolonged survival due to recent medical and surgical development, a meticulous follow-up seems to be necessary for preventing dilatation and rupture or dissection of the ascending aorta.

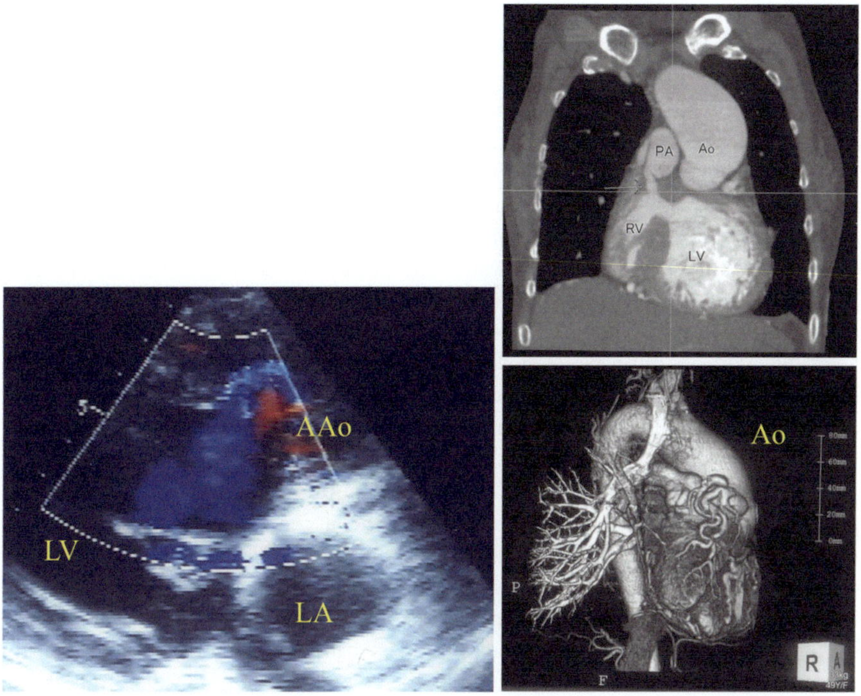

Fig. 2.7 A 50-year-old female, tricuspid atresia (1b), post-Glenn procedure, right aortic arch, moderate aortic regurgitation, ascending aortic diameter: 50 mm. *Left panel*: Severe aortic regurgitation by echo. *Right panel*: Dilated ascending aorta by MRI. *AAO* ascending aorta, *LV* left ventricle, *LA* left atrium (Courtesy by Dr. Katayama H.)

2.7 Hypertensive Pulmonary Trunk Dilatation and Cystic Medial Necrosis

Cystic medial necrosis of the pulmonary trunk is recognized in Marfan syndrome as occurring in concert with similar aortic involvement [5, 6]. However, comparing to the ascending aorta, the incidence of pulmonary trunk aneurysm in Marfan syndrome is not high [6, 17, 18]. Pulmonary trunk aneurysm in ventricular septal defect or patent ductus arteriosus and pulmonary hypertension were reported, and the pulmonary truncal wall in these patients revealed cystic medial necrosis as it was observed in Marfan's ascending aorta [38–43]. Postpartum maternal death is reported secondary to a dissecting aneurysm of the pulmonary trunk in patent ductus arteriosus and obstructive pulmonary vascular disease [44]. When pulmonary hypertension dates from birth, pulmonary trunk histology is initially indistinguishable from that of the ascending aorta [32, 45], but when pulmonary hypertension is acquired after birth, the pulmonary trunk differs significantly from the ascending aorta. Before 1 year of age, medial abnormalities are absent in hypertensive pulmonary trunks associated with nonrestrictive ventricular septal defects, but they are consistently present after the age of 5 years [45].

In the histological study [1, 46], a patient with ruptured pulmonary trunk and Eisenmenger ventricular septal defect and a patient with ruptured ascending aorta and Eisenmenger ventricular septal defect revealed cystic medial necrosis in both pulmonary trunk and ascending aortic walls. Even in cyanotic adults with decreased pulmonary blood flow and surgical excessive left to right shunt, obstructive pulmonary vascular disease with pulmonary trunk dilatation is not rare. Dissection or rupture of pulmonary trunk aneurysm in tetralogy of Fallot and Blalock-Taussig shunt is reported [47, 48]. Also, one patient with shunted tetralogy of Fallot with ruptured pulmonary trunk aneurysm and the other patient with shunted single left ventricle with pulmonary stenosis and dissected pulmonary trunk aneurysm revealed typical cystic medial necrosis in pulmonary trunk. The former patient also revealed cystic medial necrosis in ascending aortic wall [1]. It is reported that 7 of 18 patients with nonrestrictive ventricular septal defect, aging from newborn to 38 years, revealed cystic medial necrosis in the pulmonary trunk and four of seven patients revealed cystic medial necrosis in the ascending aorta simultaneously [49]. Three of 21 patients with complete transposition of the great arteries revealed cystic medial necrosis in pulmonary trunk [36]. A patient with tetralogy of Fallot with absent pulmonary valve revealed cystic medial necrosis in the pulmonary trunk [1]. It was reported that in the pulmonary trunk of tetralogy of Fallot, elastin content diminished with increase in the collagen content [50, 51]. Therefore, cystic medial necrosis in the pulmonary trunk in CHD has been considered to be partly related to pulmonary hypertension; however, there may be intrinsic abnormality in the pulmonary trunk in CHD, especially in cyanotic. However, even after repair of tetralogy of Fallot, similar medial abnormality was occasionally found [52].

2.8 Non-hypertensive Pulmonary Trunk Dilatation

Mobile congenital pulmonary valve stenosis is associated with conspicuous dilatation of the pulmonary trunk, but dysplastic pulmonary valve stenosis is accompanied by relatively little dilatation [53] despite equivalent post-stenotic turbulence, discounting turbulence per se as a pivotal factor in dilatation. Pulmonary trunk dilatation above a mobile stenotic pulmonary valve may be related to the morphology of that specific type of congenitally malformed valve rather than to its functional state. This is analogous to the proposed relationship between a bicuspid aortic valve and dilatation of the ascending aorta. Pulmonary trunk aneurysms are occasionally associated with mobile pulmonary valve stenosis [54], and fragmentation of medial elastic fibers with mucoid degeneration has been found in these aneurysms [55]. One patient was reported to be underwent pulmonary trunk aneurysmectomy with valve replacement 15 years after valvotomy for mobile congenital pulmonary stenosis; there were moderate medial abnormalities in the aneurysmal pulmonary trunk [1].

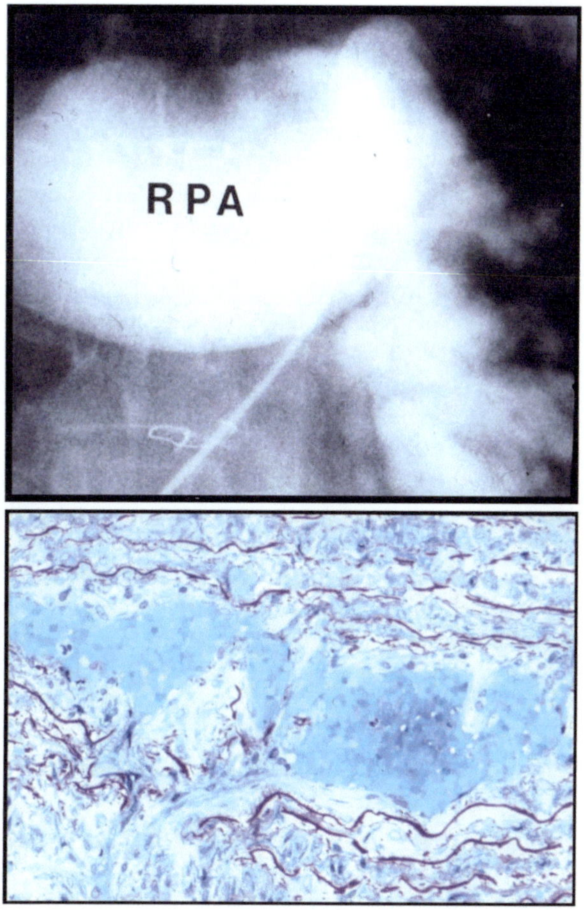

Fig. 2.8 A 26-year-old male, tetralogy of Fallot with absent pulmonary valve. *Upper panel*: Aneurysmal right pulmonary artery (RPA). *Lower panel*: Severely fragmented elastic fibers in the pulmonary arterial media. Pulmonary trunk histological severity grade 3 (polychrome stain)

When the Jatene arterial switch operation was preceded by a pulmonary artery banding, moderate to severe medial abnormalities were subsequently found in the pulmonary trunk (neoaorta) [36]. Assuming that the pulmonary trunks were initially normal, these post-banding medial abnormalities were probably acquired.

In tetralogy of Fallot with absent pulmonary valve, the pulmonary trunk and proximal branches dilate massively [56]. In utero regurgitant volume is returned to the pulmonary trunk during each right ventricular systole, phasically distending the central pulmonary arteries [56]. These aneurysmal pulmonary trunks had severe medial abnormalities (Fig. 2.8) attributed to abnormal flow patterns originating in utero. Absent pulmonary valve is often accompanied by pulmonary artery aneurysm and occasionally reveals cystic medial necrosis in the pulmonary trunk [57, 58].

2.9 Neural Crest Cell and Elastic Fiber Deficit in Great Arteries in Congenital Heart Disease

Maldevelopment of neural crest cells could be responsible for the occurrence of conotruncal anomalies (truncus arteriosus, d-transposition of the great arteries, tetralogy of Fallot with pulmonary atresia), ventricular outflow tract anomalies (bicuspid aortic valve, absent pulmonary valve), and aortic arch anomalies (coarctation of the aorta, interruption of the aorta, double aortic arch) [30, 59]. When the cardiac neural crest is removed, the rate of downstream propagation of the spatial configuration of the elastic matrix in older chick embryos is disordered [60]. Elastin, collagens I and III, and smooth muscle α-actin probably play a contractile role in outflow septation and maintaining hemodynamic characteristics of the normally developing cardiovascular system. These functional parameters are critical in determining the final phenotype of a cardiovascular malformation and occult defects in the ascending aorta and pulmonary trunk wall [60–62]. Therefore, a disorder of neural crest cell migration in early embryogenesis could possibly explain the relation between ascending aorta and pulmonary trunk dilatation with cystic medial necrosis and conotruncal, semilunar valve, and aortic arch anomalies. A partial deletion of chromosome 22q11 in patients with tetralogy of Fallot is a risk factor for aortic dilatation [63, 64].

2.10 Prevention of Aortic Dilatation and Dissection

Prophylactic beta-blockade can be effective in slowing the rate of aortic dilatation due to lowering wall stiffness of the ascending aortic wall and reducing the development of aortic complications in Marfan syndrome [65]. Also, angiotensin receptor blockers possibly slow the progression of aortic dilatation and repair the former aortic medial damage [66]. Aneurysmal expansion and dissection in the ascending aorta are most common during the third trimester, labor, and delivery in patients with or without Marfan syndrome. Half of the aortic dissection in women less than 40 years of age occurs in association with pregnancy [67]. It is reported that in pregnant women who died due to various causes unrelated to aortic complications, the elastic fibers in the ascending aorta lost its normal corrugation with increasing severity toward term [12]. In bicuspid aortic valve and coarctation of the aorta, aortic dissection is observed in their 30s and 40s [25]. In pregnant women with Marfan syndrome, preconceptual dilatation of the ascending aorta seems to be an important predictor for aortic dissection. Then it should be excluded before pregnancy [67]. Therefore, in pregnant women with bicuspid aortic valve or coarctation of the aorta with dilated aorta, administration of beta-blockade or surgical exclusion of dilatation may be recommended [68, 69]. In cyanotic CHD and large aorta without corrective surgery, ascending aorta dilatation is thought to be progressive. However, it is still controversial whether beta-blockade and angiotensin receptor blocker has prophylactic effect for progression of aortic dilatation in CHD with dilated ascending aorta or pulmonary trunk or not.

2.11 Conclusions

Cystic medial necrosis is found in the paracoarctation aorta and in the ascending aorta of bicuspid aortic valve, tetralogy of Fallot, d-transposition of the great arteries, and truncus arteriosus and is found in the pulmonary trunk of tetralogy of Fallot with absent pulmonary valve, Eisenmenger ventricular septal defect, and shunted tetralogy of Fallot or single ventricle with or without obstructive pulmonary vascular disease, encompassing a wide age range. It is suspected that great arterial dilatation in these anomalies may reflect a developmental fault in connecting tissue acting in concert with the basic CHD anomaly as observed in Marfan syndrome or annulo-aortic ectasia. Aortic medial abnormalities may be associated with or predispose to dilatation, aneurysm, and rupture and are potential cardiac surgical risks. Pulmonary trunk medial abnormalities may be associated with or predispose to dilatation and aneurysm formation in mobile pulmonary valve stenosis or tetralogy of Fallot with absent pulmonary valve. Aneurysmal hypertensive pulmonary trunks may rupture. However, three important questions still remain:

1. Whether great arterial medial abnormalities are inherent or acquired
2. Whether and to what extent CHD plays a causal or a facilitating role
3. Whether and to what extent genetic determinants are operative

References

1. Niwa K, Perloff JK, Bhuta SM et al (2001) Structural abnormalities of great arterial walls in congenital heart disease. Light and electron microscopic analyses. Circulation 103:393–400
2. Roberts CS, Roberts WC (1991) Dissection of the aorta associated with congenital malformation of the aortic valve. J Am Coll Cardiol 17:712–716
3. Mckusick VA (1972) Association of congenital bicuspid aortic valve and Erdheim's cystic medial necrosis. Lancet I 299:1026–1027
4. Dietz HC, Pyeritz RE (1995) Mutations in the human gene for fibrillin-1 (FBN1) in the Marfan syndrome and related disorders. Hum Mol Genet 4:1799–1809
5. Prejda AJ, Abraham PA, Carnes WH et al (1985) Marfan's syndrome: structural, biochemical, and mechanical studies of the aortic media. J Lab Clin Med 106:376–383
6. Sayers CP, Goltz RW, Mottaz J (1975) Pulmonary elastic tissue in general elastolysis (cutis laxa) and Marfan's syndrome. A light and electron microscopic study. J Invest Dermatol 65:451–457
7. Lindsay J Jr (1988) Coarctation of the aorta, bicuspid aortic valve and abnormal ascending aortic wall. Am J Cardiol 61:182–184
8. Mckusick VA, Logue RB, Bahnson HT (1957) Association of aortic valvular disease and cystic medial necrosis of the ascending aorta; report of four instances. Circulation 16:188–194

9. Fenoglio JJ, McAllister HAJR, DeCastro CM et al (1977) Congenital bicuspid aortic valve after age 20. Am J Cardiol 39:164–169
10. Edwards WD, Leaf DS, Edwards JE (1978) Dissecting aortic aneurysm associated with congenital bicuspid aortic valve. Circulation 57:1022–1025
11. Edwards JE (1973) Aneurysms of the thoracic aorta complicating coarctation. Circulation 48:195–201
12. Monalo-Estrell P, Barker AE (1967) Histopathologic findings in human aortic media associated with pregnancy. Arch Pathol 83:336–341
13. Schlatmann TJ, Becker AE (1977) Histologic changes in the normal aging aorta: implications for dissecting aortic aneurysm. Am J Cardiol 39:13–20
14. Carlson RG, Lillehei CW, Edwards JE (1970) Cystic medial necrosis of the ascending aorta in relation to age and hypertension. Am J Cardiol 25:411–415
15. Wang J, Nagy A, Larsson J et al (2006) Defective ALK5 signaling in the neural crest leads to increased postmigratory neural crest cell apoptosis and severe outflow tract defects. BMC Dev Biol 6:51–64
16. Erdheim J (1929) Medionecrosis aortae idiopathica. Virchows Arch (Pathol Anat) 273:186
17. Tung HL, Liebow AA (1952) Marfan's syndrome. Observations at necropsy: with special reference to medionecrosis of the great vessels. Lab Investig 1:382–406
18. McKusick V (1955) The cardiovascular aspects of Marfan's syndrome: a heritable disorder of connective tissue. Circulation 11:321–342
19. Chapman DW, Beazley HL, Peterson PK et al (1965) Annulo-aortic ectasia with cystic medial necrosis. Diagnosis and surgical treatment. Am J Cardiol 16:679–687
20. Sauvunen T, Aho HJ (1985) Annulo-aortic ectasia. Light and electron microscopic changes in aortic media. Virchows Arch [Pathol Anat] 407:279–288
21. Larson EW, Edwards WD (1984) Risk factors for aortic dissection: a necropsy study of 161 cases. Am J Cardiol 53:849–855
22. Roberts WC (1970) The congenitally bicuspid aortic valve. A study of 85 autopsy cases. Am J Cardiol 126:72–83
23. Harn RT, Roman MJ, Mogtader AH et al (1992) Association of aortic dilation with regurgitation, stenotic and functionally normal aortic valves. J Am Coll Cardiol 19:283–288
24. Becker AE, Becker MJ, Edwards JE (1970) Anomalies associated with coarctation of the aorta. Circulation 41:1067–1076
25. McCombs HL, Crocker DW (1967) Dissecting aneurysm distal to coarctation of the aorta with long survival. Am Heart J 74:675–679
26. Maron BJ, Humphries JO, Rowe RD et al (1973) Prognosis of surgically corrected coarctation of the aorta. Circulation 47:119–126
27. Forfang K, Rostad H, Sorland S et al (1979) late sudden death after surgical correction of coarctation of the aorta. Importance of aneurysm of the ascending aorta. Avta Med Scand 206:375–379
28. Mitchell IM, Pollock JCS (1990) Coarctation of the aorta and poststenotic aneurysm formation. Br Heart J 64:332–333
29. Isner JM, Donaldson RF, Fulton D et al (1987) Cystic medial necrosis in coarctation of the aorta: a potential factor contributing to adverse consequences observed after percutaneous balloon angioplasty of coarctation sites. Circulation 75:689–695
30. Kappetein AP, Gittenberge de Groot AC, Zwinderman AH et al (1991) The neural crest as a possible pathogenetic factor in coarctation of the aorta and bicuspid aortic valve. J Thorac Cardiovasc Surg 102:830–836
31. Capelli H, Ross D, Somerville J (1982) Aortic regurgitation in tetrad of Fallot and pulmonary atresia. Am J Cardiol 49:1979–1983
32. Niwa K (2013) Aortopathy in congenital heart disease in adults: aortic dilatation with decreased aortic elasticity that Impacts negatively on left ventricular function. Korean Circ J 43:215–220

33. Tan JL, Davlouros PA, McCarthy KP et al (2005) Intrinsic histological abnormalities of aortic root and ascending aorta in tetralogy of Fallot: evidence of causative mechanism for aortic dilatation and aortopathy. Circulation 112:961–968
34. Niwa K (2005) Aortic root dilatation in tetralogy of Fallot long-term after repair–histology of the aorta in tetralogy of Fallot: evidence of intrinsic aortopathy. Int J Cardiol 103:117–119
35. Marelli AJ, Perloff JK, Child JS et al (1994) Pulmonary atresia with ventricular septal defect in adults. Circulation 89:243–251
36. Takeuchi T, Imai Y, Takanashi Y et al (1996) Histological study of the great arteries in patients with arterial switch operation. Act Ped Cardiol Jpn 12:506–512
37. Egan M, Phillips A, Cook SC (2009) Aortic dissection in the adult Fontan with aortic root enlargement. Pediatr Cardiol 30:562–563
38. Boyd LJ, McGavack TH (1939) Aneurysm of the pulmonary artery. Am Heart J 18:562–578
39. Foord AG, Lewis RD (1959) Primary dissecting aneurysms of peripheral and pulmonary arteries. AMA Arch Pathol 68:553–577
40. Deterling RA Jr, Clagett OT (1947) Aneurysm of the pulmonary artery: review of the literature and report of a case. Am Heart J 34:471–499
41. Butto F, Lucas RV Jr, Edwards JE (1967) Pulmonary arterial aneurysm. A pathological study of five cases. Chest 91:237–241
42. Sardesai SH, Marshall RJ, Farrow R et al (1990) Dissecting aneurysm of the pulmonary artery in a case of unoperated patent ductus arteriosus. Eur Heart J 11:670–673
43. Natelson EA, Watts HD, Fred HL (1970) Cystic medionecrosis of the pulmonary arteries. Chest 57:333–335
44. Hankins GDV, Brekken AL, Davis LM (1985) Maternal death secondary to a dissecting aneurysm of the pulmonary artery. Obstet Gynecol 65:45S–48S
45. Tredal SM, Carter JB, Edwards JE (1974) Cystic medial necrosis of the pulmonary arteries: association with pulmonary hypertension. Arch Pathol 97:183–186
46. Niwa K, Perloff JK, Kaplan S et al (1999) Eisenmenger syndrome in adults: ventricular septal defect, truncus arteriosus, univentricular heart. J Am Coll Cardiol 34:223–232
47. Epstein S, Naji AF (1960) Pulmonary artery aneurysm with dissection after Blalock operation for tetralogy of Fallot. Am J Cardiol 5:560–563
48. Donohue BC, Binder SW, Perloff JK et al (1988) Rupture of an aneurysmal pulmonary trunk 40 years after Blalock-Taussig anastomosis. Am J Cardiol 61:477–478
49. Yamaki S, Endo M, Takahashi T (1997) Different grades of medial hypertrophy and intimal changes in small pulmonary arteries among various types of congenital heart disease with pulmonary hypertension. Tohoku J Exp Med 182:83–91
50. Farrar JF, Blomfield J, Reye RDK (1965) The structure and composition of the pulmonary circulation in congenital heart disease. J Path Bact 90:97–105
51. Johnson RJ, Ghaworth SG (1982) Pulmonary vascular and alveolar development in tetralogy of Fallot: a recommendation for early correction. Thorax 37:893–901
52. Bédard E, McCarthy KP, Dimopoulos K et al (2009) Structural abnormalities of the pulmonary trunk in tetralogy of Fallot and potential clinical implications: a morphological study. J Am Coll Cardiol 54:1883–1890
53. Koretzky ED, Moller JH, Korns ME et al (1969) Congenital pulmonary stenosis resulting from dysplasia of the valve. Circulation 40:43–53
54. Tami LF, McElderry MW (1994) Pulmonary artery aneurysm due to severe congenital pulmonic stenosis. Angiology 45:383–390
55. Maehara T, Kiso I, Hayashi I (1984) Pulmonary artery aneurysm associated with pulmonic stenosis [in Japanese]. Rinsho Kyobu Geka 4:613–618
56. Fouron JC, Sahn DJ, Bender R et al (1989) Prenatal diagnosis and circulatory characteristics in tetralogy of Fallot with absent pulmonary valve. Am J Cardiol 64:547–549
57. Rabinovitch M, Grady S, David I et al (1982) Compression of intrapulmonary bronchi by abnormally branching pulmonary arteries associated with absent pulmonary valves. Am J Cardiol 50:804–813

58. Miller RA, Lev M, Paul MH (1962) Congenital absence of the pulmonary valve. The clinical syndrome of tetralogy with pulmonary regurgitation. Circulation 26:266–278
59. Kirby ML, Waldo KL (1990) Role of neural crest cell in congenital heart disease. Circulation 82:332–340
60. Rosenquist TH, Beall AC, Modis L et al (1990) Impaired elastic matrix development in the great arteries after ablation of the cardiac neural crest. Anat Rec 226:347–359
61. Bockman DE, Redmond ME, Kirby ML (1989) Alteration of early vascular development after ablation of cranial neural crest. Anat Rec 225:209–217
62. Davies MJ, Treasure T, Richardson PD (1996) The pathogenesis of spontaneous arterial dissection. Heart 75:434–435
63. Niwa K, Siu S, Webb G et al (2002) Progressive aortic root dilatation in adults late after repair of tetralogy of Fallot. Circulation 106:1374–1378
64. John AS, McDonald-McGinn DM, Zackai EH et al (2009) Aortic root dilatation in patients with 22q11.2 deletion syndrome. Am J Med Genet A149A:939–942
65. Shores J, Berger KR, Murphy EA et al (1994) Progression of aortic dilatation and the benefit of long-term β-adrenergic blockade in Marfan's syndrome. N Engl J Med 330:1335–1341
66. Habashi JP, Judge DP, Holm TM et al (2006) Losartan, an AT1 antagonist, prevents aortic aneurysm in a mouse model of Marfan syndrome. Science 312:117–121
67. Elkayam OE, Shotan A et al (1995) Cardiovascular problems in pregnant women with the Marfan syndrome. Ann Intern Med 123:117–122
68. Anderson RA, Fineron PW (1994) Aortic dissection in pregnancy: importance of pregnancy-induced changes in the vessel wall and bicuspid aortic valve in pathogenesis. Br J Obstet Gynaecol 101:1085–1088
69. Lao TT, Sermer M, MaGee L et al (1993) Congenital aortic stenosis and pregnancy – a reappraisal. Am J Costet Gynecol 169:540–554

Chapter 3
Physiological Background

Tomoaki Murakami

Abstract From the physiological view, the aorta has two functions: conduit function and reservoir function. The typical disorder with the failure of the conduit function is aortic coarctation. On the other hand, the typical condition with the reservoir dysfunction is aging. The histological findings of the aged aorta resemble to that in the aortopathy (decrease of elastin fiber, increase of collagen, calcium deposition, and cystic medial necrosis). The aged aorta increases the systemic ventricular workload, and this is disadvantageous for the coronary perfusion. One of the possible mechanisms of the damage of the aorta is the enhanced pressure wave reflection induced by the heterogeneity or discontinuity of the aortic wall property.

Keywords Conduit function • Reservoir function • Pressure wave reflection • Cystic medial necrosis

3.1 Introduction

From the physiological view, the aorta has two functions: conduit function and reservoir function. The conduit function is easy to understand. A typical disorder with the failure of the conduit function is aortic coarctation (Fig. 3.1) [1]. The disease brings about left ventricular hypertrophy and afterload mismatch. However, the reservoir function and the problem of it are not well known. In this section, the reservoir function of the aorta will be explained.

T. Murakami, M.D., Ph.D. (✉)
Department of Cardiology, Chiba Children's Hospital, 579-1 Heta-cho, Midori-ku, Chiba 266-0007, Japan
e-mail: murat@seagreen.ocn.ne.jp

K. Niwa, H. Kaemmerer (eds.), *Aortopathy*, DOI 10.1007/978-4-431-56071-5_3

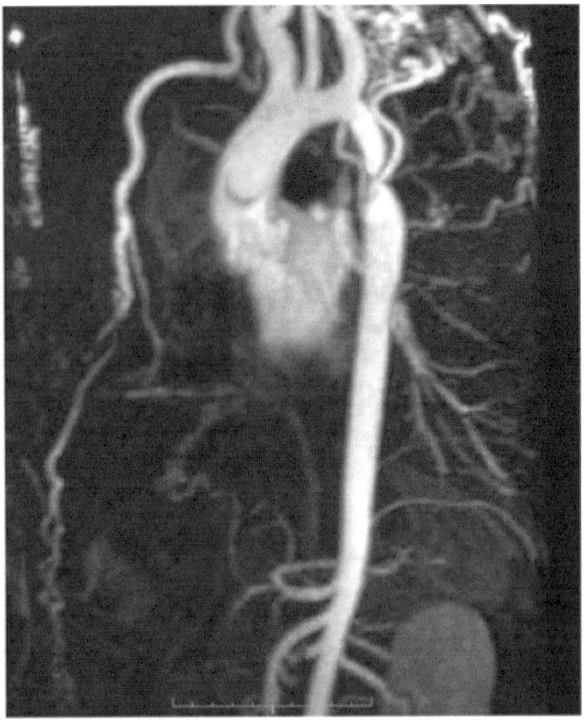

Fig. 3.1 Magnetic resonance image of a patient with conduit dysfunction of aortic arch (aortic coarctation) (Ref. [1])

3.2 Aortic Reservoir Function

The aorta is not only a simple conduit but also a functional reservoir. Figure 3.2 explains the reservoir function of the aorta [2]. During systole, the systemic ventricle ejects the blood into the aorta. However, the blood volume that runs off to organs during systole is less than half of the ejected blood. More than half of the ejected blood from the systemic ventricle is stored in the aorta during systole and runs off to the organs during diastole (Fig. 3.2a). When the reservoir function is damaged, the blood flow runoff during diastole is diminished, and the systolic blood pressure elevates, which is called isolated systolic hypertension (Fig. 3.2b). One of the most important organs that is mainly circulated during diastole is the heart. Therefore, the damage of the reservoir function is disadvantageous for the coronary circulation.

3.3 Aging of the Aorta

As with the other functions of the human body, the aortic reservoir function is deteriorating with aging. Therefore, we could study the aortic reservoir function by comparing the conditions of the function in young and old. With aging,

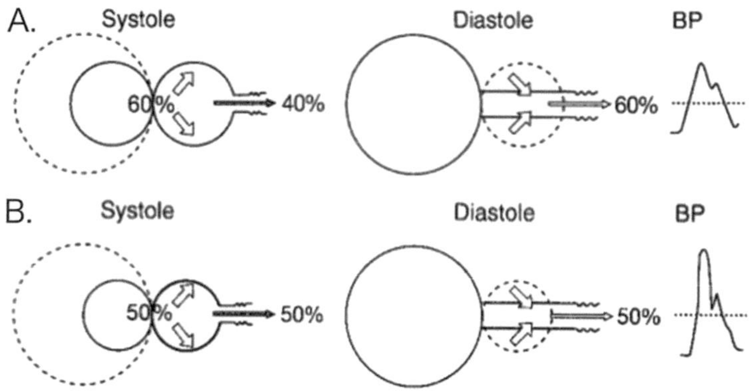

Fig. 3.2 Aortic reservoir function. Normal aorta stores more than half of the ejected blood during systole, and the stored blood runs off to the organs during diastole (**a**). The aorta with damaged reservoir function cannot store enough blood during systole. Therefore, the systolic blood pressure elevates and the diastolic blood flow decreases (**b**) (Ref. [2])

degeneration of elastin fibers in the aortic wall occurs, and collagenous material increases. Calcium deposition also occurs. The progression of the processes results in cystic medial necrosis, which is also well known as the histological characteristic of aortopathy. As a matter of course, the histological changes, the decrease of elastin fibers, and the increase of collagen cause damage to the elastic properties of the aorta. Figure 3.3 demonstrates the decreased aortic distensibility in the aging process [3]. As a result of the loss of the elasticity, the pulse wave velocity elevates with aging (Fig. 3.4) [4]. Because the ejection to the stiff aorta augments the cardiac workload, the myocardial blood flow increases (Fig. 3.5a). However, the stiff aorta, it means the damage for the reservoir function, could not increase the pooling of the blood in the aorta during systole. As a result, the myocardial flow reserve decreases with aging (Fig. 3.5b) [5].

Interestingly, it is well known that the aortic diameter enlarges with aging process (Fig. 3.6) [6]. Aortopathy is usually defined as a dilatation of the aorta. However, many reports demonstrated that the aortic root expansion and the stiffening of the aorta occur together in many clinical settings [7–10]. Moreover, it is reported that the pulse wave velocity of the dilated aorta is elevated in patients with aortopathy [11], although the increase of the diameter means the decreased pulse wave velocity based on physical laws. Therefore, it is possible that the damaged aortic distensibility precedes the dilatation of the aorta in the aortopathy. The reason why the aorta with the decreased distensibility dilates has not been fully elucidated. One of the possible mechanisms of the phenomenon is a compensation for the cardiac demand-coronary supply balance [12–14].

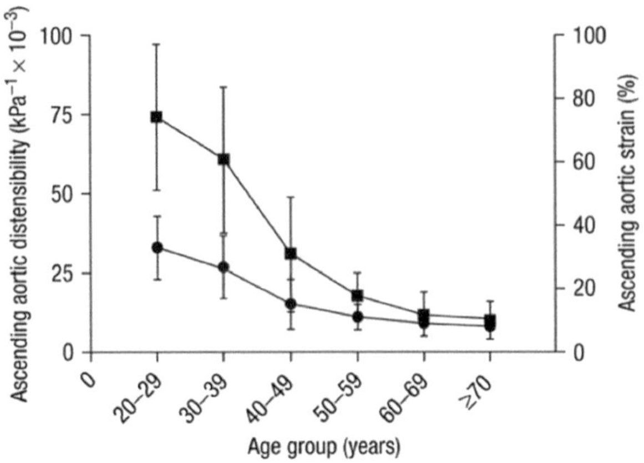

Fig. 3.3 Strain (●) and distensibility (■) of the ascending aorta decrease with aging (Ref. [3])

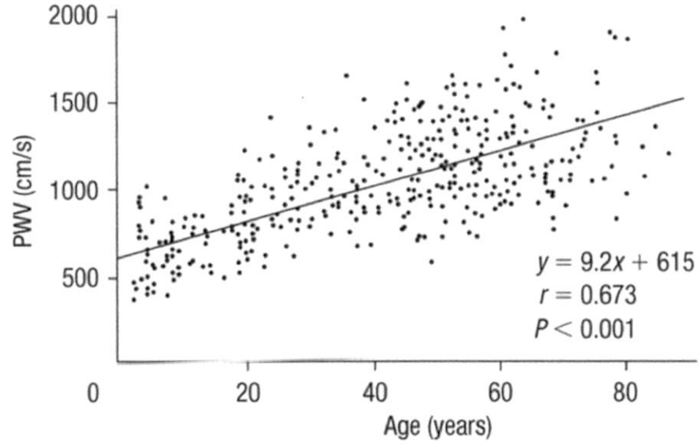

Fig. 3.4 Pulse wave velocity elevates with aging (Ref. [4])

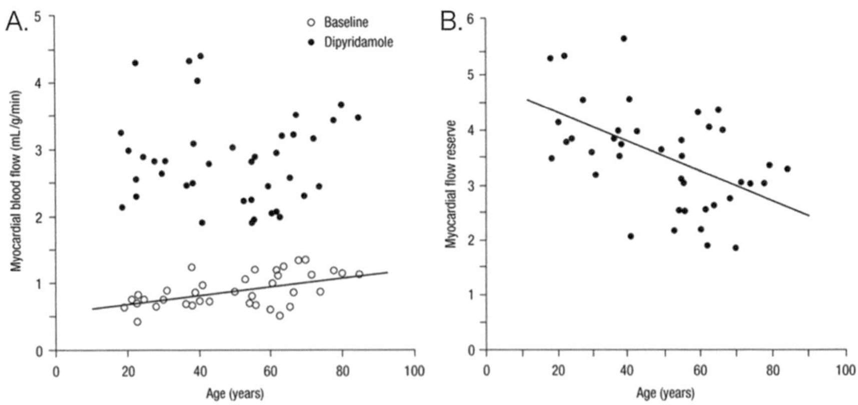

Fig. 3.5 Myocardial blood flow increases (**a**) and myocardial flow reserve decreases (**b**) with aging (Ref. [5])

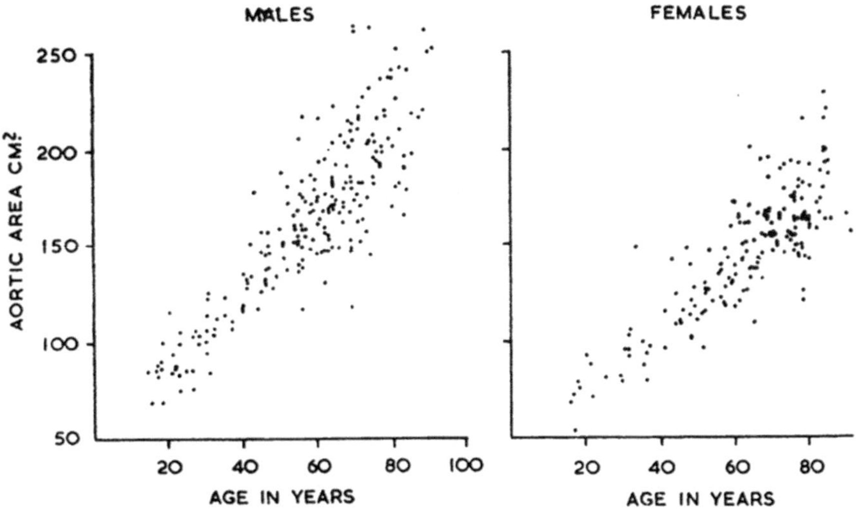

Fig. 3.6 Aortic diameter enlarges with aging (Ref. [6])

3.4 Pathophysiology of the Aortopathy

In patients with aortopathy, the change of vascular characteristics (dilation, decreased distensibility, and acceleration of pulse wave velocity) is usually limited in the ascending aorta in contrast to the aging process.

Several theories are proposed in order to explain the phenomenon.

One of the theories is that the enhanced aortic pressure augmentation caused by pressure wave reflection results in the localization of the abnormal aortic property. Aortic pressure waveform is composed of two pressure waveforms: the forward pressure wave and the reflected pressure wave. The forward pressure wave is generated by the systemic ventricular ejection, and the backward pressure is the sum of the pressure wave reflections. The pressure wave reflections arise from any discontinuity in elastic properties along the arterial tree in which there is a change (or mismatch) in impedance [15]. In young people, the reflected pressure wave returns to the heart during diastole, it means after closure of the aortic valve, because the pulse wave velocity in young is slow. Therefore, it enhances the coronary perfusion by pushing the aortic blood stored during systole. With aging, the pulse wave velocity gradually increases. It means the early return of the reflected pressure wave (in systole) impairs arterial and ventricular function. The opposite directional reflected pressure wave that returns to the heart during systole interferes with the systemic ventricular ejection and increases the workload of the systemic ventricle (Fig. 3.7).

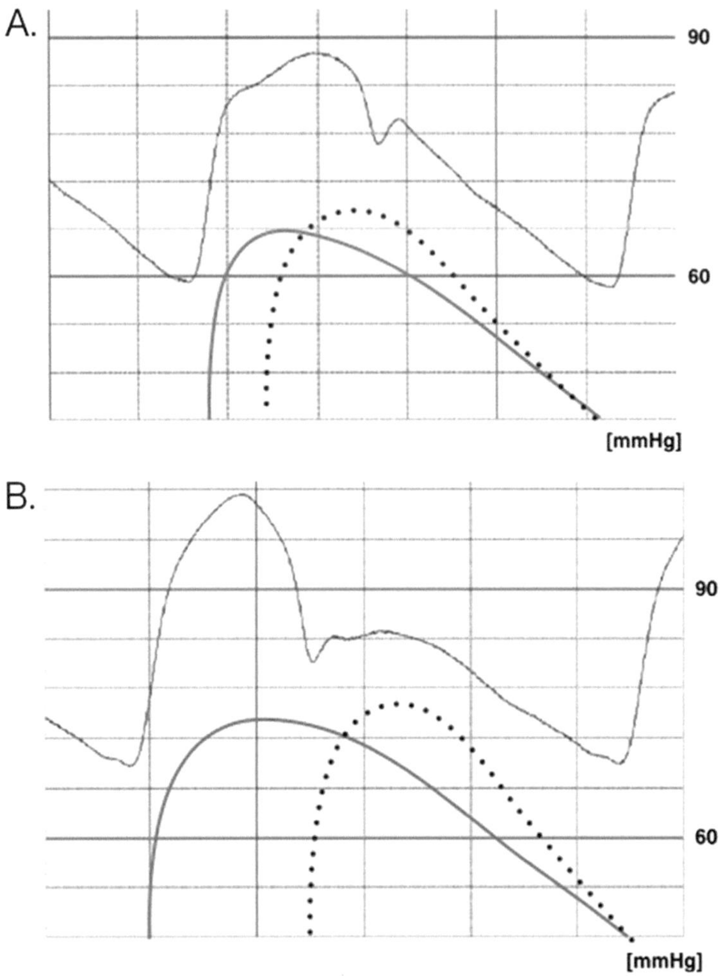

Fig. 3.7 Aortic pressure waveforms. A solid line means the forward pressure wave, and *dotted line* stands for the reflected pressure wave. Early return of the reflected pressure wave (**a**), namely, returns before closure of aortic valve, applies load to the systemic ventricle. On the other hand, late return of the reflected pressure wave (**b**) can enhance the coronary perfusion

3.5 Early Return of the Reflected Pressure Wave in Aortopathy

The mechanism of the early return of aortic pressure wave reflection in elderly people is the increase of the pulse wave velocity of the arterial tree. In congenital heart disease, the mechanism of the enhancement is not necessarily the same. In normal aortic tree, the reflecting point, which represents the integrated pressure wave reflections, exists in the region of the aortic bifurcation [16]. If there is a new

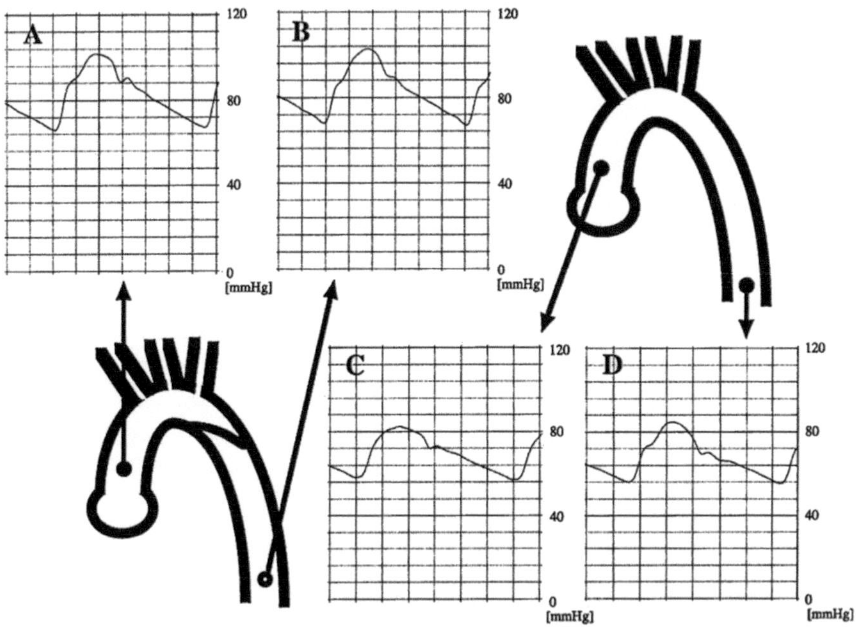

Fig. 3.8 Ascending (**a**) and descending (**b**) aortic pressure waveform in a 6-year-old patient after extended end-to-end anastomosis of the aortic arch. Ascending (**c**) and descending (**d**) aortic pressure waveform in a 6-year-old patient with normal aortic arch. The waveform A resembles D rather than C (Ref. [18])

site with impedance mismatch proximal to the aortic bifurcation, it could strongly enhance the aortic pressure augmentation. Therefore, if the heterogeneity or discontinuity of the aortic wall property that can generate a new pressure wave reflection exists proximal to the aortic bifurcation, it can damage not only the systemic ventricle but also the aorta proximal to the point of the impedance mismatch, resulting in aortic dilation [17].

In many conditions with aortic dilation, the heterogeneity of the aortic wall properties has been reported. In patients with aortic coarctation after surgical repair, the repaired site generates a new pressure wave reflection (Fig. 3.8) [18]. Moreover, it is also reported that aortic surgery is one of the risk factors for the enhancement of the pressure wave reflection [19]. In patients with a bicuspid aortic valve, it is reported that the regions of increased wall shear stress showed greater medial elastin degradation compared to adjacent areas with normal wall shear stress in the ascending aorta [20]. In patients suffering from cyanotic congenital heart disease, the shunt blood flow from systemic to pulmonary circulation increases the blood flow in the ascending aorta but not in the descending aorta. The excess blood flow in the ascending aorta could induce fatiguing effects of cyclic stress on elastin fibers and lamellae within the arterial media (elastin fracture) [15, 21]. Therefore, it makes the gap of vascular property between the ascending and the descending aorta [11]. As a result, the gap generates the new pressure wave reflection. Therefore, the heterogeneity or discontinuity of the aortic wall property should be one of the keys to the aneurysmal changes of the aorta [22].

References

1. Murakami T, Ueno M, Takeda A et al (2007) Pressure wave reflection after successful balloon dilatation of aortic coarctation. Circ J 71:1821–1822
2. London GM, Guerin AP (1999) Influence of arterial pulse and reflected waves on blood pressure and cardiac function. Am Heart J 138:S220–S224
3. Redheuil A, Yu WC, Wu CO et al (2010) Reduced ascending aortic strain and distensibility: easiest manifestations of vascular aging in humans. Hypertension 55:319–326
4. Avolio AP, Chen SG, Wang RP et al (1983) Effects of aging on changing arterial compliance and left ventricular load in a northern Chinese urban community. Circulation 68:50–58
5. Chernin J, Muller P, Chan S et al (1993) Influence of age and hemodynamics on myocardial blood flow and flow reserve. Circulation 88:62–69
6. Mitchell JR, Schwartz CJ, Zinger A (1964) Relationship between aortic plaques and age, sex and blood pressure. Br Med J 1(5377):205–209
7. Rutz T, Max F, Wahl A et al (2012) Distensibility and diameter of ascending aorta assessed by cardiac magnetic resonance imaging in adults with tetralogy of Fallot or complete transposition. Am J Cardiol 110:103–108
8. Shim CY, Cho IJ, Yang WI et al (2011) Central aortic stiffness and its association with ascending aorta dilation in subjects with a bicuspid aortic valve. J Am Soc Echocardiogr 24: 847–852
9. Niwa K (2013) Aortopathy in congenital heart disease in adults: aortic dilatation with decreased aortic elasticity that impacts negatively in left ventricular function. Korean Circ J 43:215–220
10. Murakami T, Nakazawa M, Momma K et al (2000) Impaired distensibility of neoaorta after arterial switch procedure. Ann Thorac Surg 70:1907–1910
11. Saiki H, Kojima T, Seki M et al (2012) Marked disparity in mechanical wall properties between ascending and descending aorta in patients with tetralogy of Fallot. Eur J Cardiothorac Surg 41:570–573
12. Murakami T, Takei K, Ueno M et al (2008) Aortic reservoir function after arterial switch operation in elementary school-aged children. Circ J 72:1291–1295
13. Murakami T, Niwa K (2015) Aortic stiffening and dilation: influence on coronary supply-demand balance. J Am Coll Cardiol 65:2262
14. Murakami T, Shiina Y, Niwa K (2016) Letter by Murakami et al regarding article, "segmental aortic stiffening in children and young adults with connective tissue disorders". Circulation 133:e9
15. Nichols WW, O'Rourke MF, Vlachopoulos C (2011) McDonald's blood flow in arteries, 6th edn. Hodder Arnold, London
16. O'Rourke MF (1990) Arterial stiffness, systolic blood pressure, and logical treatment of arterial hypertension. Hypertension 15:339–347
17. Raaz U, Zöllner AM, Schellinger IN et al (2015) Segmental aortic stiffening contributes to experimental abdominal aortic aneurysm development. Circulation 131:1783–1795
18. Murakami T, Takeda A (2005) Enhanced aortic pressure wave reflection in patients after repair of aortic coarctation. Ann Thorac Surg 80:995–1000
19. Murakami T, Tateno S, Kawasoe Y et al (2014) Aortic surgery is one of the risk factors for enhancement of pressure wave reflection in adult patients with congenital heart disease. Int J Cardiol 175:451–454

20. Guzzardi DG, Barker AJ, van Ooij P et al (2015) Valve-related hemodynamics mediate human bicuspid aortopathy. J Am Coll Cardiol 66:892–900
21. Murakami T, Niwa K (2015) Elastin fracture localized in ascending aorta could be one of the mechanisms of enhanced aortic pressure wave reflection in adult patients with congenital heart disease. Int J Cardiol 194:66–67
22. Murakami T, Shiina Y, Niwa K (2016) Final common pathway of aortic dilation?: heterogeneity of aortic wall property causes the aneurysmal change. J Am Coll Cardiol 67:735–736

Chapter 4
Aortopathies: Clinical Manifestation

Harald Kaemmerer and Yskert von Kodolitsch

Abstract Many native, surgically or interventionally treated patients with **congenital heart anomalies** and **genetic aortic syndromes** (GAS) (e.g., Marfan, Loeys-Dietz, Ehlers-Danlos, Turner syndrome) are at risk for the development of aortic aneurysm, dissection, or rupture, resulting from inborn anomalies of the structure and metabolism of the aortic wall.

Therefore, all caregivers should be familiar with signs and symptoms of aortopathies and imperative diagnostic and therapeutic measures.

The **diagnosis** of aortopathies largely depends on recognition of aortic dilatation prior to the development of acute complications like dissection or rupture, as well as organ involvement from complications. Clinical suspicion is crucial, as usually the growth of aortic aneurysm is asymptomatic until aortic complications occur. The **diagnostic approach** to the diagnosis of aortopathies incorporates primarily the clinical impression, the medical history, and the results of the physical examination, supplemented by sophisticated modern laboratory and imaging techniques, particularly advanced echo, MRI, and CT techniques, which have improved the clinical diagnosis substantially.

Only timely discovery provides the chance to induce prophylactic or therapeutic measures.

Keywords Aortopathy • Aortic aneurysm • Aortic dissection • Aortic rupture • Clinical diagnosis • Congenital heart disease

---

H. Kaemmerer (✉)
Klinik für Kinderkardiologie und angeborene Herzfehler, Deutsches Herzzentrum München, German Heart Center Munich, Technische Universität München, Technical University Munich, Lazarettstr. 36, D-80636 Munich, Germany
e-mail: Kaemmerer@dhm.mhn.de

Y. von Kodolitsch
Centre of Cardiology and Cardiovascular Surgery, German Aortic Center Hamburg, University Heart Center, University Medical Centre, Hamburg, Germany

K. Niwa, H. Kaemmerer (eds.), *Aortopathy*, DOI 10.1007/978-4-431-56071-5_4

4.1 Introduction

Aortic aneurysm is of outstanding importance in the context of congenital heart disease (CHD) and genetic aortic syndromes (GAS), as in the long run, many native, surgically or interventionally treated patients are at risk for the development of aortic aneurysm, dissection, or rupture.

It should be kept in mind that in many congenital heart anomalies or in genetic aortic syndromes, ectasia of the aortic root results from an inborn anomaly of the structure and metabolism of the aortic wall.

Accordingly, it has to be considered that meanwhile most patients with CHD reach adulthood and many of them mature adulthood (age 50–80) or even age beyond 80. Therefore, clinicians who provide care of adults with CHD should be aware that their patients might also develop aortopathies unrelated to the underlying congenital anomaly. Thus, caregivers have to be familiar with signs and symptoms of aortopathies and know about imperative diagnostic and therapeutic measures.

From the clinician's view, three types of thoracic aortic syndromes need particular consideration:

1. **Silent aortic syndrome (SAS)**, where aortopathy evolves from mild dilatation to acute aortic syndrome (AAS), usually through an asymptomatic increase of aortic diameter
2. **Genetic aortic syndrome (GAS)**, which comprises a growing spectrum of genetic diseases that predispose to the evolution of an aortopathy, where aneurysms already occur in adolescents and young adults
3. **Acute aortic syndrome (AAS)** that comprises several acute aortopathies that present with similar symptoms with various underlying aortic pathologies that all indicate the immediate threat of aortic rupture and death

Aortic diseases account worldwide for significant cardiovascular morbidity and mortality. A thoracic aortic aneurysm is a serious health risk because it may dissect and rupture, causing a life-threatening emergency. When detected in time, a thoracic aortic aneurysm can often be repaired with surgery or interventional techniques [1].

Contemporary awareness of **prevalence and incidence** in thoracic aortic aneurysm is predominantly based on small studies and widely indefinite. The estimated incidence of thoracic aortic aneurysms is 5–10 patients per 100,000 individuals in the population per year [2, 3]. The estimated prevalence is 3–4 % of those >65 years, and it has been increasing in the last decade and probably will continue to increase [3, 4]. Data from the USA indicate that aneurysmal disease is the 18th most common cause of death in the general western population and the 15th most common in individuals older than age 65 years, accounting for 13,843 and 11,147 deaths in these two groups, respectively [5]. Experts estimate that between 30,000 and 60,000 deaths per year in the USA are caused by aneurysmal disease [5]. The estimated prevalence of acute aortic dissection is 10–30 per million per year, or 2.6–3.5 cases per 100,000 person-years [6, 7, 8].

Table 4.1 Potential causes of aortic aneurysm

General	Advanced age
	Arteriosclerosis
	Arterial hypertension
Genetic aortic syndromes (monogenetic diseases)	
Nonsyndromic	Familial thoracic aortic aneurysm syndrome caused by mutations in the following genes
	ACTA2
	MYH11
	MMP3
	MMP9
	SMAD3
Syndromic	Marfan syndrome (FBN1)
	Loeys-Dietz syndrome (TGFBR1/TGFBR2)
	Aneurysms-osteoarthritis syndrome (*SMAD3*)
	Vascular Ehlers-Danlos syndrome (*COL3A1*)
	Polycystic kidney disease (*PKD1*, *PKD2*)
	Osteogenesis imperfecta (*COL1A1*, *COL1A2*)
	Noonan syndrome
	Turner syndrome
Congenital anomalies	
Congenital heart anomalies, isolated	Bicuspid aortic valve
	Aortic coarctation
	Conotruncal abnormalities
	Status *post operationem*
	For example:
	after Ross operation
	after arterial switch operation
Complex syndromes	
	Turner syndrome
	Williams-Beuren syndrome
	Noonan syndrome
Miscellaneous	
Infections	For example:
	HIV
	Staphylococcus species
	Salmonella
	Mycobacterium (Tbc)
	Mycotic aneurysm
Aortitis/inflammatory diseases	For example:
	Giant cell arteritis, rheumatoid arthritis, lupus erythematosus, ankylosing spondylitis, Behçet's disease, Wegener's granulomatosis, Takayasu's arteritis, retroperitoneal fibrosis (Ormond's disease)

(continued)

Table 4.1 (continued)

Trauma/strenuous activities	Deceleration injury
	Weight lifting
Pregnancy	Peripartum
Iatrogenic dissections	Catheters and guidewires
	Status *post operationem* (after aortotomy, vascular clamp)
Drugs	Chronic corticosteroid
	Cocaine

Causes of thoracic aortic aneurysm are given in Table 4.1.

4.2 Silent Aortic Syndrome (SAS)

The **clinical diagnosis** of aortopathy largely depends on recognition of aortic dilatation (SAS) prior to the development of acute complication (AAS) like dissection or rupture, as well as organ involvement from complications. Clinical suspicion is crucial, as usually the growth of aortic aneurysm is asymptomatic until aortic complications occur.

The **diagnostic approach** to the diagnosis of aortopathies incorporates primarily the clinical impression, the medical history, and the results of the physical examination.

A comprehensive **medical history** is useful in consideration of disorders connected with aortic aneurysm. The review of risk factors for aortic disease includes family history, disorders at risk for aortic involvement, and congenital heart defects but also arteriosclerosis, arterial hypertension, specific infections, or inflammatory disease (Table 4.2) [6].

It is of vital importance to identify individuals with GAS early before AAS develops. For example, Marfan syndrome can be identified according to typical stigmata, where prediction models are available to identify Marfan syndrome with the help of simple clinical signs such as skin striae or arachnodactyly. Similarly, Loeys-Dietz syndrome may be suspected in persons with a bifid uvula.

An educated **physical examination** may help to detect marked aneurysm still in the asymptomatic state (SAS). The occasional patient with marked thoracic aneurysm may experience dysphagia from esophageal compression, hoarseness from injury of the recurrent laryngeal nerve, cough, shortness of breath, and back pain. Moreover, a pulsatile sternum can indicate a retrosternal aneurysm.

Sometimes in aneurysm of the ascending aorta and the aortic arch, the Oliver-Cardarelli sign occurs. This tracheal tug consists of a pulsation of the larynx to one side synchronous with ventricular systole, which can be felt in the upright patient when the larynx is palpated between the thumb and index finger.

An abdominal aortic aneurysm may with limited accuracy be palpable as epigastric mass [9, 10, 11].

Table 4.2 Signs and symptoms of silent aortic syndrome (SAS) [11, 14, 15]

Finding	Explanation
Symptoms	
Chest pain	Location is also possible in the back, shoulders
Dyspnea and shortness of breath	Usually only mild and felt as substernal oppression, rarely due to oppression of the trachea or bronchi
Cough	Linked to involvement of recurrent laryngeal nerve
Upper venous congestion	Oppression of vessels such as the superior vena cava, the pulmonary artery, or the innominate vein can lead to visible enlargement of the veins, cyanosis, and swelling of upper extremity
Hoarseness and dysphonia	Injury of the recurrent laryngeal nerve
Dysphagia	Esophageal compression by aneurysm; symptom is closely allied to dysphonia
Horner's syndrome	Ptosis, miosis, and exophthalmus due to paralysis of the superior cervical ganglion
Atypical	Loss of weight and appetite, palpitations, fever, cyanosis
Physical signs	
Pulsatile sternum	Due to a large retrosternal aneurysm
Tracheal tug (Oliver-Cardarelli sign)	Aneurysm of the ascending aorta and the aortic arch. This tracheal tug consists of a pulsation of the larynx to one side synchronous with ventricular systole, which can be felt in the upright patient when the larynx is palpated between the thumb and index finger
Dullness on percussion	Sub- and parasternal dullness in proximal aortic aneurysms and left interscapular or left subscapular dullness
Aortic diastolic murmur	Due to aortic valve regurgitation
Palpation of epigastric mass	Abdominal aneurysm

This basic **diagnostic armamentarium** has meanwhile been supplemented by sophisticated modern imaging techniques, particularly advanced echo, MRI, and CT techniques, which have improved the clinical diagnosis substantially. Each method has relative advantages and disadvantages, but all have high sensitivity and specificity.

4.2.1 Thoracic Aortic Aneurysm (TAA)

The aneurysm of the sinuses of Valsalva that previously had been described as **anulo-aortic ectasia** denotes a dilatation of the proximal aorta at the level of the aortic root that may transcend the aortic ridge and involve also the ascending part of the aorta. Clinically, ectasia (dilatation) is defined by a transverse diameter exceeding 1.5 times the expected size. Proximal aortic aneurysm was also identified with diameters of the aorta, which is at least 50 % larger than normal [6, 12].

Assessing the absolute size of the aorta, it is reasonable to refer the diameter to body size, weight, and body surface area, as well as the gender and age of a person.

As a rule of thumb, in an average-sized adult, an aortic aneurysm is an enlargement of at least 4.0 cm in diameter, and usually the abdominal aorta is as thick as the patient's thumb.

Ectasia (dilatation) or aneurysm formation of the aortic root is often seen in patients with congenital heart anomalies, such as bicuspid aortic valve (BAV) or coarctation of the aorta (CoA), or with GAS, such as Marfan, Loeys-Dietz, and Ehlers-Danlos syndrome.

4.2.1.1 Clinical Presentation of Thoracic Aortic Aneurysm (TAA)

Most thoracic aortic aneurysms are asymptomatic and may be diagnosed incidentally on echo or chest X-ray, or if compression of adjacent structures occur or complications develop, e.g., dissection and rupture.

Thoracic aneurysms are rarely diagnosed by physical examination (Table 4.2).

Chest pain is not uncommon in patients with aneurysmal dilatation of the aortic anulus, chronic aortic dilatation, aortic wall thinning, and aortic distension [13].

Physical findings may be absent, but signs and symptoms may appear from mass effect. Once the dilated aorta compresses adjacent structures (e.g., superior vena cava, esophagus, trachea, or recurrent laryngeal nerve), a superior vena cava syndrome, stridor, dysphagia, or hoarseness may occur.

Progressive ectasia of the aortic root and aortic sinuses can lead to aortic valve regurgitation. Narrowing of the coronary artery ostia may lead to myocardial ischemia and even infarction. A sluggish blood flow can predispose to atheroma, thrombus formation, and peripheral embolization.

4.3 Acute Aortic Syndrome (AAS)

For the identification of patients at **risk for acute aortic syndrome** (AAS), the early clinical detection of aortopathies is of outstanding importance. Only timely discovery provides the chance to induce prophylactic or therapeutic measures.

Pain is the central feature of an AAS which comprises aortic dissection (AD), intramural hematoma (IMH), and penetrating atherosclerotic ulcer (PAU) (Fig. 4.1) [4, 7]. Among these disorders, AD occurs more often (62–88 % of all patients with AAS) than IMH (10–30 %) and PAU (2–8 %) [7].

Acute aortic pain is caused by aortic distention or disruption due to tears, intramural hematoma, dissection, ulceration, or rupture, while **chronic aortic pain** is associated with aortic dilatation, distension, and dissection [13].

The annual incidence of AAS is not so high, but mortality is extreme and the most frequently fatal condition for patients with chest pain [16].

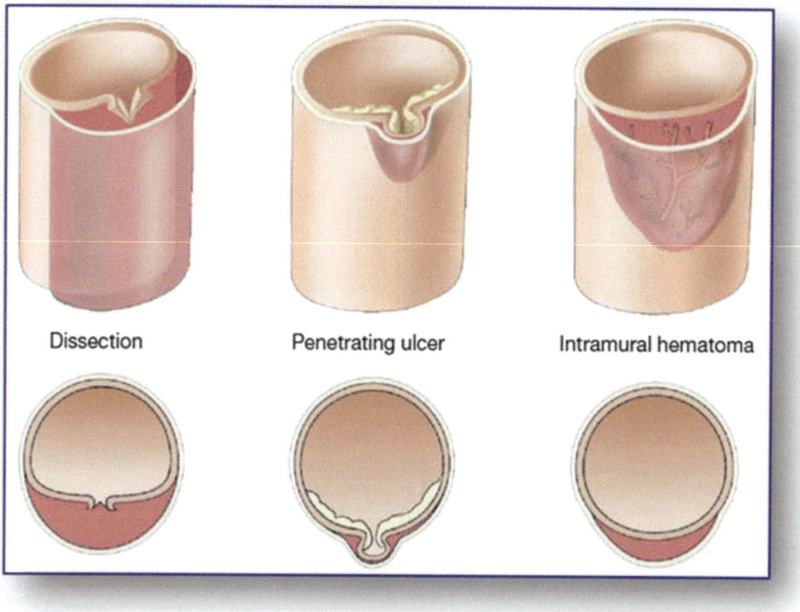

Fig. 4.1 Aortic pathologies that all cause acute aortic syndrome (AAS): schematic of aortic dissection (*left*), intramural hematoma (*middle*), and penetrating ulcer (*right*) (From: Elefteriades JA. Thoracic aortic aneurysm: reading the enemy's playbook. Current problems in cardiology 2008;33:203–77) [4]

4.3.1 Overt Aortic Dissection (OAD)

Acute aortic dissection **results from** a tear in the aortic intima. Blood enters through this tear into the medial layer of the aortic wall, propagates along the media, and forms a second blood-filled channel within the aortic wall, resulting in a "true lumen" and the "false lumen," a channel within the media (Figs. 4.1 and 4.2) [17].

Elderly hypertensive individuals (> 65 years), particularly male, are **predisposed**. Risk factors for OAD in patients < 40 years of age are connective tissue disorders (e.g., Marfan, Loeys-Dietz, Ehlers-Danlos, Turner syndrome) or congenital heart anomalies (e.g., aortic coarctation, bicuspid aortic valve disease) [7] Fig. 4.3.

4.3.1.1 Clinical Presentation of Overt Aortic Dissection (OAD)

Clinical criteria for aortic dissection are poorly defined (Table 4.3) [18].

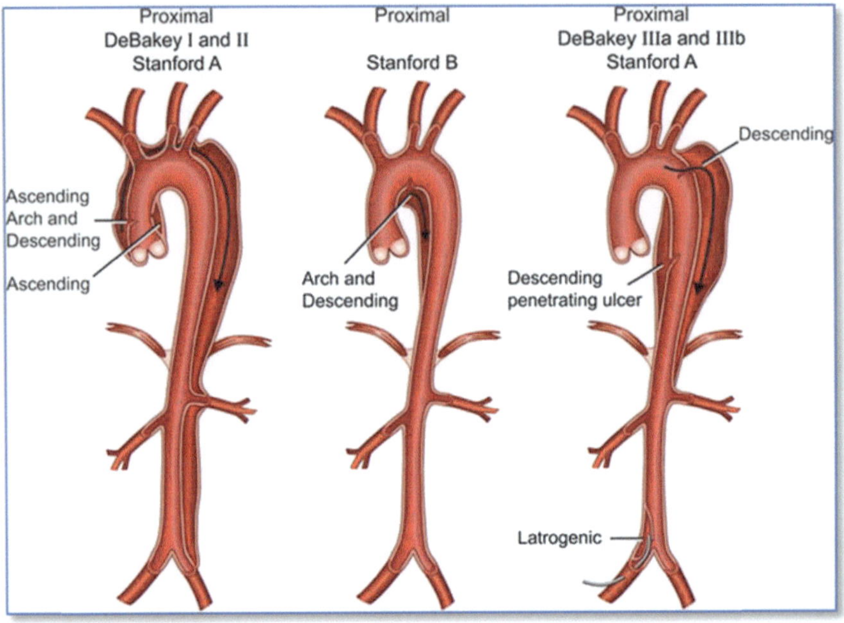

Fig. 4.2 Aortic dissection according to the DeBakey and Stanford classifications
Stanford-classification
Type A: All dissections involving the ascending aorta, regardless of the site of origin
Type B: Dissection does not involve the ascending aorta
DeBakey classification
Type I: Dissection originates in the ascending aorta and propagates at least to the aortic arch
Type II: Dissection originates in the ascending aorta and involves only the ascending aorta
Type III: Dissection originates in the descending aorta and propagates down the aorta (rarely retrogrades to the aortic arch and the ascending aorta) (From Ref. [17])

Patients with OAD often present as an emergency with severe chest pain and a tearing sensation in their anterior or posterior chest, the neck, the throat, the back, the interscapular, the abdomen, or the legs [16, 19].

Typically the pain starts abruptly and can vary in intensity. The pain of acute aortic dissection may be pulsatile, varying in intensity with each heartbeat and pulse, perhaps because of intermittent changes in wall tension, wall stress, and neuropathic transmission [13, 20].

Patients are often hypertensive, but they may be also normo- or hypotensive.

Depending on the degree and extent of the dissection, occlusion of aortic branches and end-organ ischemia may also be present and induce myocardial infarction, cerebral ischemia/stroke, abdominal organ ischemia, limb ischemia, or paraplegia (due to involvement of the largest anterior segmental medullary artery, i.e., artery of Adamkiewicz, A. radicularis magna) [21].

The pain can radiate or migrate [16]. The site of the painful complaints can indicate the localization of the aortic dissection, such as anterior chest pain in type I

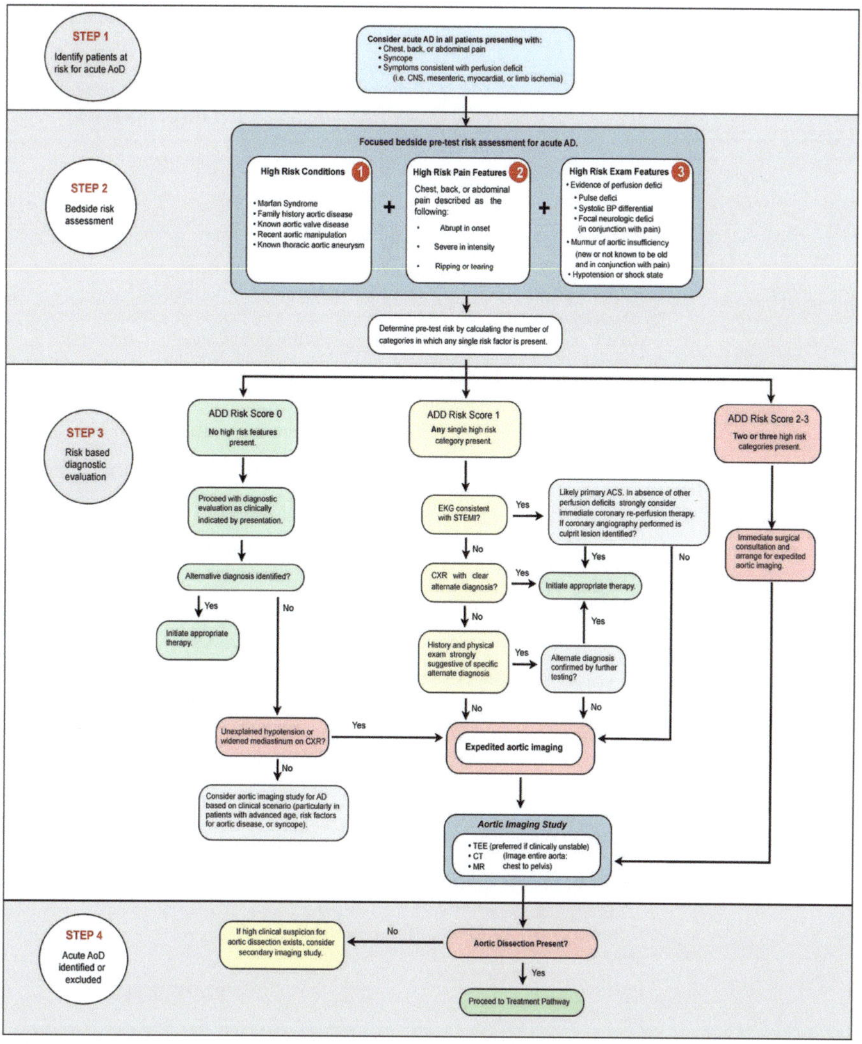

Fig. 4.3 Guideline-based evaluation pathway for the identification of acute aortic dissection at initial presentation [47, 18, 40]. (*ACS* acute coronary syndrome, *ADD* aortic dissection detection, *BP* blood pressure, *CNS* central nervous system, *CT* computed tomography, *CXR* chest X-ray, *MRI* magnetic resonance imaging, *STEMI* ST segment elevation myocardial infarction, *TEE* transesophageal echocardiogram) (From Ref. [47])

or II dissection and backache in type I or III aortic dissection extending into the descending thoracic aorta [13]. However, the correlation of pain localization and site of aortic dissection is not so strong, and there may be many exceptions [6].

As independent predictors of acute aortic dissection, von Kodolitsch et al. identified a sudden tearing or ripping pain, a mediastinal and/or aortic widening on chest radiography, and pulse differentials and/or blood pressure differentials.

Table 4.3 Clinical signs and symptoms in acute aortic syndrome/aortic dissection (AAS)

			Comment
Pain	Location	Chest, anterior	Site may relate vaguely to the involved section of the aorta
		Chest, posterior	
		Neck	
		Back	
		Epigastrium	
		Abdomen	
		Legs	
	Onset	Acute, abrupt	Acute or increasing pain suggests expansion with the risk of dissection
		Increasing	
		Chronic	
	Type	Intense, often tearing or sharp	Maximum at the time of dissection.
			n.b.: Dissection may be painless
Blood pressure			Hypertensive
			Normotensive
			Hypotensive
			Shock
			n.b.: Pseudo-hypotension due to peripheral vascular problems
Acute aortic regurgitation			If a proximal dissection involves the aortic valve
Thromboembolic events		Arterial emboli	Cerebral, coronary, visceral arteries, peripheral arteries
Compression/eroding of local structures	Recurrent laryngeal nerve	Hoarseness	
	Pericardium	Tamponade	
	Coronary artery	Myocardial infarction	
	Pulsus paradoxus		Strongly suggests tamponade
	Pulsus deficit		Strongly suggests loss of perfusion
	Superior vena cava distention		Strongly suggests tamponade acute left to right shunt (fistula)
	Trachea	Cough, stridor, dyspnea	Suggests aortobronchial fistula
	Bronchi	Hemoptysis	
	Left-sided pleural effusion	Cough, dyspnea	Sign of rupture
			Hematothorax
	Esophagus	Hematemesis	Suggests aortoesophageal fistula
		Dysphagia	
	Vertebral body	Back pain	
Systemic symptoms		Fever	

The probability of dissection was low with absence of all the three variables (7 %), intermediate with isolated findings of pain or mediastinal widening (31 and 39 %, respectively), and high with isolated pulse or blood pressure differentials or any combination of the three variables (≥83 %) [18].

However, it should be underlined that aortic dissection can also occur *without any* pain or with completely atypical complaints. This may be just the case in patients with connective tissue disease (e.g., Marfan syndrome), after previous heart surgery or in older patients with neurologic disorders [13, 22].

Signs of rupture, like mediastinal hematoma and pleural or pericardial effusions, are seen more frequently in women [23].

In persons younger than 40 years, dissection occurs in 7 %, typically linked to hereditary disorders (e.g., Marfan syndrome), congenital heart anomalies, previous cardiac surgery, or pregnancy [6, 24].

Particularly in type A dissection, prolapse of the aortic valve or dilation of the aortic root or of the aortic anulus can give rise to aortic valve regurgitation. Acute aortic pain and auscultatory finding of an aortic diastolic murmur should raise strong clinical suspicion of type A aortic dissection.

Dissections involving the coronary ostia, commonly the right coronary ostium, result in acute myocardial ischemia and infarction.

Extension of the dissection into the pericardial space may prompt pericardial effusion and tamponade, a common reason for syncope, hypotension, and death.

Pleural effusion or mediastinal hemorrhage may occur. Mediastinal hemorrhages can compress the superior cervical ganglion, causing Horner's syndrome, or the left laryngeal recurrent nerve, producing vocal cord paralysis or hoarseness [19]. This is, however, more often seen in chronic aneurysm of the aortic arch.

In descending aortic dissections, also the ischemia-induced malperfusion of kidneys, the mesenteric circulation, or the lower extremities can be seen. Compromise of spinal artery perfusion may result in paraplegia.

Fever can occur due to release of pyrogenic substances from the aortic wall [19, 25].

In aortic dissection some **major problems**, including pericardial tamponade, tension hematothorax, aortoenteric fistulae, or aortocaval fistulae, can obscure the clinical presentation (Table 4.3) [26].

Tension Hematothorax After aneurysm rupture hemodynamic instability can occur due to a tension hematothorax resulting from intrathoracic blood expanding into the parietal pleura. The patient is in shock from the acute blood loss, from the increased intrathoracic pressure causing decreased cardiac output, respiratory distress, hypoxia, and acute loss of lung volume. No breath sounds can be heard on the involved side of the chest [26, 27].

Aortoenteric Fistula An aortoenteric fistula is a connection between an aortic segment and an adjacent portion of the gastrointestinal tract, most commonly the duodenum.

Some patients with abdominal aortic aneurysm may present with massive GI bleeding and be in shock. In the presence of a GI bleeding in a patient with known abdominal aortic aneurysm, an aortoenteric fistula should be considered [26, 28, 29].

After the clinical suspicion, esophagogastroduodenoscopy is indicated to localize the bleeding source and a computed tomography with contrast and arteriography to define the relationship between the GI tract and the aorta [28, 30, 29, 31].

Aortocaval Fistula Aortocaval fistulae are harmful complications of abdominal aortic aneurysm, wherein an aortic aneurysm erodes and ruptures into the inferior vena cava.

Thereby blood shunts from the high-pressure arterial system to the low-pressure venous system causing venous hypertension and an increased cardiac preload. The venous hypertension may worsen renal perfusion and trigger renal failure [20]. Clinical presentation depends upon the fistula size, anatomical position, and acute or chronic onset.

Minor fistulae may remain asymptomatic, while major fistulae give rise to systemic venous hypertension and stasis (bilateral pedal edema in the lower half of the body, hematuria, intestinal bleeding), high-output cardiac failure, shock, or renal failure [32].

Physical sign can be an abdominal thrill, accompanied by a continuous murmur [32, 33]. Doppler echo, CT, MRI, and aortography are the diagnostic modalities of choice.

4.3.2 Intramural Hematoma (IMH)

Intramural hematoma (IMH) is defined as an atypical form of aortic dissection without a loss of intimal continuity, an entry tear, or an intimal flap. The pathogenesis is unclear. IMH has been called "mediastinal apoplexy" because IMH is considered to originate from a spontaneous rupture of the vasa vasorum with localized or propagating hemorrhage into the medial layer of the aortic wall [34]. Alternatively, IMH may arise from a penetrating atherosclerotic ulcer that erodes the medial vasa vasorum. This type of IMH usually causes only localized intramural hematoma [6]. Intramural hematoma can weaken the aortic wall and may progress to an outward rupture of the aortic wall or to an inward intima disruption, leading to aortic dissection. Therefore, IMH has been called a precursor of OAD [35].

IMH are typically seen in older patients with arterial hypertension or after blunt chest trauma with aortic wall injury. Other predisposing factors are arterial hypertension or GAS such as Marfan syndrome [6].

Intramural hematoma seems to arise mostly in the ascending or descending aorta and rarely in the aortic arch. Their length and their distal extension may be more limited as compared to OAD [36, 35].

4.3.2.1 Clinical Presentation

The usual presenting symptoms of IMH are almost indistinguishable from OAD, a severe pain, localized central thoracic, with radiation to the back or the abdomen in a middle- to older-aged male patient with a history of arterial hypertension [13].

Notably, according to the data of the International Registry of Aortic Dissection (IRAD), patients with IMH describe more severe initial pain compared with patients with OAD but present less likely with ischemic leg pain, pulse deficits, or aortic valve regurgitation [37].

Many patients with IMH develop complications like pericardial, pleural, or mediastinal effusions, tamponade, coronary artery compression, aortic regurgitation, and rupture [6].

4.3.3 Penetrating Atherosclerotic Ulcer (PAU)

In the early stages of a penetrating atherosclerotic ulcer (PAU), just the intima is ulcerated, but the process may progress further into the media, inducing a hematoma within the media [38]. The penetrating atherosclerotic ulcer can resolve, stay stable, but can also cause aortic aneurysms, aortic dissection, and even aortic rupture [39].

Penetrating aortic ulcers are located commonly in the descending aorta, where atherosclerosis is more prevalent.

4.3.3.1 Clinical Presentation

PAU typically occurs in older individuals with generalized atherosclerosis such as coronary artery disease. Affected persons are usually males with cardiovascular risk factors including arterial hypertension, hyperlipidemia, and smoking. PAU are also frequently associated with chronic obstructive pulmonary disease [39].

Some patients may be asymptomatic and the diagnosis is made incidentally. Classically patients present with symptoms of an acute aortic syndrome or dissection, i.e., acute intense chest pain, often described as tearing, ripping, migrating, or pulsating [39].

4.4 Abdominal Aortic Aneurysm (AAA)

Approximately 75 % of aortic aneurysms develop in the abdominal aorta, where aortic atherosclerosis is more common than in the thoracic aorta [40]. AAA is usually caused by atherosclerosis and more common in men and in individuals aged

65 years or older. There is a familial predisposition, and relatives of affected patients have an increased risk for developing also an AAA.

4.4.1 *Clinical Presentation*

AAA usually remains asymptomatic until rupture.

In lean individuals, AAA can be diagnosed as a pulsatile mass on physical examination by abdominal palpation. Typically, AAA is detected during routine abdominal ultrasound.

If symptoms occur, they can include localized abdominal pain and deep pain in the back or side, in the groin, or in the legs. Sudden beginning of severe abdominal and back pain may indicate impending rupture [1].

The pain pattern can vary upon the site where rupture occurred or where the dissection spread, e.g., in the retroperitoneum, peritoneum, duodenum, bronchus, or vena cava [41]. The history of pain can be associated with aortic thrombosis, lower extremity thromboembolism, syncope, or shock if the aneurysm has ruptured.

4.5 Diagnostic Approach to Acute Aortic Syndrome and Differential Diagnosis

The differential diagnosis of an acute aortic syndrome comprises conditions such as acute coronary syndrome, pericarditis, pulmonary embolism, pleuritis, pneumothorax, esophagitis or esophageal rupture/perforation, cholecystitis, pancreatitis, or renal colic [19].

Because of the complex etiology, symptoms of an acute aortic syndrome are clinically often indistinguishable. In almost all cases, the presumptive diagnosis has to be ensured by modern imaging techniques [19].

Besides the clinical examination and modern imaging modalities, additional technical basic methods are used.

4.5.1 *Electrocardiogram (ECG)*

In every patient with acute chest pain with and without suspected thoracic aortic dissection, a 12-lead ECG should be acquired, mainly in order to rule out an acute coronary syndrome.

However, the ECG often shows normal results or nonspecific abnormalities. In the IRAD study, nearly half of the patients had a normal ECG and none had signs of acute myocardial infarction [37]. However, up to 1–2 % of patients with AD may have acute ST elevation [42].

4.5.2 Chest X-Ray (CXR)

Chest radiography has a sensitivity of 64 % and a specificity of 86 % for AAS [43].

Hence, in the setting of unclear chest pain, chest radiography may indicate presence of an enlarged aorta size, where signs such as abnormal aortic contour, widening of the aortic silhouette, abnormal cardiac contour, or pleural or pericardial effusions may raise the clinical suspicion of acute aortic dissection or other pathologies of AAS [6, 43].

In any case, a normal chest X-ray cannot exclude the presence of aortic dissection, as 12–15 % of patients with acute aortic dissection will have a normal chest X-ray [42].

4.5.3 Serum Biomarkers

Biomarkers for the biochemical detection of acute aortic dissection have been described, including smooth muscle myosin heavy chain (smMHC), smooth muscle troponin (calponin), and soluble elastin fragments (sELAF). Some biomarkers may help to accelerate diagnosis, but currently no biochemical test exists that can reliably identify dissection. They all have difficulties in recognizing and differentiating patients with dissection, intramural hematoma, and acute penetrating ulcers. To some degree, C-reactive protein and creatine kinase isoenzyme can be elevated [44, 45].

D-dimer is meanwhile an essential biomarker in aortic dissection. D-dimer levels increase during the acute phase dissection and also relate to complications.

By contrast, D-dimer levels remain normal in the case of intramural hematoma and in patients with a thrombosed false lumen. **OAD** can be ruled out reliably depending on cutoff values [46].

4.6 Current Guidelines

The American Heart Association and the American College of Cardiology published in 2010 guidelines for the diagnosis and management of patients with thoracic aortic disease. The clinical risk markers proposed are highly sensitive and important clinical tools for a staged approach to diagnosis and management of acute aortic dissection [47].

In 2014 the European Society of Cardiology Guidelines on the diagnosis and treatment of aortic disease appeared, focusing on acute aortic syndromes, aortic aneurysms, genetic and congenital diseases, aortic inflammation, and aortic tumors [48]. Their commandments [49] encompass:

- Modern imaging of the total aorta requiring standardized and measurements and reports
- Scanning of the abdominal aorta for abdominal aortic aneurysms that should be performed in all elderly patients undergoing transthoracic echocardiography
- Standard values for all imaging techniques
- A flowchart for the emergency decision-making in acute aortic syndromes
- Diagnostic steps and therapeutic options for aortic dissection, intramural hematoma, penetrating aortic ulcer, and traumatic aortic injury
- Management recommendations for the optimal treatment and selection of endovascular or open surgery
- New information on genetic and congenital aortic diseases with detailed recommendations, particularly for genetic testing
- The need to set up aortic teams and centers for the acute and for the intensive follow-up of patients with aortic diseases

References

1. Isselbacher EM (2005) Thoracic and abdominal aortic aneurysms. Circulation 111:816–828
2. Abraha I, Romagnoli C, Montedori A, Cirocchi R2009 Thoracic stent graft versus surgery for thoracic aneurysm. Cochrane Database Syst Rev :CD006796
3. Booher AM, Eagle KA. Diagnosis and management issues in thoracic aortic aneurysm. Am Heart J 2011;162:38–46, e1
4. Elefteriades JA (2008) Thoracic aortic aneurysm: reading the enemy's playbook. World J Surg 32:366–374
5. Elefteriades JA, Farkas EA (2010) Thoracic aortic aneurysm clinically pertinent controversies and uncertainties. J Am Coll Cardiol 55:841–857
6. Hutchison S (2008) Aortic intramural hematoma. In: Aortic diseases. Acute Aortic Dissection Philadelphia, Saunders Elsevier, pp 113–30
7. Clough RE, Nienaber CA (2015) Management of acute aortic syndrome. Nat Rev Cardiol 12:103–114
8. Clouse WD, Hallett JW Jr, Schaff HV et al (2004) Acute aortic dissection: population-based incidence compared with degenerative aortic aneurysm rupture. Mayo Clin Proc 79:176–180
9. Fink HA, Lederle FA, Roth CS, Bowles CA, Nelson DB, Haas MA (2000) The accuracy of physical examination to detect abdominal aortic aneurysm. Arch Intern Med 160:833–836
10. Karkos CD, Mukhopadhyay U, Papakostas I, Ghosh J, Thomson GJ, Hughes R (2000) Abdominal aortic aneurysm: the role of clinical examination and opportunistic detection. Eur J Vasc Endovasc Surg 19:299–303
11. Lynch RM (2004) Accuracy of abdominal examination in the diagnosis of non-ruptured abdominal aortic aneurysm. Accid Emerg Nurs 12:99–107
12. Hutchison S (2008) Thoracic aortic aneurysms. In: Aortic diseases. Acute Aortic Dissection Philadelphia, Saunders Elsevier, pp 195–214

13. Wooley CF, Sparks EH, Boudoulas H (2008) Aortic pain. In: Boudoulas H, Stefanadis C (eds) The aorta. Informa Healthcare, New York, pp 78–87
14. Joyce JW, Fairbairn JF 2nd, Kincaid OW, Juergen JL (1964) Aneurysms of the thoracic aorta. A clinical study with special reference to prognosis. Circulation 29:176–181
15. Boyd L (1924) A study of four thousand reported cases of aneurysm of the thoracic aorta. Am J Med Sci 168:654–657
16. Hagan PG, Nienaber CA, Isselbacher EM et al (2000) The International Registry of Acute Aortic Dissection (IRAD): new insights into an old disease. JAMA 283:897–903
17. Nienaber CA, Powell JT (2012) Management of acute aortic syndromes. Eur Heart J 33:26–35b
18. von Kodolitsch Y, Schwartz AG, Nienaber CA (2000) Clinical prediction of acute aortic dissection. Arch Intern Med 160:2977–2982
19. Garcia-Lopez A, Zamorano J (2008) Intramural hematoma and atherosclerotic ulcer. In: Boudoulas H, Stefanadis C (eds) The aorta. Informa Healthcare, New York, pp 193–200
20. Wittels K. Aortic emergencies. Emerg Med Clin North Am 2011;29:789–800, vii.
21. Macura KJ, Corl FM, Fishman EK, Bluemke DA (2003) Pathogenesis in acute aortic syndromes: aortic dissection, intramural hematoma, and penetrating atherosclerotic aortic ulcer. AJR Am J Roentgenol 181:309–316
22. Kaemmerer H, Oechslin E, Seidel H et al (2005) Marfan syndrome: what internists and pediatric or adult cardiologists need to know. Expert Rev Cardiovasc Ther 3:891–909
23. Nienaber CA, Fattori R, Mehta RH et al (2004) Gender-related differences in acute aortic dissection. Circulation 109:3014–3021
24. Januzzi JL, Isselbacher EM, Fattori R et al (2004) Characterizing the young patient with aortic dissection: results from the International Registry of Aortic Dissection (IRAD). J Am Coll Cardiol 43:665–669
25. Fredman C, Serota H, Deligonul U, Barner H, Pearson A, Kern MJ (1990) Ascending aortic aneurysm masquerading as fever, altered mental status, and mediastinal mass. Am Heart J 119:408–410
26. White A, Broder J (2012) Acute aortic emergencies–part 1: aortic aneurysms. Adv Emerg Nurs J 34:216–29; quiz 30–1
27. Pizon A, Bissell BJ, Gilmore N (2012) Rupture of an ascending and descending thoracic aortic aneurysm causing tension hemothorax: a case report. J Emerg Med 43:625–626
28. Doney MK, Vilke GM (2012) Case report: aortoenteric fistula presenting as repeated hematochezia. J Emerg Med 43:431–434
29. Thomson VS, Gopinath KG, Joseph E, Joseph G (2009) Primary aorto-enteric fistula: a rare complication of abdominal aortic aneurysm. J Postgrad Med 55:267–269
30. Sakalihasan N, Limet R, Defawe OD (2005) Abdominal aortic aneurysm. Lancet 365:1577–1589
31. Xiromeritis K, Dalainas I, Stamatakos M, Filis K (2011) Aortoenteric fistulae: present-day management. Int Surg 96:266–273
32. Akwei S, Altaf N, Tennant W, MacSweeney S, Braithwaite B (2011) Emergency endovascular repair of aortocaval fistula–a single center experience. Vasc Endovasc Surg 45:442–446
33. Psathas ED, Lioudaki S, Doulaptsis M, Charalampoudis P, Klonaris C, Verikokos C (2012) Clinical manifestations of aortocaval fistulas in ruptured abdominal aortic aneurysm: report of two cases. Case Rep Surg 2012:123081
34. von Kodolitsch Y, Nienaber CA (1998) Intramural hemorrhage of the thoracic aorta: diagnosis, therapy and prognosis of 209 in vivo diagnosed cases. Z Kardiol 87:797–807
35. Nienaber CA, von Kodolitsch Y, Petersen B et al (1995) Intramural hemorrhage of the thoracic aorta. Diagnostic and therapeutic implications. Circulation 92:1465–1472
36. Kaji S, Akasaka T, Katayama M, et al. 2003 Long-term prognosis of patients with type B aortic intramural hematoma. Circulation 108(Suppl 1):II307–II311.
37. Evangelista A, Mukherjee D, Mehta RH et al (2005) Acute intramural hematoma of the aorta: a mystery in evolution. Circulation 111:1063–1070

38. Hayashi H, Matsuoka Y, Sakamoto I et al (2000) Penetrating atherosclerotic ulcer of the aorta: imaging features and disease concept. Radiographics 20:995–1005
39. Lansman SL, Saunders PC, Malekan R, Spielvogel D (2010) Acute aortic syndrome. J Thorac Cardiovasc Surg 140:S92–7–discussion S142–S146
40. LF H, GL B, JA B et al (2010) 2010 ACCF/AHA/AATS/ACR/ASA/SCA/SCAI/SIR/STS/SVM guidelines for the diagnosis and management of patients with thoracic aortic disease: executive summary. A report of the American College of Cardiology Foundation/American Heart Association Task Force on Practice Guidelines, American Association for Thoracic Surgery, American College of Radiology, American Stroke Association, Society of Cardiovascular Anesthesiologists, Society for Cardiovascular Angiography and Interventions, Society of Interventional Radiology, Society of Thoracic Surgeons, and Society for Vascular Medicine. Catheter Cardiovasc Interv 76:E43–E86
41. Lewiss RE, Egan DJ, Shreves A. Vascular abdominal emergencies. Emerg Med Clin North Am 2011;29:253–272, viii.
42. Braverman AC (2010) Acute aortic dissection: clinician update. Circulation 122:184–188
43. von Kodolitsch Y, Nienaber CA, Dieckmann C et al (2004) Chest radiography for the diagnosis of acute aortic syndrome. Am J Med 116:73–77
44. Ranasinghe AM, Bonser RS (2010) Biomarkers in acute aortic dissection and other aortic syndromes. J Am Coll Cardiol 56:1535–1541
45. Suzuki T, Distante A, Eagle K (2010) Biomarker-assisted diagnosis of acute aortic dissection: how far we have come and what to expect. Curr Opin Cardiol 25:541–545
46. Segreto A, Chiusaroli A, De Salvatore S, Bizzarri F (2014) Biomarkers for the diagnosis of aortic dissection. J Card Surg 29:507–511
47. Rogers AM, Hermann LK, Booher AM et al (2011) Sensitivity of the aortic dissection detection risk score, a novel guideline-based tool for identification of acute aortic dissection at initial presentation: results from the international registry of acute aortic dissection. Circulation 123:2213–2218
48. Erbel R, Aboyans V, Boileau C et al (2014) 2014 ESC guidelines on the diagnosis and treatment of aortic diseases: document covering acute and chronic aortic diseases of the thoracic and abdominal aorta of the adult. The task force for the diagnosis and treatment of aortic diseases of the European Society of Cardiology (ESC). Eur Heart J 35:2873–2926
49. Erbel R (2014) The 'Ten commandments' for European Society of Cardiology guidelines on aortic diseases. Eur Heart J 35:2990

Chapter 5
Genetics of Marfan Syndrome, Related Disorders, and Bicuspid Aortic Valve

Takayuki Morisaki and Hiroko Morisaki

Abstract Recently, the genetic study of aortic diseases such as Marfan syndrome has been advanced, leading to not only identifying responsible genes but also providing better understanding of the pathophysiology and possible new therapeutic targets. Genes identified for aortic diseases include *FBN1*, *TGFBR1*, *TGFBR2*, *SMAD3*, *TGFB2*, *TGFB3*, *SKI*, *EFEMP2*, *COL3A1*, *FLNA*, *ACTA2*, *MYH11*, *MYLK*, *SLC2A10*, and *NOTCH1* as well as others. Their dysfunction is mainly connected with altered function of transforming growth factor-β (TGF-β) signaling pathways, as well as that of the extracellular matrix and smooth muscle contractile apparatus, resulting in progression of structural damage to aorta and great vessels including aortic aneurysms and dissections. Furthermore, it has been shown that the TGF-β signaling pathway plays a key role in the pathogenesis of Marfan syndrome and related disorders, which may be important for development of strategies for medical and surgical treatment of thoracic aortic aneurysms and dissections.

Keywords Aortic aneurysm • Aortic dissection • Valve diseases • Transforming growth factor-β (TGF-β) • Extracellular matrix • Smooth muscle

5.1 Introduction

Aortic diseases including aortic aneurysms and dissections account for 1–2 % of all deaths in Western countries [1]. There are two types of aortic aneurysms based on their location: thoracic aortic aneurysm (TAA) and abdominal aortic aneurysm (AAA). It was reported that the incidence of TAA and dissection (TAAD) is about 10 per 100,000 person-years [2]. In TAA, approximately 20 % of patients have a

T. Morisaki, M.D., Ph.D. (✉)
Department of Clinical Engineering, Tokyo University of Technology School of Health Sciences, 5-23-22 Nishi-Kamata, Otaku, Tokyo, Japan
e-mail: tmorisaki-tky@umin.ac.jp

H. Morisaki
Department of Clinical Engineering, Tokyo University of Technology School of Health Sciences, 5-23-22 Nishi-Kamata, Otaku, Tokyo, Japan

Department of Medical Genetics, Sakakibara Heart Institute, Fuchu, Tokyo, Japan

K. Niwa, H. Kaemmerer (eds.), *Aortopathy*, DOI 10.1007/978-4-431-56071-5_5

positive family history, while 10–20 % of patients with AAA also have such a positive history. However, most patients with AAA also have various risk factors for cardiovascular events, such as smoking, hyperlipidemia, hypertension, sex, and age [3]. Therefore, AAA is thought to be a multifactorial disease with several genes and loci identified to have a positive association with the disease.

In this chapter, we especially focus on Marfan syndrome, related disorders, and bicuspid aortic valve in TAAD [4]. It is thought that excessive matrix degradation is involved in the development of TAAD, though the exact pathological mechanisms are not yet fully understood. An imbalance between matrix metalloproteinases (MMPs) and their inhibitors is thought to induce medial degeneration and aneurysm development. In addition, some other conditions including hypertension can lead to thickening and fibrosis of the intimal layer, and degradation and apoptosis of smooth muscle cells, resulting in wall weakness and eventually development of aneurysms, dissections, and ruptures.

Over the past more than two decades after discovery of the *FBN1* gene as a causative factor for Marfan syndrome (MFS), it has become clear that genetic factors are also at the basis of TAAD formation. Studies of the human syndromic form of TAAD including MFS and its counterparts in mice have provided a better understanding of the cause of the disease condition, including the finding that the transforming growth factor-β (TGF-β) signaling pathway plays a key role in the pathogenesis of TAAD. Since the genes for Marfan related to other syndromic aneurysmal conditions (Loeys-Dietz syndrome, arterial tortuosity syndrome, autosomal recessive cutis laxa, aortic osteoarthritis syndrome, others) have been identified, it is now considered that there is ample evidence showing that dysregulation of TGF-β signaling is the common pathogenic process in aortic diseases. In addition, recent findings have led to new therapeutic strategies for patients with Marfan and related diseases.

5.2 Marfan Syndrome (MFS)

5.2.1 MFS: Syndromic TAAD and TGF-β Signaling

MFS (OMIM #154700) is an autosomal dominant connective tissue disorder first described by Antoine Marfan [5] and with a prevalence of about 1 per 5000 individuals [6]. It was found to be caused by mutations in the *FBN1* gene encoding fibrillin-1, a large glycoprotein and component of extracellular matrix microfibrils. MFS is a systemic disorder affecting skeletal (increased height, disproportionately long limbs and digits, anterior chest deformity, joint laxity, vertebral column deformity, narrow highly arched palate with crowding of teeth), ocular (myopia, increased axial globe length, corneal flatness, ectopia lentis), and cardiovascular (dilatation of aorta, especially aortic root, aortic regurgitation, mitral valve prolapse, mitral regurgitation) systems. Other phenotypes of MFS are dural ectasia, striae distensae, inguinal hernias, pneumothorax, and pulmonary emphysema, though cardiovascular phenotypes, especially TAA, are the most important causes of morbidity and mortality in MFS patients. In most cases, the primary dilatation occurs at the aortic root, especially at the level of the sinus of Valsalva.

For clinical diagnosis of MFS, first the Berlin [7], later the Ghent [8], and most recently the revised Ghent nosology [9] (Table 5.1) were proposed. The revised Ghent nosology is thought to facilitate accurate recognition of MFS and differential diagnosis from other related but distinct disorders, thereby improving patient management as well as counseling. Four possible sets of findings can lead to a diagnosis of MFS in a patient: aortic root dilatation (Z-score >2) and ectopia lentis, aortic root dilatation with an FBN1 mutation, aortic root dilatation with sufficient systemic findings (score of ≥7 on systemic scale), and ectopia lentis with an *FBN1* mutation that has been previously associated with aortic root dilatation. As compared with the previous nosology, the revised Ghent nosology adds more weight to genetic information, especially the relevant *FBN1* mutation.

Scoring of systemic features

Systemic features	Score
Wrist and thumb sign (wrist or thumb sign)	3 (1)
Pectus carinatum deformity – (pectus excavatum or chest asymmetry)	3 (1)
Hindfoot deformity (plain pes planus)	2 (1)
Pneumothorax	2
Dural ectasia	2
Protrusio acetabuli	2
Reduced US/LS and increased arm/height and no severe scoliosis	1
Scoliosis or thoracolumbar kyphosis	1
Reduced elbow extension	1
Facial features (3/5) (dolichocephaly, enophthalmos, downslanting palpebral fissures, malar hypoplasia, retrognathia)	1
Skin striae	1
Myopia >3 diopters	1
Mitral valve prolapse (all types)	1

Maximum total, 20 points; score ≥7 indicates systemic involvement

Criteria for causal FBN1 mutation

Mutation	Conditions
Segregation	Mutation previously shown to segregate in Marfan family
De novo	De novo (with proven paternity and absence of disease in parents) mutation (one of the five following categories)
Nonsense	Nonsense mutation
Deletion/ Insertion	In-frame and out-of-frame deletion/insertion
Splice site mutation	Splice site mutations affecting canonical splice sequence or shown to alter splicing on mRNA/cDNA level

(continued)

Mutation	Conditions
Missense	Missense affecting/creating cysteine residues
	Missense affecting conserved residues of the EGF consensus sequence ((D/N) X(D/N)(E/Q)Xm(D/N)Xn(Y/F) with m and n representing variable number of residues; D aspartic acid, N asparagine, E glutamic acid, Q glutamine, Y tyrosine, F phenylalanine)
	Other missense mutations: segregation in family if possible + absence in 400 ethnically matched control chromosomes, if no family history absence in 400 ethnically matched control chromosomes
Linkage	Linkage of haplotype for n ≥ 6 meioses to the FBN1 locus

Table 5.1 Revised Ghent nosology [9]

General criteria	
	Condition
In the absence of family history	(1) Ao (Z≥2) and EL = MFS
	(2) Ao (Z≥2) and *FBN1* = MFS
	(3) Ao (Z≥2) and Syst (≥7pts) = MFS[a]
	(4) EL and *FBN1* with known Ao = MFS
In the presence of family history	(5) EL and FH of MFS (as defined above) = MFS
	(6) Syst (≥7 pts) and FH of MFS (as defined above) = MFS*
	(7) Ao (Z≥2 above 20 years old, ≥3 below 20 years old) + FH of MFS (as defined above) = MFS*
Others	EL with or without Syst and with an *FBN1* not known with Ao or no *FBN1*= ELS
	Ao (Z< 2) and Syst (≥5) without EL = MASS
	MVP and Ao (Z<2) and Syst (<5) without EL = MVPS

Ao aortic diameter at the sinuses of Valsalva above indicated Z-score or aortic root dissection, *Z* Z-score, *EL* ectopia lentis, *Syst* systemic score (see below), *FBN1* fibrillin-1 mutation, *FBN1 with known Ao FBN1* mutation that has been identified in an individual with aortic aneurysm; *FBN1 not known with Ao FBN1* mutation that has not previously been associated with aortic root aneurysm/dissection; *ELS* ectopia lentis syndrome, *MASS* myopia, mitral valve prolapse, aortic root dilatation, striae, skeletal findings, aortic aneurysm syndrome, *MVPS* mitral valve prolapse syndrome, *MFS* Marfan syndrome

and after *TGFBR1/2*, collagen biochemistry, and *COL3A1* testing if indicated, other conditions/genes will emerge with time

[a]Caveat: without discriminating features of SGS, LDS, or vEDS

5.2.2 MFS: FBN1 and TGF-β Signaling Pathways (Fig. 5.1)

Fibrillin-1 regulates the TGF-β signaling pathway by interacting with latency-associated peptide (LAP), which is a protein derived from the N-terminal region of the TGF-β gene product and latent TGF-β-binding protein (LTBP) [10]. TGF-β interacts with LAP to form a complex termed small latent complex (SLC), which is bound by LTBP to form a larger complex called large latent complex (LLC) and then secreted to the extracellular matrix. Then, TGF-β remains in the extracellular

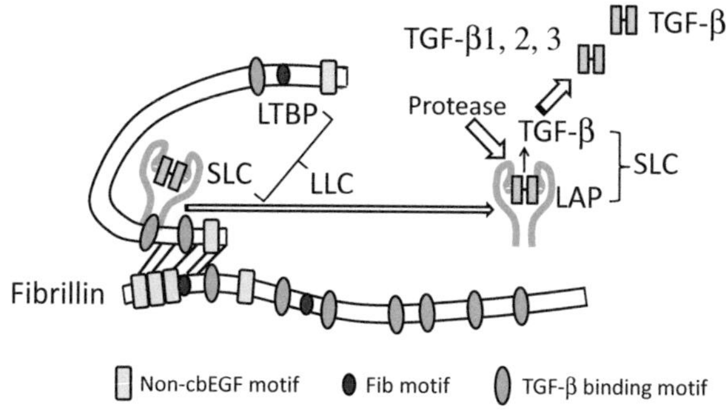

Fig. 5.1 FBN1 and TGF-β signaling pathways. Fibrillin-1 regulates the TGF-β signaling pathway by associating with LLC, consisting of LTBP and SLC. Active, free TGF-β molecules (TGF-β1, TGF-β2, TGF-β3) will be released by protease cleavage of inactive SLC molecules bound to LAP. *LLC* large latent complex, *SLC* small latent complex, *LAP* latency-associated peptide, *LTBP* latent TGF-β-binding protein

matrix in an inactivated complex with LTBP and LAP, and this inactive complex regulates mediation of TGF-β signaling. Since fibrillin-1 interacts with LTBP and LAP to regulate the active level of TGF-β, its dysfunction results in activation of TGF-β signaling [11]. Therefore, it was initially thought that upregulation of TGF-β signaling occurred in canonical (SMAD-dependent) pathways. However, recent findings have shown changes in noncanonical (SMAD-independent) TGF-β pathways involving mitogen-activated protein kinases (MAPK), including extracellular signal-regulated kinase (ERK)1/2, p38, and Jun N-terminal kinase (JNK). As a result, increased TGF-β signaling via both canonical and noncanonical pathways contributes to aortic lesion formation. As shown in the following sections, increased TGF-β signaling is also critical for pathogenic changes in other related genetic aortopathies.

5.2.3 *FBN1 Mutations in MFS*

In 1990, the genetic locus for MFS was mapped to chromosome 15 by linkage analysis [12]. Thereafter, the first fibrillin gene mutation was found in an MFS patient in 1991, and it was confirmed that mutations in the *FBN1* gene on chromosome 15 are responsible for MFS [13]. Since then, more than 1500 *FBN1* mutations have been identified in MFS patients. Several lines of evidence were also shown that many *FBN1* mutant alleles cause MFS phenotypes through a dominant-negative effect [14], though there is a considerable number of patients with mutations resulting in haploinsufficiency due to gene deletion, splicing mutations, or nonsense mutations causing nonsense-mediated mRNA decay (NMD) [15] (Fig. 5.2). Therefore, decreased protein synthesis as well as the dominant-negative effect by the mutant protein is thought to be a pathogenic mechanism for MFS

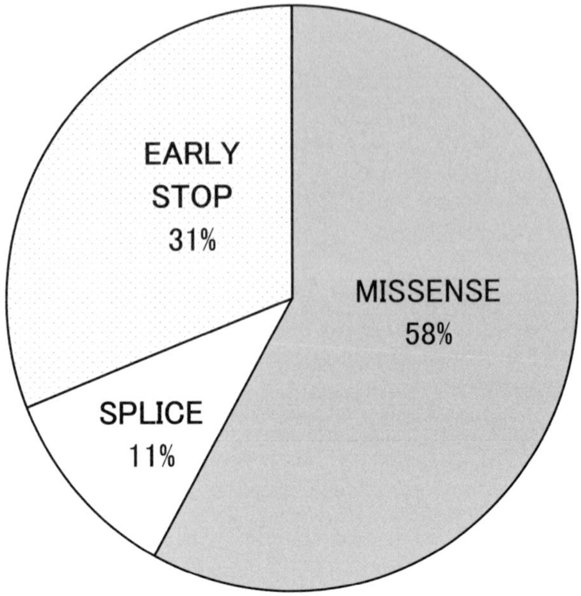

Fig. 5.2 NMD and haploinsufficiency. About 30 % of FBN1 mutations resulted in haploinsufficiency, while about 60 % of mutations resulted in qualitative changes of fibrillin-1 molecules and about 10 % of mutations resulted in splicing defect [4]

[16]. In addition, the function of fibrillin-1 was shown to be closely related to regulation of TGF-β signaling pathways, as noted in the previous section.

5.3 Loeys-Dietz Syndrome (LDS)

5.3.1 LDS and Related Disorders

Loeys-Dietz syndrome (LDS: OMIM #609192, #610168) is an autosomal dominant disorder with an aortic disease and widespread systemic involvement that shows both similarities and differences as compared with MFS [17]. LDS was originally described as a disorder with the triad of arterial tortuosity and aneurysms, hypertelorism, and bifid uvula or cleft palate, though a wide range of variable phenotypes associated with this disorder were recognized [18]. The syndrome was originally reported as that caused by mutations in the TGF-β receptor 1 and 2 genes (*TGFBR1, TGFBR2*), and diagnosis is confirmed by genotyping. Some patients have craniofacial involvement consisting of cleft palate, craniosynostosis, or hypertelorism, though those features do not appear in all. Bifid uvula may also be present in some, but not in all patients. Some reports have indicated that the natural history is characterized by aggressive arterial aneurysms, while some patients show milder aortic phenotypes.

Mutations in the *TGFBR2* gene in patients with the type 2 variant of MFS, MFS without ocular involvement, were also reported [19]. Most LDS patients develop aortic root aneurysms, while a previous study showed that the mean age at death was 26 years old (range 0.5–47 years) and caused by such factors as thoracic aortic dissection, abdominal aortic dissection, and intracerebral bleeding [17]. Based on this, it is recognized that LDS patients tend to experience more aggressive vascular events. However, it is also known that LDS has a large variability of phenotypes including vascular lesions, since some affected patients show severe and rapid aortic events with typical craniofacial features, while others show mild aortic lesions without craniofacial or skeletal features.

5.3.2 LDS and Related Disorders: TGF-β Signalopathies (Fig. 5.3)

Most LDS patients demonstrate missense mutations in the serine/threonine kinase domain of the TGF-β receptors, suggesting loss of function in these molecules as the pathogenic mechanism. Also, there were several reports of dysregulation of TGF-β signaling. In histochemical studies, increased TGF-β and MAPK signaling in aortic lesions of affected patients as well as in *Tgfbr2* knockout mice was found [20].

Recently, three additional genes were identified as responsible for LDS-like syndromic aortopathy: *SMAD3*, *TGFB2*, and *TGFB3*. *SMAD3* mutations were initially described in relation to aneurysm-osteoarthritis syndrome [21], though some patients with an *SMAD3* mutation do not show such prominent osteoarthritis. *TGFB2* mutations have also been described in patients with mild systemic features of MFS or LDS [22, 23]. Very recently, *TGFB3* mutations were also reported in patients with syndromic types of thoracic aortic aneurysms similar to those seen in MFS and LDS [24], though one patient with a de novo *TGFB3* mutation showed MFS and LDS features with no evidence of vascular disease [25].

In most of these gene mutations, immunohistochemical staining reveals an increase of phosphorylated SMAD2 in aortic tissues, indicating that TGF-β signaling has been changed to increase the downstream molecules. Therefore, in addition to the receptors, intracellular signaling molecules as well as their ligands are now considered to be responsible for the common pathogenic changes toward MFS- or LDS-related phenotypic features. Nevertheless, it remains unknown how dysfunction or haploinsufficiency status of these molecules results in increased TGF-β signaling even if such a change causes loss of function. Although the precise mechanisms involved in these changes are uncertain, it is considered that negative feedback and noncanonical stimulus may lead to the increase in TGF-β signaling. Indeed, previous results showed that haploinsufficient *Tgfbr2* mice as well as cranial neural crest cell-specific *Tgfbr2*-deficient mice recapitulate human phenotypes, such as aortic dilatations or craniofacial deformities, along with increased noncanonical (phosphorylated extracellular signal-regulated kinase) TGF-β signaling pathways [20, 26].

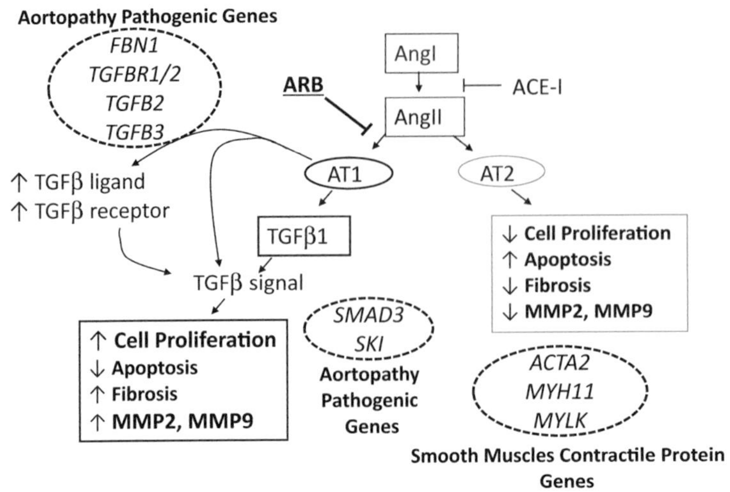

Fig. 5.3 TGF-β signalopathies. Several genes (*FBN1*, *TGFBR1*, *TGFBR2*, *TGFB2*, *TGFB3*, *SMAD3*, and *SKI*) associated with Marfan and related disorders are indeed closely connected with the TGF-β signaling pathways. Changes in the signal regulatory function promote pathological progress of vessels. Also, genes for smooth muscle contractile proteins (*ACTA2*, *MYH11*, *MYLK*) were depicted

Shprintzen-Goldberg syndrome (SGS: OMIM 182212), which results in craniosynostosis, skeletal changes (arachnodactyly, camptodactyly, scoliosis, joint hypermobility), and aortic aneurysms, shows considerable phenotypic overlap with MFS and LDS, and affected patients have been found to have mutations in the v-ski avian sarcoma viral oncogene homolog gene, SKI [27]. The oncogene *SKI* encodes a protein that plays important roles in the negative feedback loop of the TGF-β signaling pathway. Therefore, not only signaling molecules but also molecules affecting the TGF-β signaling pathway, as well as possibly others, may play additional key roles in MFS- or LDS-like phenotypes including aortopathy.

Autosomal recessive cutis laxa type 1B and arterial tortuosity syndrome, two other rare recessive connective tissue disorders, were shown to have autosomal recessive gene mutations in *EFEMP2* [28], which codes FBLN4 proteins. FBLN4 binds to LTBP1 and regulates the latency of TGF-β cytokine. Indeed, upregulated TGF-β signaling has been found in both fibroblasts of patients with *FBLN4* mutations and of the aortic walls in *Fbln-4* hypomorphic mice [28, 29].

5.4 Vascular Ehlers-Danlos Syndrome (vEDS)

5.4.1 vEDS and Gene

The vascular type of Ehlers-Danlos syndrome (vascular EDS, vEDS, type 4 EDS: OMIM #130050), caused by a defect of type III collagen (*COL3A1*) [30], is a disorder featuring cutaneous, skeletal, and vascular abnormalities, including vascular rupture and easy bruising, though affected individuals usually do not show skin hyperextensibility. Clinical features include rupture of the middle-sized arteries, the bowels, or the uterus. Therefore, general care and follow-up examinations are critical for management of vEDS patients upon the diagnosis, and determination of the *COL3A1* mutation is critical for affected individuals and their family members. There is no evidence indicating that *COL3A1* mutations change TGF-β pathway regulation, while it was reported that celiprolol can reduce the risk for vascular events in patients with vEDS [31].

5.4.2 EDS-Like Features and FLNA

It was also reported that EDS-like phenotypes are associated with *FLNA* mutations [32]. The *FLNA* gene encodes filamin A, an intermediate filament connecting the contractile apparatus of vascular smooth muscle cells to the cell membrane [33]. Also, filamin A has numerous interaction partners, including membrane receptors, signaling proteins, and transcription factors. *FLNA* mutations are well known to be associated with periventricular nodular heterotopias (OMIM #300049), though patients with those mutations may also exhibit aortic root dilatation, mitral valve disease, and joint hypermobility even without demonstrating periventricular nodular heterotopias.

5.5 TAAD with Bicuspid Aortic Valves

In 1–2 % of the population, a bicuspid aortic valve (BAV) is present, frequently associated with aortic valve stenosis, insufficiency, and dilatation of ascending aorta which may cause aortic dissection. The valve calcification was also often observed in BAV. Mutations in the signaling and transcription regulator NOTCH1 were reported to cause a spectrum of developmental aortic valve anomalies and severe valve calcification in nonsyndromic aortopathy pedigrees [34]. In 2008, two heterozygous missense variants of *NOTCH1* in six probands among 91 unrelated patients with congenital aortic valve stenosis, bicuspid aortic valve, coarctation of the aorta, and/or hypoplastic left heart syndrome were reported [35]. Since the NOTCH1 variant was also present in an unaffected parent, the report suggested that these variants represent susceptibility alleles but are not the direct cause to perturb cardiac development. About the BAV, it was also reported that a genome-wide screen in 353 BAV individuals with or without associated cardiovascular malformation from 38 families obtained significant linkage peaks in 18q22, 5q15-21, and 13q33-qter [36] besides 9q34 and 17q24.

5.6 Other Types of Syndromic TAAD

In addition to syndromic TAAD described above, aortic aneurysms and/or dissection have also been found in other rare genetic syndromes. Sometimes, patients were not recognized to have distinct syndromic features but showed TAAD events as the main clinical features. In these cases, other signaling pathways besides the TGF-β pathway seem to be involved. For example, aortic aneurysms have been described to sporadically occur in association with mutations involving the rat sarcoma (RAS)-ERK signaling pathway, including Noonan syndrome pathogenic genes such as *PTPN11* [37] and the neurofibromatosis gene, *NF1* [38]. The fact that these genes play roles in TAAD indicates that the RAS and noncanonical TGF-β signaling pathways are involved in aortic aneurysms, as shown in MFS and LDS.

Also, the Notch signaling pathway, which is involved in Alagille syndrome [39] as well as in BAV as indicated above, and genes encoding collagens or enzymes involved in collagen maturation (*COL1A1/A2*, *COL4A1*, *COL4A3/4/5*, *PLOD3*) have been shown to be associated with aortic aneurysm development. In addition, aortic aneurysm has been implicated to have an association with autosomal dominant polycystic kidney disease (ADPKD) [40], and aortic aneurysms and/or dissections of the thoracic aorta occur more frequently in patients with ADPKD.

5.7 Nonsyndromic TAAD

In addition to the genes involved in syndromic types of TAAD, several other genes have been identified in nonsyndromic familial TAAD (FTAAD), while *ACTA2* mutations have been found to be responsible for approximately 15 % of patients with FTAAD [41]. The *ACTA2* gene encodes a smooth muscle-specific isoform of the α-actin protein and is involved in contractile function of vascular smooth muscles. Patients with an *ACTA2* mutation also show other vascular diseases, such as coronary artery disease and stroke, as well as several functional disorders of smooth muscles including vasculopathy, congenital mydriasis, patent ductus arteriosus, and thoracic aortic aneurysm. In addition, some specific *ACTA2* missense mutations (p.Arg179His, p.Arg258His, p.Arg258Cys) have been reported to be accompanied with a moyamoya-like cerebral arterial disorder [42, 43]. Livedo reticularis and iris flocculi were also found in patients with the p.Arg149Cys *ACTA2* missense mutation [33].

Mutations in *MYH11* were also found in patients with FTAAD and patent ductus arteriosus [44]. *MYH11* encodes a myosin heavy chain involved in the contractile function of vascular smooth muscles. In addition, *MYLK* mutations were found in a minority of FTAAD patients [45]. The *MYLK* gene encodes myosin light-chain kinase, which regulates the calcium-calmodulin-binding capacity of vascular smooth muscles by phosphorylating myosin.

Interestingly, upregulation of TGF-β signaling in the aortic walls of TAAD patients with *ACTA2* or *MYH11* mutations was reported [46]. This phenomenon suggests interactions between the smooth muscle contractile apparatus and cell surface integrins that regulate TGF-β activity. However, aortic events in patients with a dysfunction of smooth muscle contractile proteins seem somewhat different as compared to those in patients with a dysfunction of the TGF-β pathway, such as MFS or LDS, since FTAAD patients with an *ACTA2* or *MYH11* mutation demonstrate enlargement of the entire ascending aorta, not restricted to the sinus of Valsalva. Therefore, there may be some differences regarding the pathophysiological processes involved in dysfunction of the smooth muscle contractile apparatus and those of the TGF-β pathway.

5.8 Therapy for TAAD

After identification of the genes causing TAAD as shown above, clinical management stratification is based on the phenotypes related to the underlying genetic mutation. For example, LDS patients with a *TGFBR1* or *TGFBR2* mutation have greater risk for aortic and arterial aneurysms than other TAAD patients and are thought to need more extensive imaging follow-up examinations to prevent vascular events. As for patients with *ACTA2* mutations, the risk of coronary artery disease or stroke should be evaluated to prevent those events. The current guidelines of the American College of Cardiology [47] recommend prophylactic surgery based on different scenarios according to the underlying gene since the different clinical courses are expected in patients with different gene mutations.

Medical management strategy for TAAD patients aims to control blood pressure and reduce aortic wall stress, generally by β-blocker treatment. In addition, calcium channel blockers and angiotensin-converting enzyme inhibitors or angiotensin receptor blockers may be considered. In a study of MFS and related disorders, the discovery of the key role of TGF-β signaling pathway in the pathogenesis of Marfan syndrome mice prompted investigation of the effects of anti-TGF-β treatment by a TGF-β-neutralizing antibody and losartan, an angiotensin II type I receptor antagonist, in a mouse model [48]. Results showed beneficial effects of losartan on aortic root dilatation and elastic fiber fragmentation by reduction of TGF-β signaling [44]. Since losartan is an established drug for treatment of hypertension, investigations of its usefulness in MFS patients have begun. An initial preliminary study showed improved effectiveness for reducing progressive aortic root dilatation by losartan added to β-blocker therapy as compared with β-blocker therapy alone

[49]. However, the largest clinical trial to date to assess the efficacy of losartan as compared with a β-blocker found no better outcome in MFS patients who received losartan therapy [50]. However, there are several lines of evidence showing involvement of the TGF-β pathway in MFS, LDS, and related disorders. Therefore, treatments aimed to block noncanonical components of the TGF-β signaling pathway are anticipated and proposed. In addition, changes in the VSMC contractile apparatus or MMP proteins are thought to have other important pathogenic roles in genetic aortic diseases. Based on these mechanisms, other alternative therapeutic targets will also have to be considered. Further delineation of the genes and pathways responsible for aortopathies with unknown mechanisms is also needed.

5.9 Conclusion

Since the discovery of *FBN1* and *COL3A1* mutations in patients with MFS or vEDS in the late twentieth century, several genes responsible for genetic aortic diseases have been identified, and understanding of the related pathophysiological mechanisms has progressed very much. However, progress for developing new strategies to cure these diseases remains rather slow, despite the rapid understanding of the physiological roles of genes involved in these aortic diseases. Therefore, additional studies are needed for development of novel therapeutic strategies for these aortic diseases.

References

1. Lindsay ME, Dietz HC (2011) Lessons on the pathogenesis of aneurysm from heritable conditions. Nature 473:308–316
2. Ramanath VS, Oh JK, Sundt TM 3rd, Eagle KA (2009) Acute aortic syndromes and thoracic aortic aneurysm. Mayo Clin Proc 84:465–481
3. Blanchard JF, Armenian HK, Friesen PP (2000) Risk factors for abdominal aortic aneurysm: results of a case-control study. Am J Epidemiol 151:575–583
4. Morisaki T, Morisaki H (2016) Genetics of hereditary large vessel diseases. J Hum Genet 61:21–26
5. Marfan AB (1896) Un cas de deformation congenitale des quatre membres, plus prononcee aux extremites, caracterisee par l'allongement des os avec un certain degre d'amincissement. Bull Mem Soc Med Hop Paris 13:220–226
6. Pyeritz RE, McKusick VA (1979) The Marfan syndrome. New Engl J Med 300:772–777
7. Beighton P, De Paepe A, Danks D et al (1988) International nosology of heritable disorders of connective tissue, Berlin, 1986. Am J Med Genet 29:581–594
8. De Paepe A, Devereux RB, Dietz HC et al (1996) Revised diagnostic criteria for the Marfan syndrome. Am J Med Genet 62:417–426
9. Loeys BL, Dietz HC, Braverman AC et al (2010) The revised Ghent nosology for the Marfan syndrome. J Med Genet 47:476–485
10. Annes JP, Munger JS, Rifkin DB (2003) Making sense of latent TGFβ activation. J Cell Sci 116:217–224

11. ten Dijke P, Arthur HM (2007) Extracellular control of TGFbeta signalling in vascular development and disease. Nat Rev Mol Cell Biol 8:857–869
12. Kainulainen K, Steinmann B, Collins F et al (1991) Marfan syndrome: no evidence for heterogeneity in different populations, and more precise mapping of the gene. Am J Hum Genet 49:662–667
13. Dietz HC, Cutting GR, Pyeritz RE et al (1991) Marfan syndrome caused by a recurrent de novo missense mutation in the fibrillin gene. Nature 352:337–339
14. Aoyama T, Francke U, Gasner C et al (1995) Fibrillin abnormalities and prognosis in Marfan syndrome and related disorders. Am J Med Genet 58:169–176
15. Faivre L, Collod-Beroud G, Loeys BL et al (2007) Effect of mutation type and location on clinical outcome in 1013 probands with Marfan syndrome or related phenotypes and FBN1 mutations: an international study. Am J Hum Genet 81:454–466
16. Judge DP, Biery NJ, Keene DR et al (2004) Evidence for a critical contribution of haploinsufficiency in the complex pathogenesis of Marfan syndrome. J Clin Invest 114:172–181
17. Loeys BL, Schwarze U, Holm T et al (2006) Aneurysm syndromes caused by mutations in the TGF-beta receptor. N Engl J Med 355:788–798
18. Loeys BL, Chen J, Neptune ER et al (2005) A syndrome of altered cardiovascular, craniofacial, neurocognitive and skeletal development caused by mutations in TGFBR1 or TGFBR2. Nat Genet 37:275–281
19. Mizuguchi T, Collod-Beroud G, Akiyama T et al (2004) Heterozygous TGFBR2 mutations in Marfan syndrome. Nat Genet 36:855–860
20. Li W, Li Q, Jiao Y, Qin L et al (2014) Tgfbr2 disruption in postnatal smooth muscle impairs aortic wall homeostasis. J Clin Invest 124:755–767
21. van de Laar IM, van der Linde D, Oei EH et al (2012) Phenotypic spectrum of the SMAD3-related aneurysms-osteoarthritis syndrome. J Med Genet 49:47–57
22. Boileau C, Guo DC, Hanna N et al (2012) TGFB2 mutations cause familial thoracic aortic aneurysms and dissections associated with mild systemic features of Marfan syndrome. Nat Genet 44:916–921
23. Lindsay ME, Schepers D, Bolar NA et al (2012) Loss-of-function mutations in TGFB2 cause a syndromic presentation of thoracic aortic aneurysm. Nat Genet 44:922–927
24. Bertoli-Avella AM, Gillis E, Morisaki H et al (2015) Mutations in a TGFβ ligand, TGFB3, cause syndromic aortic aneurysms and dissections. J Am Coll Cardiol 65:1324–1336
25. Rienhoff HY Jr, Yeo CY, Morissette R et al (2013) A mutation in TGFB3 associated with a syndrome of low muscle mass, growth retardation, distal arthrogryposis and clinical features overlapping with Marfan and Loeys-Dietz syndrome. Am J Med Genet 161A:2040–2046
26. Iwata J, Hacia JG, Suzuki A et al (2012) Modulation of noncanonical TGF-β signaling prevents cleft palate in *Tgfbr2* mutant mice. J Clin Invest 122:873–885
27. Doyle AJ, Doyle JJ, Bessling SL et al (2012) Mutations in the TGF-β repressor SKI cause Shprintzen-Goldberg syndrome with aortic aneurysm. Nat Genet 44:1249–1254
28. Renard M, Holm T, Veith R et al (2010) Altered TGFbeta signaling and cardiovascular manifestations in patients with autosomal recessive cutis laxa type I caused by fibulin-4 deficiency. Eur J Hum Genet 18:895–901
29. Huang J, Davis EC, Chapman SL et al (2010) Fibulin-4 deficiency results in ascending aortic aneurysms: a potential link between abnormal smooth muscle cell phenotype and aneurysm progression. Circ Res 106:583–592
30. Superti-Furga A, Gugler E, Gitzelmann R et al (1988) Ehlers-Danlos syndrome type IV: a multi-exon deletion in one of the two COL3A1 alleles affecting structure, stability, and processing of type III procollagen. J Biol Chem 263:6226–6232
31. Ong KT, Perdu J, De Backer J et al (2010) Effect of celiprolol on prevention of cardiovascular events in vascular Ehlers-Danlos syndrome: a prospective randomised, open, blinded-endpoints trial. Lancet 376:1476–1484

32. Sheen VL, Jansen A, Chen MH et al (2005) Filamin A mutations cause periventricular heterotopia with Ehlers-Danlos syndrome. Neurology 64:254–262
33. Fox JW, Lamperti ED, Ekşioğlu YZ et al (1998) Mutations in filamin 1 prevent migration of cerebral cortical neurons in human periventricular heterotopia. Neuron 21:1315–1325
34. Garg V, Muth AN, Ransom JF et al (2005) Mutations in NOTCH1 cause aortic valve disease. Nature 437:270–274
35. McBride KL, Riley MF, Zender GA et al (2008) NOTCH1 mutations in individuals with left ventricular outflow tract malformations reduce ligand-induced signaling. Hum Mol Genet 17:2886–2893
36. Martin LJ, Ramachandran V, Cripe LH et al (2007) Evidence in favor of linkage to human chromosomal regions 18q, 5q and 13q for bicuspid aortic valve and associated cardiovascular malformations. Hum Genet 121:275–284
37. Tartaglia M, Mehler EL, Goldberg R et al (2001) Mutations in PTPN11, encoding the protein tyrosine phosphatase SHP-2, cause Noonan syndrome. Nat Genet 29:465–468
38. Wallace MR, Marchuk DA, Andersen LB et al (1990) Type 1 neurofibromatosis gene: identification of a large transcript disrupted in three NF1 patients. Science 249:181–186
39. Oda T, Elkahloun AG, Pike BL et al (1997) Mutations in the human Jagged1 gene are responsible for Alagille syndrome. Nat Genet 16:235–242
40. Roodvoets AP (1980) Aortic aneurysms in presence of kidney disease. Lancet 1:1413–1414
41. Guo DC, Pannu H, Tran-Fadulu V et al (2007) Mutations in smooth muscle alpha-actin (ACTA2) lead to thoracic aortic aneurysms and dissections. Nat Genet 39:1488–1493
42. Guo DC, Papke CL, Tran-Fadulu V et al (2009) Mutations in smooth muscle alpha-actin (ACTA2) cause coronary artery disease, stroke, and Moyamoya disease, along with thoracic aortic disease. Am J Hum Genet 84:617–627
43. Roder C, Peters V, Kasuya H et al (2011) Analysis of ACTA2 in European Moyamoya disease patients. Eur J Paediatr Neurol 15:117–122
44. Zhu L, Vranckx R, Khau Van Kien P et al (2006) Mutations in myosin heavy chain 11 cause a syndrome associating thoracic aortic aneurysm/aortic dissection and patent ductus arteriosus. Nat Genet 38:343–349
45. Wang L, Guo DC, Cao J et al (2010) Mutations in myosin light chain kinase cause familial aortic dissections. Am J Hum Genet 87:701–707
46. Renard M, Callewaert B, Baetens M et al (2013) Novel MYH11 and ACTA2 mutations reveal a role for enhanced TGFβ signaling in FTAAD. Int J Cardiol 165:314–321
47. Hiratzka LF, Bakris GL, Beckman JA et al (2010) 2010 ACCF/AHA/AATS/ACR/ASA/SCA/SCAI/SIR/STS/SVM Guidelines for the diagnosis and management of patients with thoracic aortic disease: a report of the American College of Cardiology Foundation/American Heart Association Task Force on Practice Guidelines, American Association for Thoracic Surgery, American College of Radiology, American Stroke Association, Society of Cardiovascular Anesthesiologists, Society for Cardiovascular Angiography and Interventions, Society of Interventional Radiology, Society of Thoracic Surgeons, and Society for Vascular Medicine. J Am Coll Cardiol 55:e27–e129
48. Habashi JP, Judge DP, Holm TM et al (2006) Losartan, an AT1 antagonist, prevents aortic aneurysm in a mouse model of Marfan syndrome. Science 312:117–121
49. Brooke BS, Habashi JP, Judge DP et al (2008) Angiotensin II blockade and aortic-root dilation in Marfan's syndrome. N Engl J Med 358:2787–2795
50. Lacro RV, Dietz HC, Sleeper LA et al (2014) Atenolol versus losartan in children and young adults with Marfan's syndrome. N Engl J Med 371:2061–2071

Part II
Diagnosis and Management

Chapter 6
Imaging: Echo, CT and MRI

Kenneth Guo, Narayan Lath, and Ju Le Tan

Abstract Rapid advances in imaging technology with ever-increasing capabilities of ultrasound transducers, number of detector rows and x-ray tubes in CT, increasing field strength and newer sequences in MRI, and a plethora of highly capable imaging modalities are now available to optimally image the thoracic aorta. Each of these has their advantages and weaknesses and is used not only for the initial assessment of aortopathies but also plays a vital part in serial monitoring, treatment planning, and assessing posttreatment complications. Choice of a particular imaging modality should be guided by the clinical issue at hand and also affected by ease of availability, cost, and field of coverage.

Keywords Aortopathy • Congenital heart

6.1 Introduction

6.2 Imaging Modalities, Methods, and Technical Considerations

6.2.1 Echocardiography

Transthoracic echocardiography (TTE) is cheap, widely available, and in most cases able to provide good visualization of the aortic root and proximal ascending aorta (pAAo) and to a lesser extent the aortic arch (AoA), descending thoracic aorta (DTAo), and abdominal aorta (AbdAo) especially in adults with challenging echo

K. Guo (✉) • J.L. Tan
Department of Cardiology, National Heart Centre Singapore, 5 Hospital Drive, 169609 Singapore, Singapore
e-mail: Kenneth_guowq@yahoo.com.sg

N. Lath
Department of Diagnostic Radiology, Singapore General Hospital, Singapore, Singapore

K. Niwa, H. Kaemmerer (eds.), *Aortopathy*, DOI 10.1007/978-4-431-56071-5_6

windows. In addition, TTE also provides concomitant information and assessment of cardiac chambers and other valvular or non-valvular pathologies commonly associated with aortopathy such as bicuspid aortic valve, aortic regurgitations, coarctation of the aorta, etc.

6.2.1.1 Standard Imaging Planes in TTE

Left Parasternal Long-Axis View (PLAX View)

This is the best view (Figs. 6.1a, 6.1b, and 6.1c) for visualizing the aortic root and the proximal ascending aorta. The left lung and sternum often obscure the midportion of the ascending aorta which is best visualized from a higher PLAX echo window one intercostal space up (Figs. 6.2a and 6.2b). The 2015 American Society of Echocardiography (ASE) and European Association of Cardiovascular Imaging (EACI) Guidelines [1] recommended the measurement of the *aortic valve annulus* (hinge point of the right coronary cusp (RCC) to the fibrous trigone between the left coronary cusp (LCC) and non-coronary cusp (NCC)) at *mid/peak systole* using *the inner edge to inner edge (I-I) convention* such as used by MDCT.

However, for the measurements of the aortic root and the rest of the aorta, the recommendation was to use back the *leading-edge-to-leading-edge (L-L) convention at end diastole in a plane perpendicular to the long axis of the aorta* as the currently available long-standing reference values for the aorta (Table 6.1) were based on the L-L convention [2–4].

Aortic root dilatation at the level of the Sinus of Valsalva (SOV) is defined as greater than 95 % confidence interval of the distribution in a large reference population. This

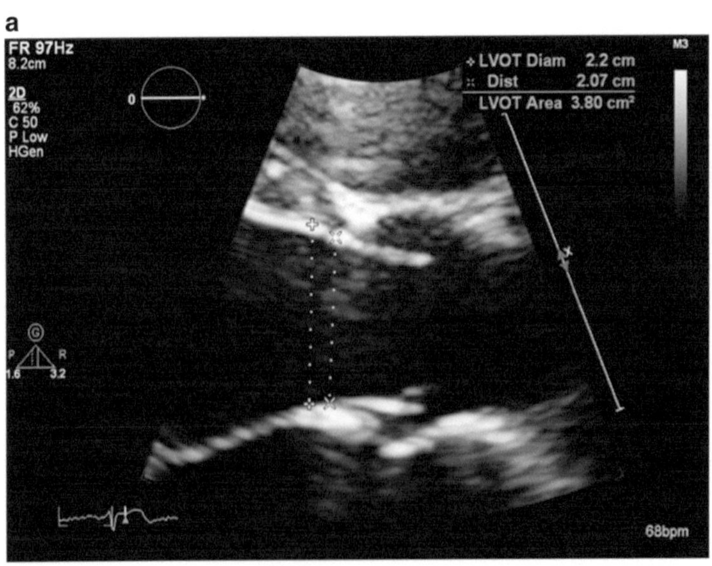

Fig. 6.1a PLAX zoom view at peak/mid-systole to measure the aortic annulus and LVOT

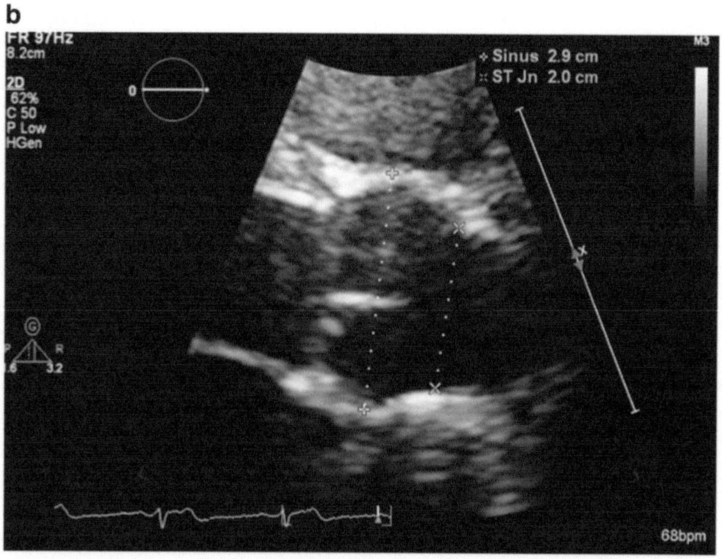

Fig. 6.1b PLAX zoom view at end diastole to measure the SOV and STJ

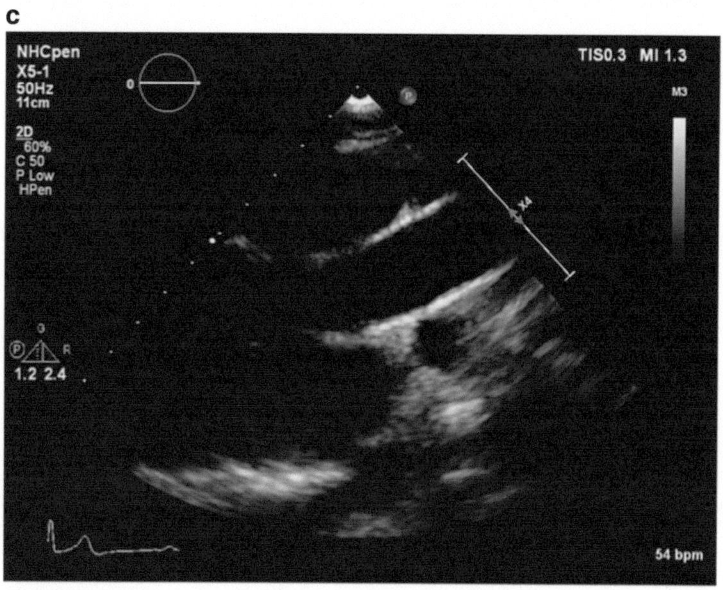

Fig. 6.1c High PLAX view at end diastole to measure the proximal and mid-ascending aorta

varies according to different age range (from children to adults above the age of 40) and their BSA; the commonly used reference range is published by Roman, et al. [2].

In addition, direct two-dimensional (2D) measurements of the aorta are now preferable to M-mode measurements because of possible inaccuracies arising from cardiac motion during acquisition of the M-mode images.

a

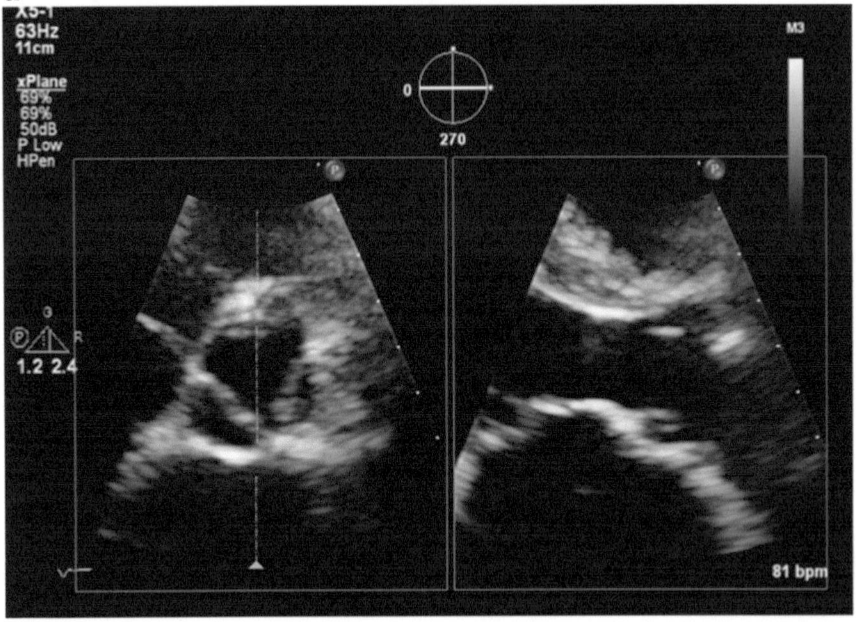

Fig. 6.2a Simultaneous biplane (X-plane) orthogonal images from the 3D matrix transducer confirming that the measured PLAX aortic annulus dimension is through the correct anteroposterior (AP) plane from the right coronary cusp (RCC) to the fibrous trigone between the left coronary cusp (LCC) and non-coronary cusp (NCC)

b

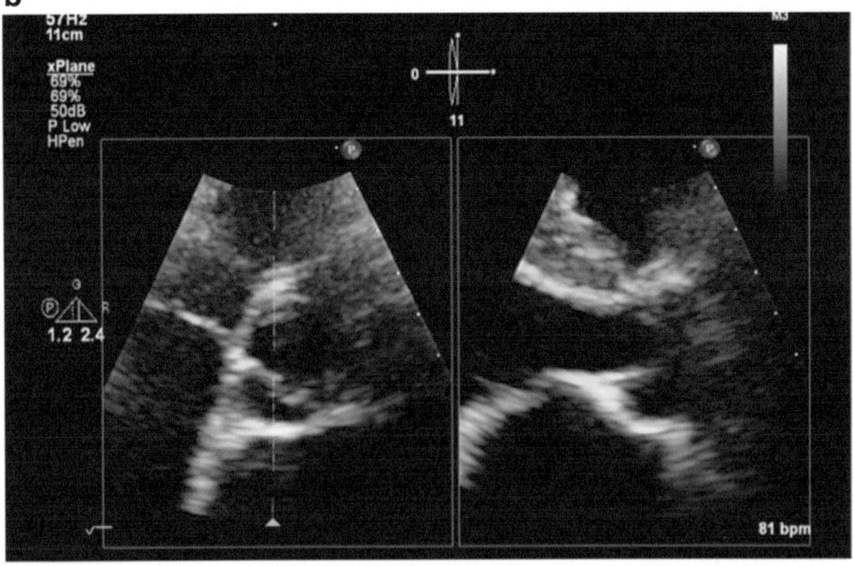

Fig. 6.2b Incorrect aortic annulus measurement taken from an eccentric oblique plane

Table 6.1 Dimensions of the aorta in normal adult population

	Absolute values (cm)		Indexed values (cm/m2)	
Aortic regions	Men	Women	Men	Women
Aortic annulus	2.6 ± 0.3	2.3 ± 0.2	1.3 ± 0.1	1.3 ± 0.1
Sinus of Valsalva	3.4 ± 0.3	3.0 ± 0.3	1.7 ± 0.2	1.8 ± 0.2
Sinotubular junction	2.9 ± 0.3	2.6 ± 0.3	1.5 ± 0.2	1.5 ± 0.2
Proximal ascending aorta	3.0 ± 0.4	2.7 ± 0.4	1.5 ± 0.2	1.6 ± 0.3

This table is adapted from Roman et al. [2] and Hiratzka et al. [4]

Left Parasternal Short-Axis View (PSAX View)

Aortic Annulus

Simultaneous biplane (X-plane) orthogonal images from the 3D matrix transducer using an initial PSAX view can be helpful for confirmation that the measured PLAX aortic annulus dimension is through the correct anteroposterior (AP) plane from the right coronary cusp (RCC) to the fibrous trigone between the left coronary cusp (LCC) and non-coronary cusp (NCC) as depicted in Fig. 6.2a. Errors can arise from incorrect measurements taken from an eccentric oblique plane as shown in Fig. 6.2b. In some patients, the aortic root is more elliptical in structure, and the AP plane dimension is often smaller than the medial–lateral dimension.

Aortic Root

Not uncommonly the dilatation at the level of SOV may be eccentric involving one particular cusp more than others. The SAX view allows the direct measurement of the SOV from one cusp to another. Data from other imaging modalities such as CMR has shown that measuring the diameter of the SOV using the sinus to sinus method (from the middle of one cusp to the middle of another cusp) resulted in a mean 2–3 mm larger diameter than the sinus to commissure method (from the middle of one cusp to the commissure between the two cusps) [5]. It is important to report where the largest aortic SOV dimension was obtained in the serial follow-up of patients with dilated aortic root for meaningful comparisons to previous and for future echo follow-up studies.

Other Echo Views

The aortic root and the proximal ascending aorta may also be visualized in other echo windows such as the apical long axis (apical three chamber) as shown in Fig. 6.3a and apical five chamber (Fig. 6.3b). The mid- to distal part of the ascending aorta and the aortic arch can be visualized in the modified suprasternal view (transducer tilted slightly to the right), and the distal ascending aorta, the aortic arch, and the descending thoracic aorta are best visualized in the suprasternal window as shown in Fig. 6.3c and 6.3d, respectively. The abdominal aorta

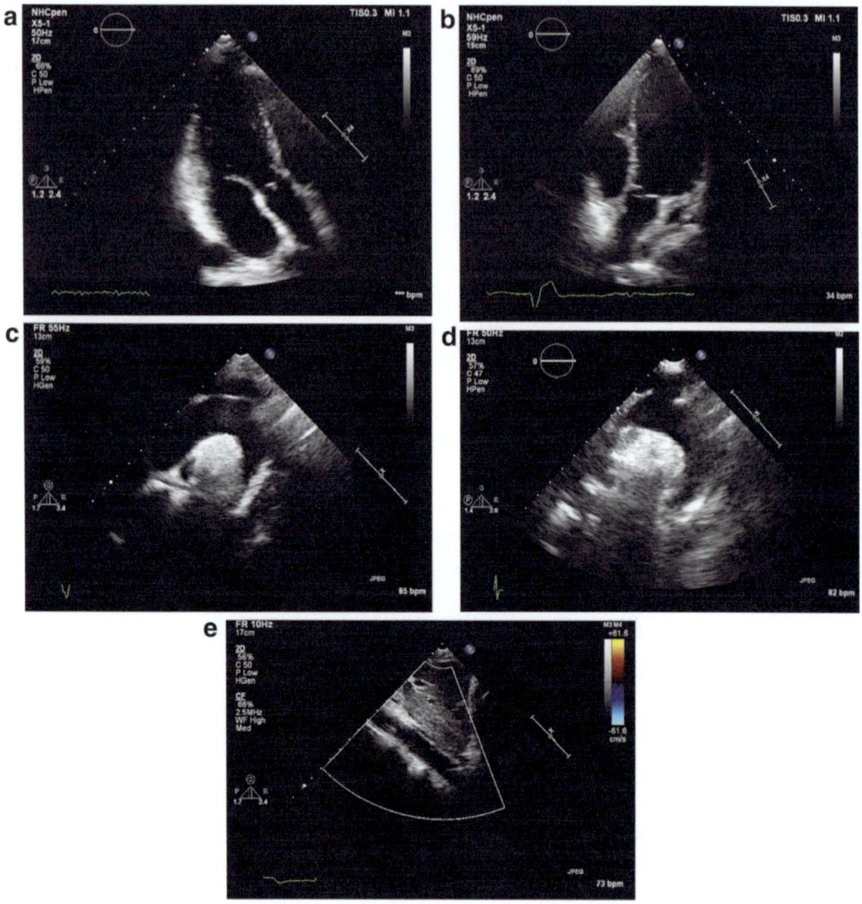

Fig. 6.3 (**a–e**) View of different aortic segments from the various echo windows such as the apical three-chamber view (**a**), apical five-chamber view (**b**), modified suprasternal view (**c**), suprasternal view (**d**), and subcostal view (**e**)

(Fig. 6.3e) is best seen from the subcostal view to the left of the inferior vena cava in sagittal (superior–inferior) alignment.

6.2.2 Transesophageal Echocardiography (TEE) and Three-Dimensional (3D) Echocardiography in Aortopathy

The most important TEE views are the mid-esophageal TEE long-axis view (between 120 and 150°) and the short-axis views (30–60°) to visualize the aortic valve, aortic root, and proximal ascending aorta as shown in Figs. 6.4a and 6.4b,

a

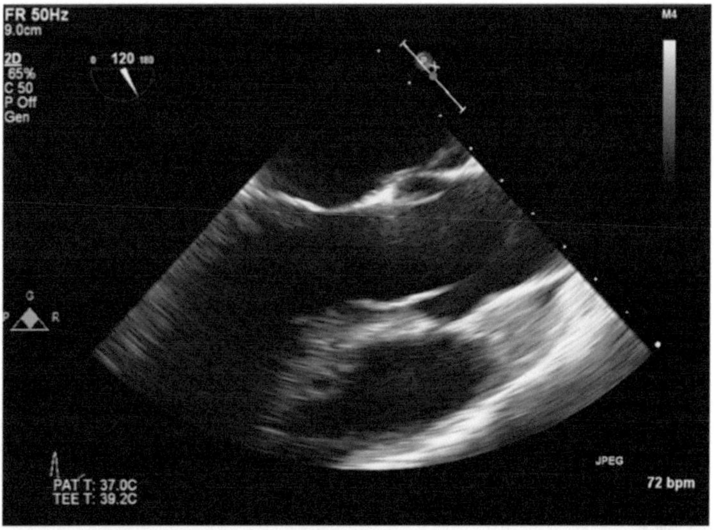

Fig. 6.4a High TEE long-axis view at 120° showing the aortic valve, the aortic root, and the ascending aorta

b

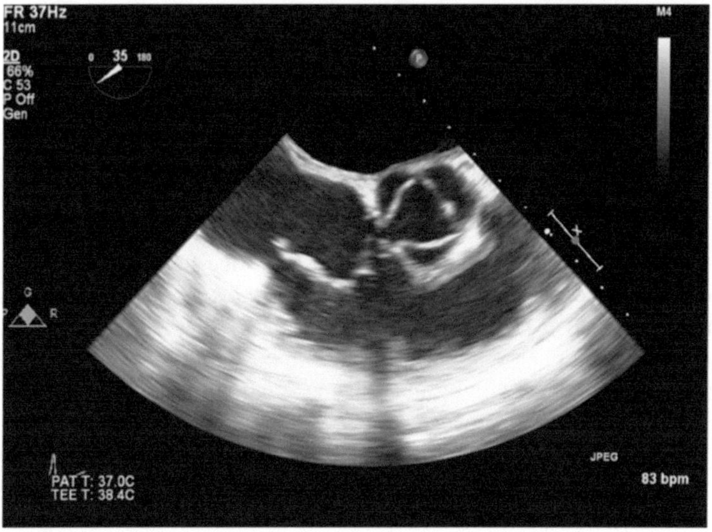

Fig. 6.4b High TEE short-axis view at 35° showing the en face view of the aortic valve

respectively. With minimal manipulation and rotation of the transducer array, a continuum of transverse and longitudinal image planes of the descending thoracic aorta can be obtained as shown in Fig. 6.4c (simultaneous transverse and longitudinal plane of the descending thoracic aorta using X-plane). The TEE probe can

c

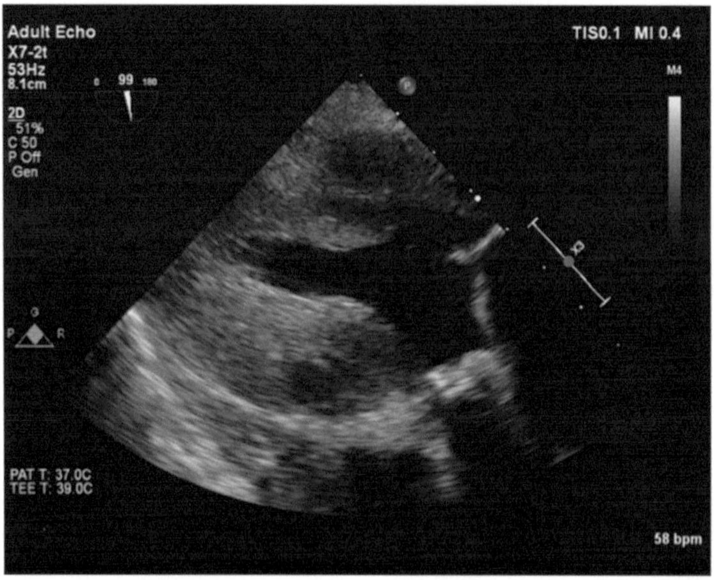

Fig. 6.4c Deep transgastric view at 99° showing the aortic valve, aortic root, and proximal Asc Ao in a patient with post bioprosthetic aortic valve replacement for severe aortic stenosis

then be advanced or withdrawn to image the lower thoracic/upper abdominal aorta or the upper thoracic aorta, respectively. To image the aortic arches, the TEE probe is rotated posteriorly and withdrawn slowly from the mid-esophagus at 0°. The right brachiocephalic and the left common carotid branches are difficult to see, but the left subclavian artery takeoff can usually be seen.

It is important to be wary of occasional reverberation artifacts in the ascending thoracic aorta presenting as linear horizontal lines due to reverberation from the motion of the posterior wall of the ascending aorta as shown in Fig. 6.4d. Extra precaution should also be taken when measuring the descending thoracic aortic diameter (transverse plane) in patients with tortuous aortas as the transverse cut is often in an oblique plane with resultant overestimation of the aortic diameter.

TEE has added advantage over TTE in imaging the aorta because of its superior image quality (especially in adult patients with poor windows) and the ability to image the aortic valve, aortic root, and nearly all the ascending and descending thoracic aorta except for a blind area (area between the distal ascending aorta and the proximal aortic arch due to interposition of the trachea and right bronchus).

A summary of the different echo modalities and windows for optimal visualizations of the various aortic segments are as shown in Table 6.2.

Real-time three-dimensional imaging of the aortic root with cropping along the long axis may help in understanding the true shape, size, and dilatation of the LVOT, aortic annulus, SOV, and Sino-tubular junction (STJ).

d

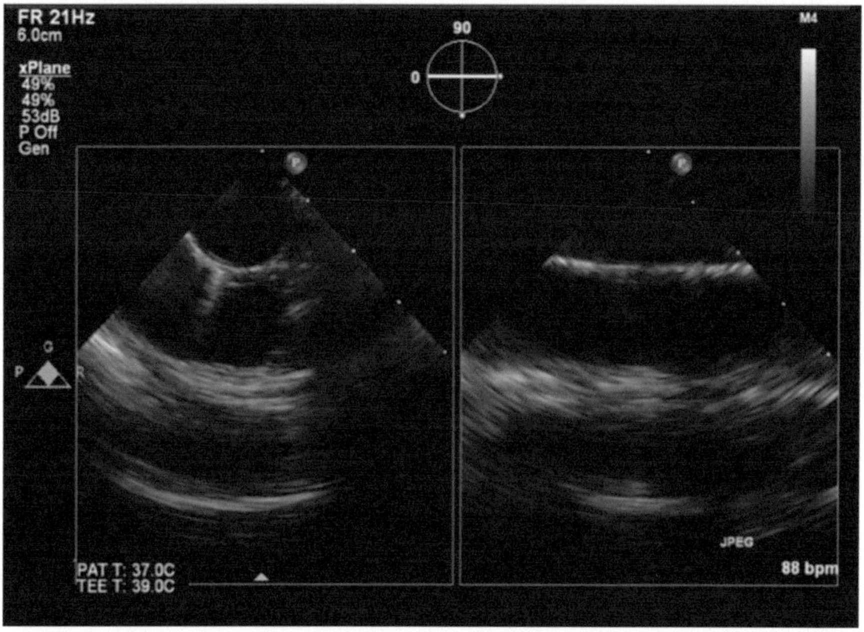

Fig. 6.4d Transverse and longitudinal plane of the descending thoracic aorta

6.2.3 Pulse Wave, Continuous Wave, and Tissue Doppler Echocardiography in Aortopathy

Pulse wave (PW) Doppler allows measurement of blood velocity at a single point and may be used (in the absence of aliasing) to confirm and differentiate multiple areas of discrete stenosis such as subaortic, valvular, or supra-aortic stenosis. It is also helpful in differentiating the severity of aortic regurgitation by looking for the presence of pan-diastolic flow reversal in the thoracic or abdominal aorta. Continuous wave (CW) Doppler is used in the assessment of peak pressure gradient across aortic coarctation.

TDI of the upper ascending aortic wall in early diastole for evaluation of aortic elastic properties is possible but to date remains more in the research arena and not widely used clinically [6].

6.2.4 Computed Tomography (CT)

Multi-detector row CT (MDCT) is one of the most used techniques in the assessment of aortopathies. Its major advantages are excellent spatial and temporal

Table 6.2 Different echo modalities and windows for optimal visualizations of the various aortic segments

	Segments of the aorta adequately visualized in adults					
Echo modes and views	Aortic valve	Aortic root	Ascending aorta	Aortic arch	Desc thoracic aorta	Abdominal aorta
(A) TTE						
(i) PLAX and SAX	X	X	X			
(ii) A3C and A5C	X	X	X			
(iii) Subcostal	X	X	X			X
(iv) Suprasternal			X	X	X	
(B) TEE						
(i) Upper esophagus			X (mid)	X	X	
(ii) Mid-esophagus	X	X	X (prox)		X	
(iii) Deep transgastric	X	X	X	X (prox)		X

Key: *Desc* descending, *prox* proximal, *TTE* transthoracic echocardiogram, *PLAX* parasternal long axis, *SAX* short axis, *A3C* apical three chamber, *A5C* apical five chamber

resolution, widespread availability, and ability to image the entire aorta within seconds. Furthermore, it elegantly shows the aortic lumen and wall, resulting in precise and reproducible measurements. Current scanners with higher detector rows allow acquisition of isotropic volumetric datasets, which can be reconstructed in any plane for optimal display and measurements of a structure.

6.2.4.1 CT Angiography

CT Angiography (CTA) acquisition uses iodinated contrast medium (ICM) delivered at rate of 3–5 mL/s by a power injector and usually followed by a saline bolus. The injection site (right vs left, arm vs leg vein) needs consideration, particularly when assessing arch pathologies or Fontan pathways. Optimal contrast enhancement in area of interest is ascertained by "bolus tracking" or "test injection" methods.

6.2.4.2 ECG Gating

On conventional non-ECG-gated CT, outline of the ascending aorta is indistinct due to cardiac motion, resulting in inaccurate measurements and appearance of "pseudo-dissection." ECG "gating" eliminates these artifacts and also allows proximal coronary arterial assessment in the same setting. ECG gating can be "retrospective" or "prospective," of which the latter results in significantly lower radiation doses [7].

6.2.4.3 Challenges and Comparison with Other Modalities

Main drawbacks of CT are the need for ICM administration and ionizing radiation exposure. ICM may cause allergic reactions and need cautious use in patients with renal impairment. Ionizing radiation exposure in CT may limit its use in younger people, especially when serial follow-up is needed. Various newer dose reduction techniques are used in modern CT scanners to significantly reduce effective dose, some of which include prospective ECG triggering, ECG-based tube current modulation, lower peak kilovoltage (kVp), and iterative reconstruction algorithms [8, 9]. Compared to other modalities such as TTE and MRI, CT lacks flow assessment capabilities which are useful in assessment of aortic insufficiency and shunts.

6.2.4.4 Measurements

There is still some inconsistency in methods used in different modalities in measuring the aorta, like leading edge to leading edge used in TEE [1] vs external diameters in CT/MRI [4] and sinus to sinus vs sinus to commissure at SOV level. It is thus important to note the method used and follow it on subsequent studies for comparison. Standardized levels for measurements of aortic diameters are shown in Fig. 6.5, adapted from Hiratzka et al. The upper limits of normal are 3.7 cm for the

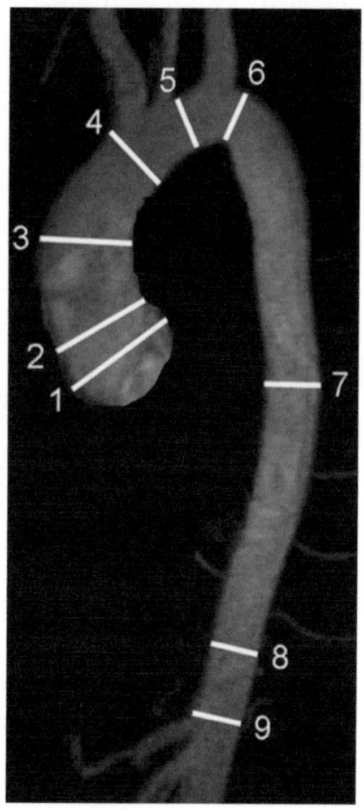

Fig. 6.5 Anatomic landmarks for standardized reporting of diameters of the aorta (Adapted from Hiratzka et al.)

aortic root at the sinuses, 3.6 cm for the ascending aorta, and 2.5 cm for the descending thoracic aorta by CT [1, 10, 11].

6.2.5 *Magnetic Resonance Imaging (MRI)*

MRI is well suited for the diagnosis of aortic diseases, given its ability to delineate the intrinsic contrast between blood flow and vessel wall. Key indicators for decision-making can be reliably obtained through MRI. Spin-echo black-blood sequences outline the shape and diameter and show intimal flaps nicely [12]. Gradient echo sequences show changes in the diameters during the cardiac cycle and blood flow turbulences. Contrast-enhanced MRI can show the aorta and its branches rapidly, without the need for ECG gating. Gadolinium-enhanced sequences are used to differentiate slow flow from thrombus in the false lumen.

6.2.5.1 Quantitative Analysis

Multilevel measurements of aortic diameters through MRI are obtained on double oblique multi-planar images perpendicular to blood flow at standardized levels [4]. See Fig. 6.5, adapted from Hiratzka, et al. These measurements should be obtained at diastole if possible. The diameters of sinuses or sinotubular junction may not be measured on un-gated images since motion artifacts can lead to blurring and may result in the under- or overestimation of the diameters. These require ECG-gated acquisitions, either from contiguous stack of cines aligned to transect the axis of the aortic root, or three-dimensional balanced steady state-free precession (b-SSFP) images acquired in late diastole. Three-dimensional b-SSFP gives sharp-edge profiling and is easy to acquire and post process. It also shows good interobserver correlation [13]. Volume-rendered techniques may be used for demonstration purposes, but not for detailed analysis.

6.2.5.2 Analysis of the Aortic Wall

Assessment of the aortic wall thickness and irregularities is best achieved by reviewing the turbo spin-echo images.

6.2.5.3 Advantage over Computed Tomography

Cardiac MRI avoids the use of radiation in young patients, who may require repeated scans over their lifetime. Its main advantage is its ability to allow tissue characterization and the analysis of flow and dynamic movement of cardiovascular structures.

6.2.5.4 Challenges

The usual technical difficulties faced when performing cardiac MRI examinations are further amplified in young adults with congenital heart disease. Optimal image quality may be compromised because of the smaller size of structures and the reduced time for image acquisition due to inability or difficulty when breath-holding for patients who have intellectual disability.

Due to the variety of morphology presented to us, it is advised that a trained cardiologist or radiologist be present during the scan so that the appropriate planning of the sequences and imaging planes can be done during the visit.

Potential of gadolinium nephrotoxicity appears to be lower than for CT contrast agents and should be avoided with a glomerular filtration rate of less than 30 ml/min/1.73 m^2.

6.2.5.5 Spatial Resolution

Smaller fields of views (FOVs) and the use of thinner slice are required to image small anatomical structures. The resultant reduction in signal-to-noise ratio can be compensated by increasing the number of acquisitions, removing parallel imaging features, or using a coarser matrix.

6.2.5.6 Strategies to Reduce Motion Artifact

This can be overcome by using the following techniques: manual shimming techniques, increasing the number of acquisitions, respiratory compensation methods, or acquiring data using real-time imaging sequences.

6.2.5.7 Consideration of Prior Implants

The presence of implants and devices has been evaluated extensively in scanners with static magnetic fields of 1.5 tesla or less. In addition to the challenges posed due to distortion of the image around the implant, deleterious effects such as heating, dislodgement, and acoustic damage must also be considered. These effects can be further amplified if scanning is done in a 3-tesla environment. Further information specific to the safety of implants can be obtained through "The LIST" found at www.MRIsafety.com.

6.3 Imaging of the Aorta in Specific Congenital Heart Disease

6.3.1 *Marfan Syndrome*

6.3.1.1 Echo

TTE is the main imaging modality for the diagnosis and follow-up of patients with Marfan syndrome where the dilatation of the aorta occurs mainly in the aortic root (Fig. 6.6a, b) at the level of the SOV with relative sparing of the STJ and proximal

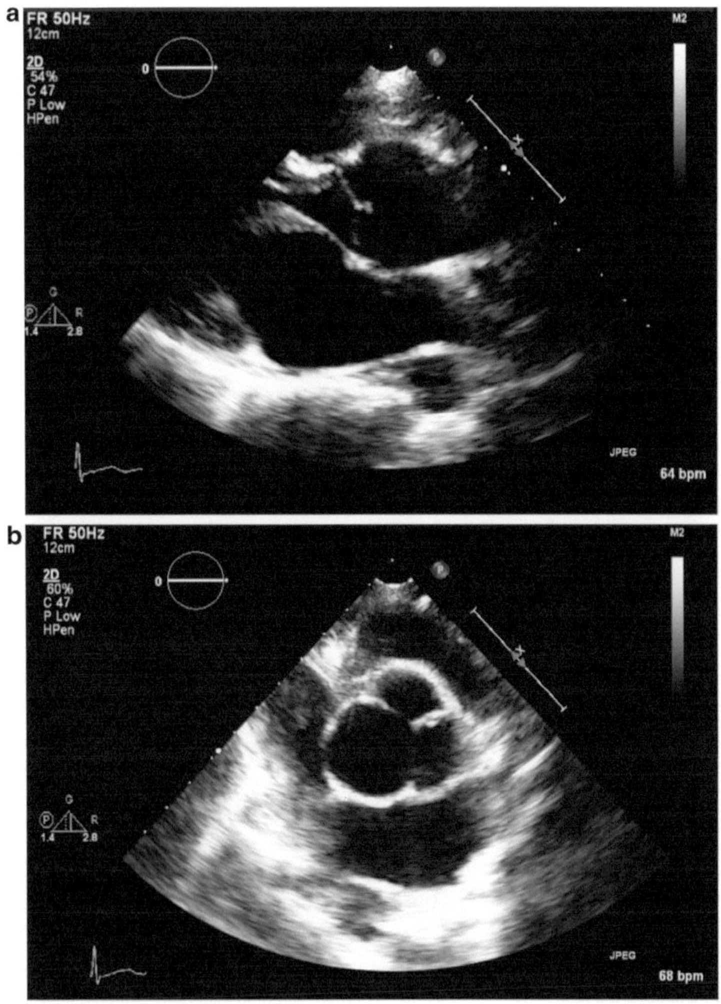

Fig. 6.6 (**a**, **b**) PLAX view (**a**) and PSAX view (**b**) showing dilated aortic root involving mainly the SOV (*onion shaped*) with relative sparing of the STJ and Asc Ao which is typical for Marfan syndrome

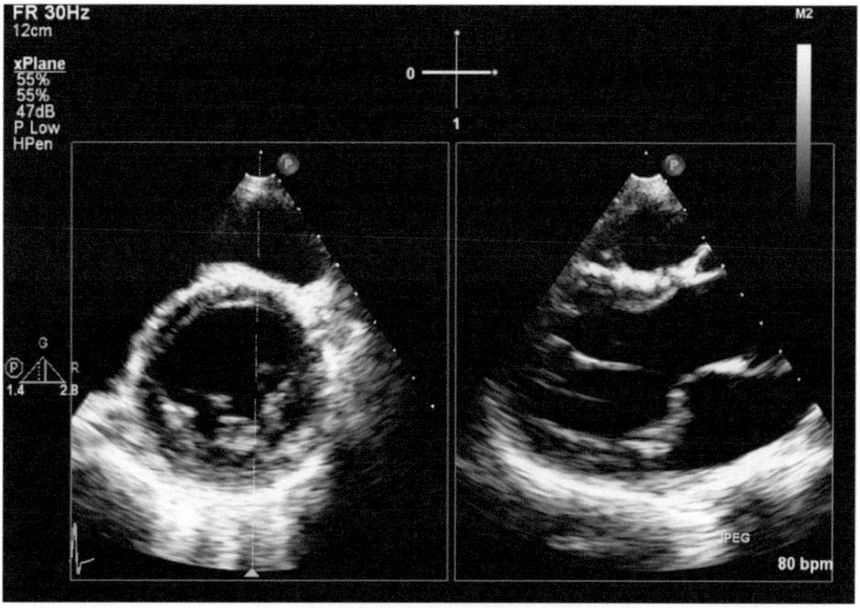

Fig. 6.7 Myxomatous mitral valve with mitral valve prolapse in a patient with Marfan syndrome

ascending aorta. An aortic root z-score (at the level of the SOV) greater than 2 is one of the major Ghent criteria needed for diagnosis [14].

ASE 2015 guidelines [1] recommend an annual follow-up echo assessment for dilated aortic root <45 mm and six monthly echo for aortic root > 45 mm. Annual TTE for follow-up after aortic root replacement is also recommended.

TTE is also useful for looking at other associated complications arising from dilated aortic root such as aortic regurgitation, aortic dissection, and other cardiac lesions such as mitral valve prolapse (Fig. 6.7), mitral regurgitation, mitral annular calcification in patients aged less than 40, dilatation of the pulmonary artery, etc. Nollen et al. have shown that in some Marfan patients with dilated aortic root, there may be concomitant dilatation in their pulmonary arteries with the dilatation occurring mainly at the pulmonary root level rather than the main pulmonary trunk [15].

In Marfan patients presenting with acute chest pain, TEE is more sensitive than TTE for the diagnosis of aortic dissection (Fig. 6.8a, b) and for visualization of the dissection flap, but TTE can also provide a quick and immediate assessment of any significant complications such as aortic regurgitation, pericardial effusion or hemopericardium, regional wall motion abnormalities due to compromised coronary artery flow from dissection flap, etc.

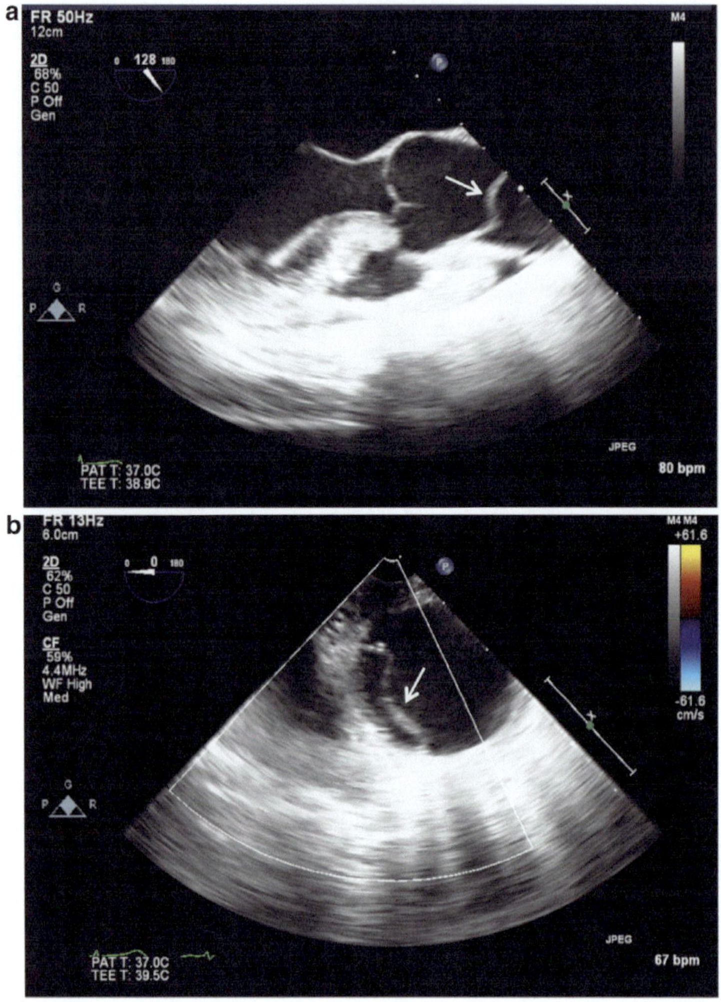

Fig. 6.8 (**a**, **b**) Type A aortic dissection in a Marfan syndrome patient, with flap seen in the ascending aorta (**a**) and descending thoracic aorta (**b**)

6.3.1.2 CT

CT demonstrates typical aortic root dilatation (Fig. 6.9a, b) as seen on TTE. In addition, CT readily shows acute complications such as dissection (Fig. 6.9c, d), periaortic hematoma and hemopericardium in aortic rupture, and extension of dissection flap into coronaries. Systemic nonvascular imaging findings such as pectus, kyphoscoliosis, dural ectasia, etc. can also help suggest presence of underlying connective tissue disorder [1]. Aortic insufficiency, which results from a dilated root, is better assessed by TTE/MRI.

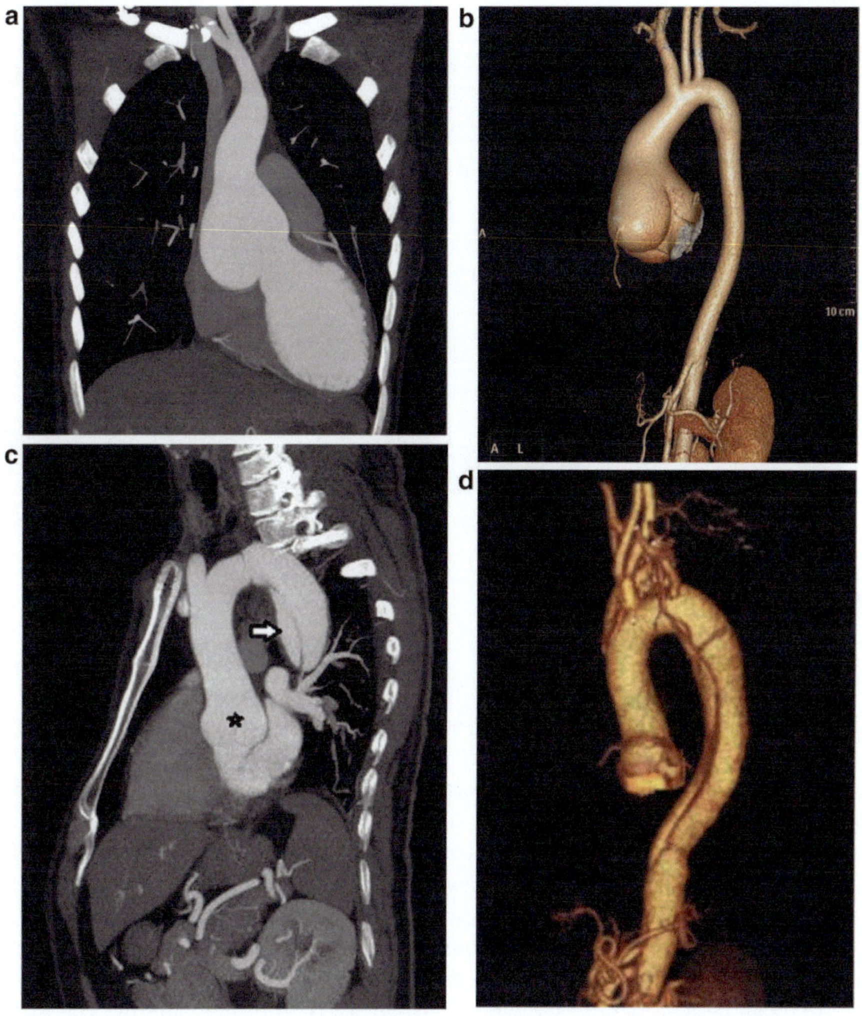

Fig. 6.9 (**a**–**d**) Coronal thick MIP (**a**) and VRT (**b**) images from ECG-gated CT aortogram in a Marfan syndrome patient showing dilated aortic sinuses with relative sparing of the Asc Ao. Sagittal MPR (**c**) and VRT (**d**) CT images from another Marfan patient showing mildly dilated aortic sinuses (* in **c**) with type B aortic dissection (*arrow* **c**)

6.3.1.3 Cardiac MRI

The mechanism and degree of aortic regurgitation can be determined. In addition to quantifying aortic dilatation or dissection (Fig. 6.10), including the identification of the true and false lumen (Fig. 6.11), additional information can be obtained, e.g., presence of dural ectasia, left ventricular volumes and systolic function, and differentiation from Loeys–Dietz syndrome thorough the presence of tortuous head, neck, and arch vessels.

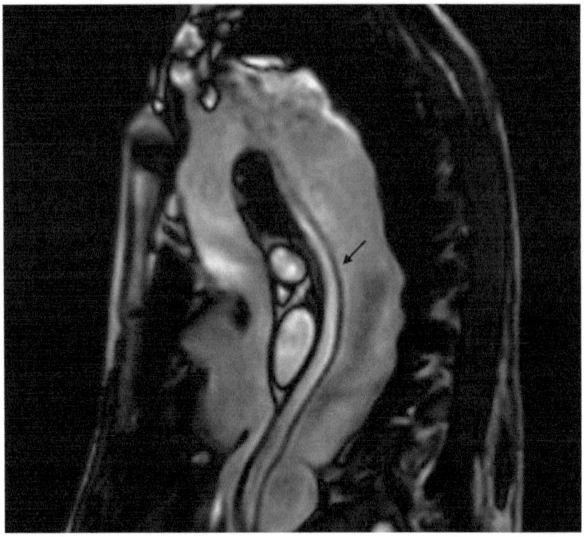

Fig. 6.10 Extent of dissection flap (shown by *arrow*) in a patient with Marfan syndrome

6.3.2 Bicuspid Aortic Valve

6.3.2.1 Echo

BAV is the most common congenital heart defects in the adult ACHD population, and bicuspid aortopathy is present in 20–84 % of these patients [16, 17]. The pattern of aortic dilatation in BAV is often diverse, affecting some or nearly all of the aortic segments from the aortic root to the aortic arch. Valvular lesions such as aortic stenosis or aortic regurgitation and coarctation of the aorta are commonly associated and may be present in varying degree of severity. Coronary artery anomalies such as anomalous origin of the left circumflex artery from the right coronary cusp may also occur, and hence attempt should be made to visualize and report the origin of the left and right coronary arteries in patients with BAV.

TTE can help to identify the types of BAV based on fusion patterns. The most common fusion pattern seen in BAV involves the right and left cusps (R-L fusion pattern, Type 1 typical pattern) and less commonly fusion of the right and non-coronary cusps (R-N fusion pattern, Type 2 atypical pattern). The least common pattern is the type involving the fusion of the left and non-coronary cusps (L-N fusion pattern, Type 3) as shown in Fig. 6.12. Sometimes, there is no raphe and the leaflets may be asymmetrical in size.

Type 1 pattern is associated with aortic stenosis and dilatation of the tubular ascending aorta (predominantly along its convex segment). Type 2 pattern involves mainly the tubular ascending aorta with extension into the transverse aortic arch and relative sparing of the aortic root. Type 3 is rare, associated with aortic regurgitation and involving mainly the aortic root only with sparing of the tubular ascending aorta and aortic arch [16].

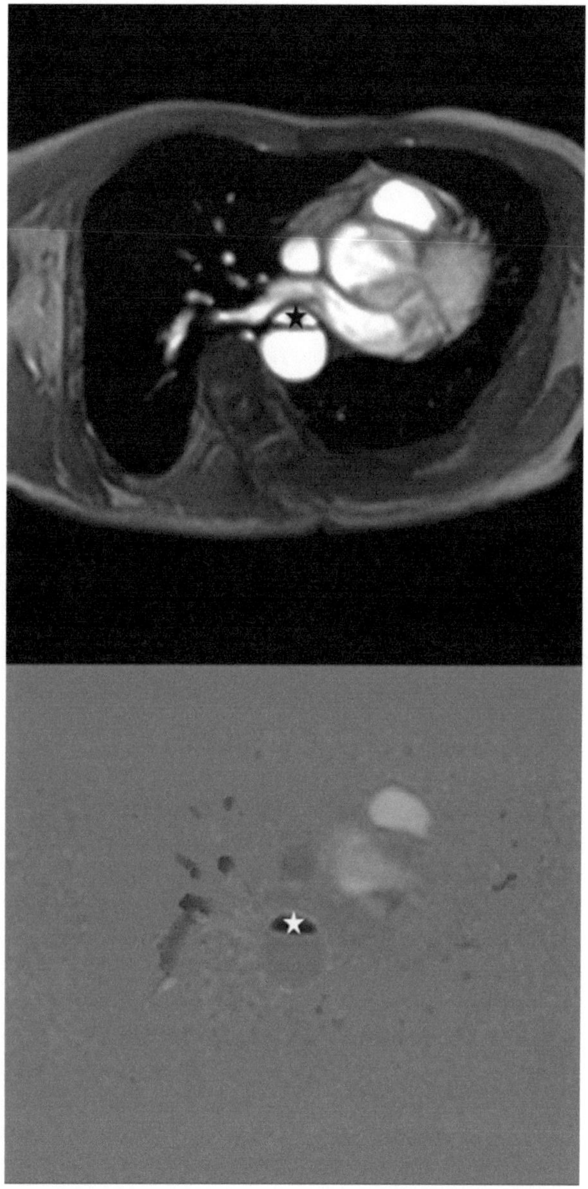

Fig. 6.11 Identification of the smaller true lumen (*) with correlation from velocity-encoded images

In BAV patients with dilated aorta <45 mm and no family history of aortic dissection, annual serial echocardiogram is recommended. If the aorta is >45 mm, a shorter six monthly follow-up is advisable. However, in patients with stable nonprogressive aortic dilatation, TTE follow-up for the aortopathy may be individualized [1].

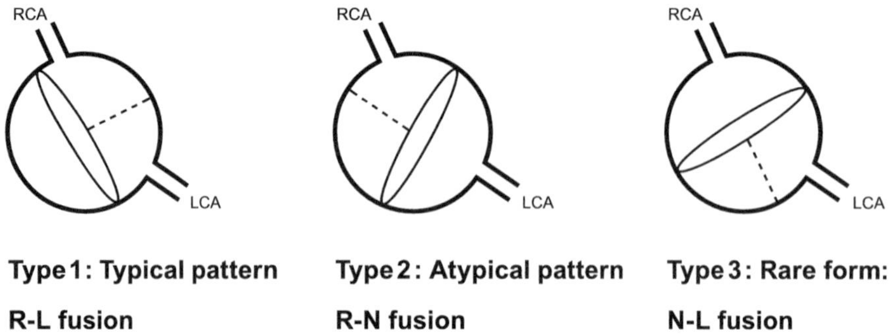

Fig. 6.12 Different BAV phenotypes

6.3.2.2 CT

BAV phenotypes may predict associated patterns of aortic dilatation. Fazel et al. [18] have described four distinct patterns of aortic dilatation in patients with BAVs with dilatation of the tubular ascending aorta and SOV occurring more frequently. Dilatation of the aortic arch and descending thoracic aorta can also occur but is less common [1]. Patients with BAVs may also have coexisting coronary artery anomalies and coarctation [1] which should always be looked for.

6.3.2.3 Cardiac MRI

The degree of aortic dilatation or dissection and presence of coarctation can be determined. Cardiac MRI will allow views of the aortic valve (Fig. 6.13), presence of aortic regurgitation (Fig. 6.14), and aorta to be obtained without interference from calcification. A study of patients with confirmed BAV found that 10 % of the patients were misidentified as having tricuspid valve using transthoracic echocardiogram, and 28 % had a nondiagnostic study, in comparison with 4 % and 2 %, respectively, with cardiac MRI [19]. The use of sophisticated 4D flow cardiac MRI in patients with fusion of the right and left coronary leaflets has been shown to produce a right-anteriorly directed helical systolic flow jet with marked peripheral skewing toward the ascending aorta convexity [20], which may explain the larger aortic root dimension and asymmetric dilatation of the mid-ascending aorta.

6.3.3 Coarctation of the Aorta

6.3.3.1 Echo

In aortic coarctation, the narrowing of the aorta most commonly occurs just distal to the left subclavian artery in the juxta-ductal region. CoA is also associated with a form of vasculopathy resulting in higher risk for aneurysmal formation in the

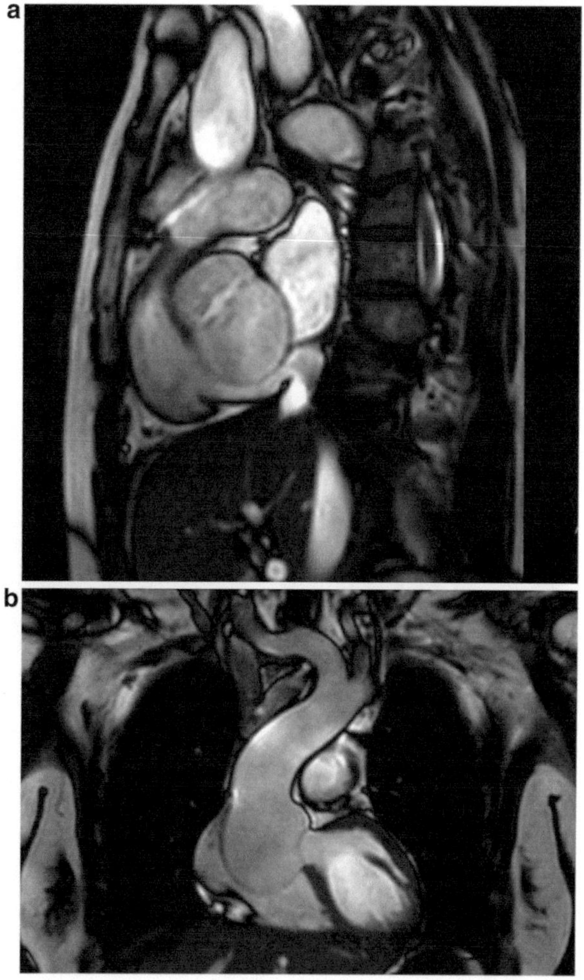

Fig. 6.13 (**a**, **b**) Asymmetric dilatation of the aortic sinuses in a patient with bicuspid aortic valve

ascending aorta, at the site of previous CoA repair, and risk for intracranial aneurysm. BAV is common in CoA patients and may be present in >50 % of these patients.

Echo evaluation of CoA patients should include the following:

- Echo measurements of all the segments of the aorta
- Evaluation of CoA severity at the descending thoracic aorta with CW Doppler to record peak CoA gradient and presence of diastolic tail (Fig. 6.15a)
- PW or CW Doppler at the abdominal aorta (diaphragmatic level) to see the presence of continuous systolic and diastolic flow suggesting systolic and diastolic gradients across a tight CoA or continuous flow from the presence of multiple collaterals due to tight CoA (Fig. 6.15b) [21]
- Evaluation of aortic valve for bicuspid aortic valve and aortic stenosis or regurgitation

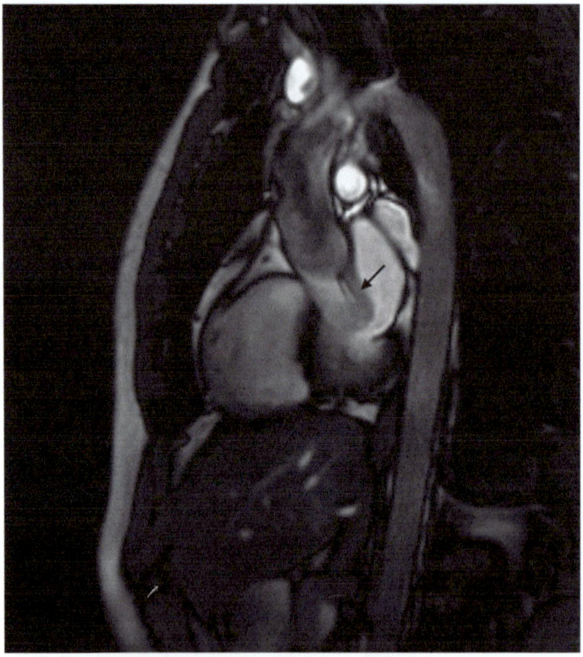

Fig. 6.14 Presence of aortic regurgitation (*arrow*) in a patient with bicuspid aortic valve

a

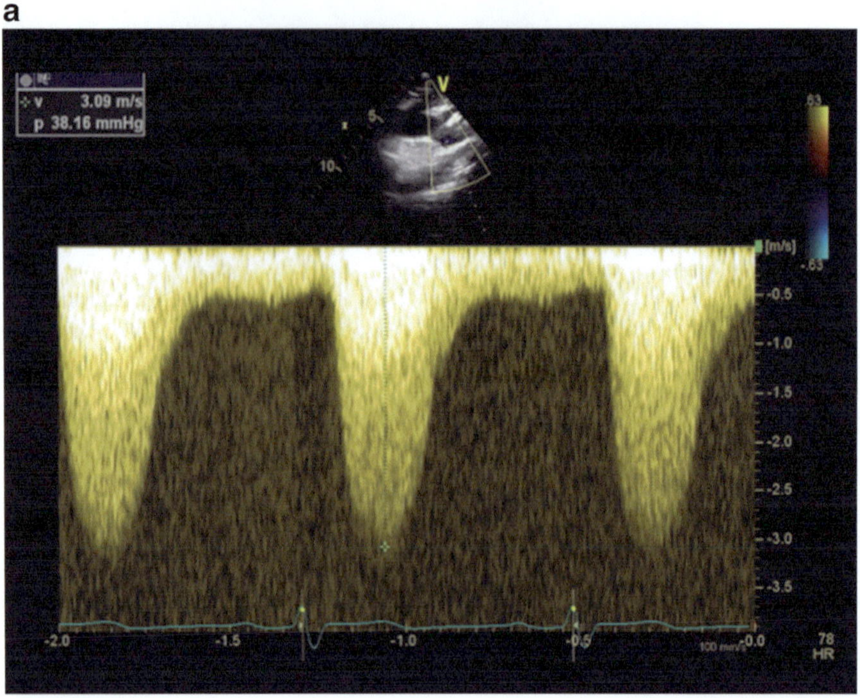

Fig. 6.15a CW Doppler of a patient with CoA demonstrating a peak gradient of 38 mmHg and a long diastolic tail with end-diastolic velocity of 0.5 m/s

b

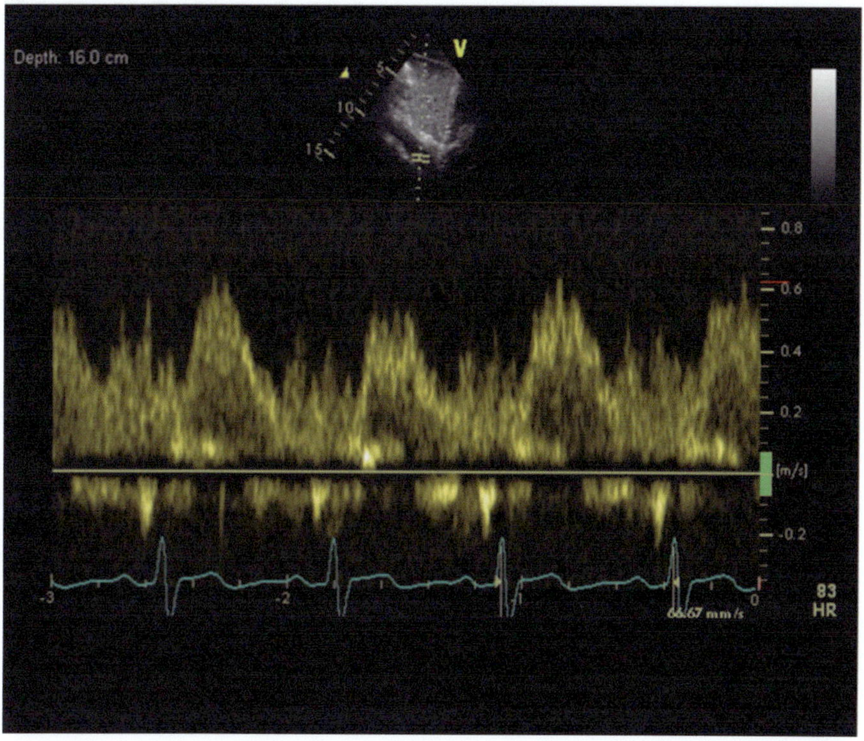

Fig. 6.15b CW Doppler of a patient with continuous systolic and diastolic flow at the abdominal aortic level

6.3.3.2 CT

Both CT and MRI show site and length of CoA segment, degree of narrowing, extent of collaterals (Fig. 6.16a), and associations such as ascending aortopathy-related dilatation and BAV [1]. MRI, however, provides additional coarctation and collateral flow-related information. Posttreatment complications such as recurrent coarctation, dissection, and aneurysm formation at coarctation repair site (Fig. 6.16b, c), and patients who may have an ascending to descending aortic bypass graft (Fig. 6.16d) are well assessed.

6.3.3.3 Cardiac MRI

Multi-planar reconstruction of acquired 3D images allows for accurate assessment of the diameter of the coarctation site (see Fig. 6.17). Complex anatomy can also be depicted using 3D-volume rendering (see Fig. 6.18).

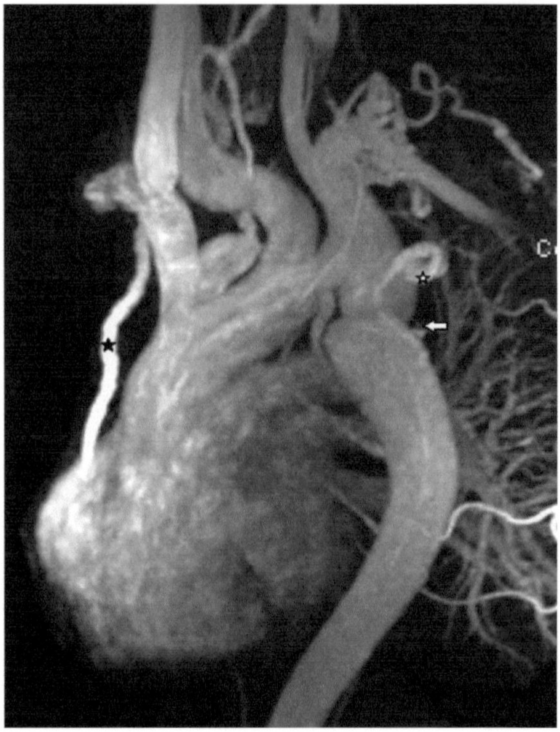

Fig. 6.16a Thick MIP images showing post-ductal CoA (*arrow*) with prominent and tortuous intercostal and internal mammary (*) arteries

The presence and degree of collaterals can be determined. The peak coarctation velocity can be measured, and the presence of diastolic prolongation of forward flow can be shown.

Velocity-encoded cine MR imaging has shown great promise for the functional assessment of hemodynamic compromise in aortic coarctation. Using this phase contrast technique, a magnetic gradient is used to phase encode the velocity of flow [22]. Data obtained from through-plane acquisitions can be used to measure peak flow velocity (v) across the area of maximal narrowing. The pressure gradient can be estimated using the modified Bernoulli eq. 4 $(v)^2$. A study suggests a pressure gradient of 15 mmHg obtained through this method as a threshold for timely intervention [23]. Velocity-encoded cine MR imaging allows the measurement of blood from the heart and great vessels as well as the quantification of collateral flow, pressure gradients, stenosis, and flow dynamics. This technique allows the ability to visualize the moving anatomy with high spatial resolution and accuracy without the use of radiographic contrast agents.

The direct depiction of enlarged collateral vessels is a reliable indicator of the hemodynamic significance of aortic coarctation [24]. The presence of retrograde blood flow through the intercostal arteries toward the descending aorta suggests collateral flow. The volume of collateral perfusion to the lower body can be obtained by determining the amount of blood flow increase from the proximal to the distal descending aorta [25].

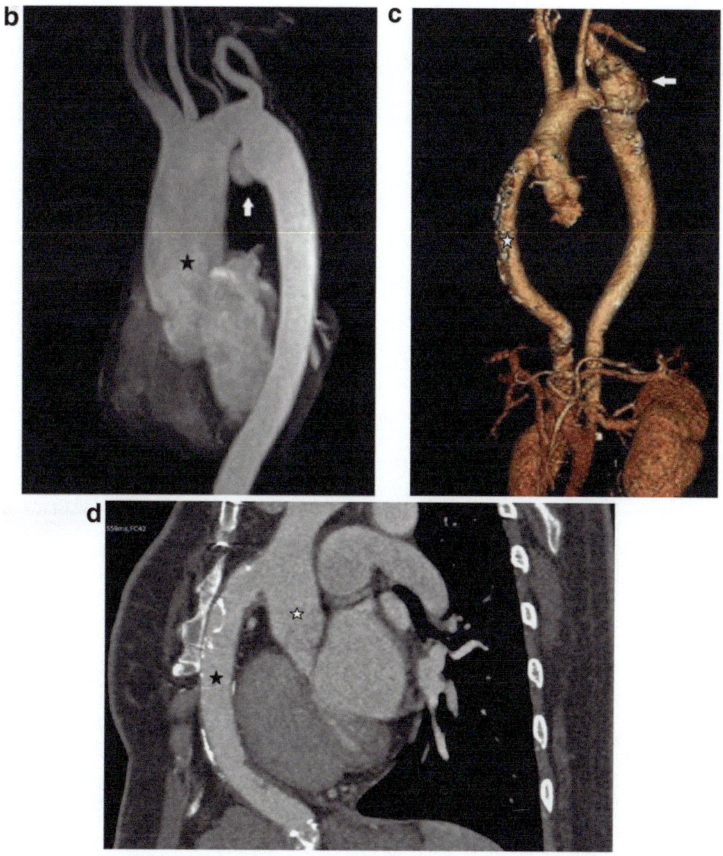

Fig. 6.16b–d Coronal MPR CT image (**b**) in a post CoA repair patient showing a small aneurysm at the post repair site (*arrow* in **b**) and dilatation involving the SOV and ascending aorta (* in **b**). VRT (**c**) and coronal MPR (**d**) images from a different post CoA repair case show a large complex aneurysm at repair site in arch (*arrow* **c**) and a patent jump graft (* in **d**) from the ascending to abdominal aorta

6.3.4 Repaired Tetralogy of Fallot

6.3.4.1 Echo

In TOF patients, dilatation of the aorta occurs more frequently in the proximal aortic root comprising the aortic annulus and SOV (Fig. 6.19a) and to a lesser extent the distal portion comprising the sinotubular junction and proximal ascending aorta (Fig. 6.19b) [26]. In this study by Chong et al., aortic root dilatation correlated with increased aortic stiffness and decreased aortic strain and distensibility.

In the largest cross-sectional multicenter study on aortic dilatation in TOF patients to date, Mongeon et al. reported the prevalence of aortic root dilatation at 28.9 % if an absolute cutoff value of ≥40 mm at level of SOV was used, but

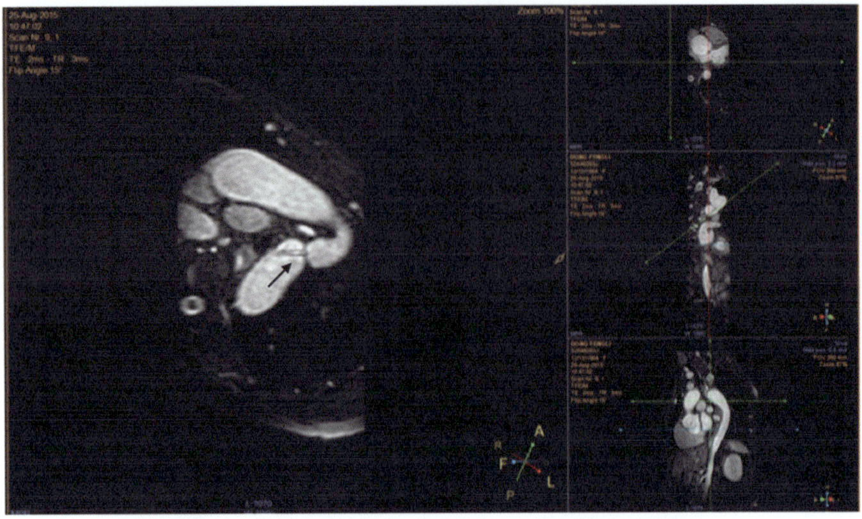

Fig. 6.17 Measurement of the diameter of the coarctation site using multi-planar reconstruction with 3D images. *Arrow* depicts dephasing due to the tight coarctation

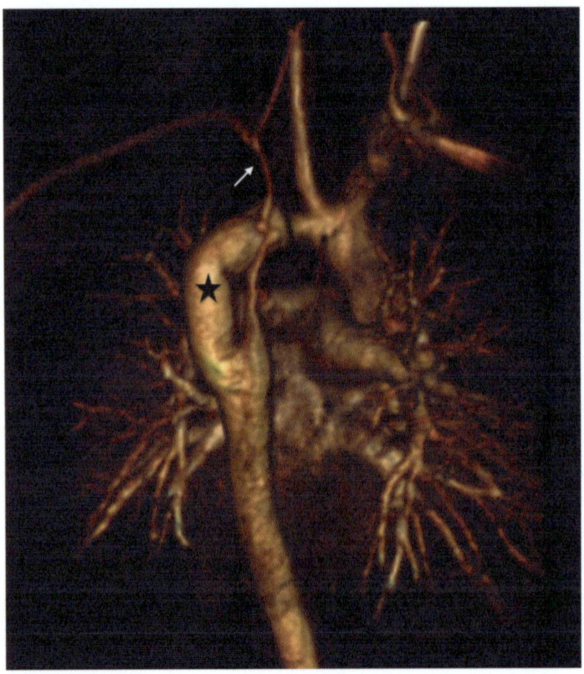

Fig. 6.18 Volume-rendered image of a patient who is status post repair of a tight coarctation segment with a jump graft. Notice the patent jump graft (*) and atretic left subclavian artery (*white arrow*)

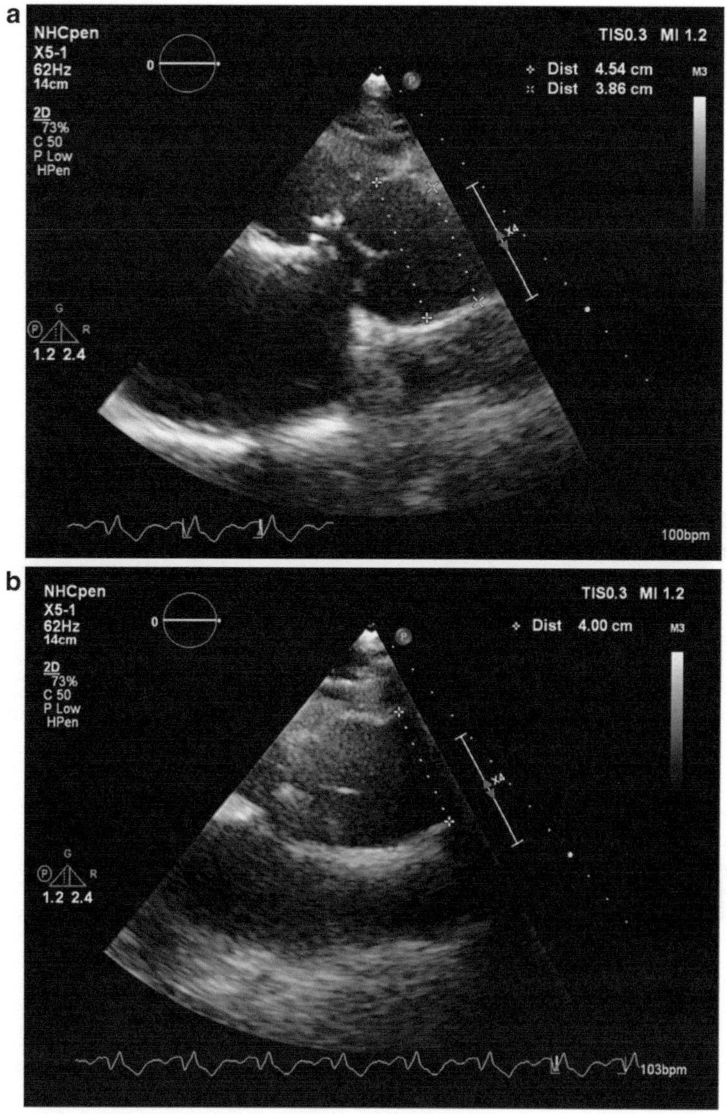

Fig. 6.19 (**a**, **b**) PLAX view showing dilatation involving the SOV and STJ (**a**) and also the proximal ascending aorta (**b**) in an adult post-op TOF patient

prevalence was only 6.6 % if an observed-to-expected aortic root diameter cutoff ratio of >1.5 was used instead. The prevalence of aortic root dilatation ≥ 45 mm was 9.7 % and that of aortic root diameter ≥ 50 mm was 2.3 %. In addition, the overall prevalence of moderate or severe aortic regurgitation in this study was low at 3.5 %. Right-sided aortic arch and age at repair were not associated with aortic root dilatation by multivariate analysis, and no independent predictor was identified to predict aortic root dilatation [27].

6.3.4.2 CT

Aortic root and ascending aorta dilatation (Fig. 6.20a, b), if present, are as well assessed in MRI.

6.3.4.3 Cardiac MRI

In addition to quantifying the presence of a right aortic arch (Fig. 6.21), aortic root dilatation, or aortic valve regurgitation (Figs. 6.22a and 6.22b), additional information can be obtained, e.g., left ventricular volumes and systolic function and the presence of additional ventricular septal defects.

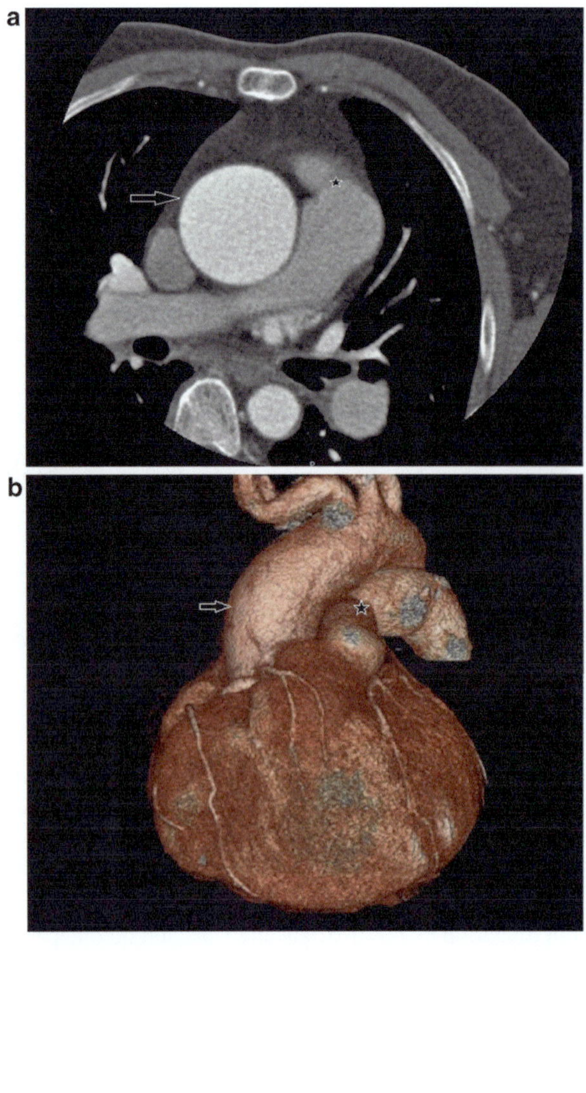

Fig. 6.20 (**a**, **b**) Axial (**a**) and VRT (**b**) images from an adult post-op TOF patient showing dilatation involving the SOV as well as proximal ascending aorta (Note RVOT repair site indicated by (*) and also good delineation of the proximal coronary arteries in this ECG-gated study)

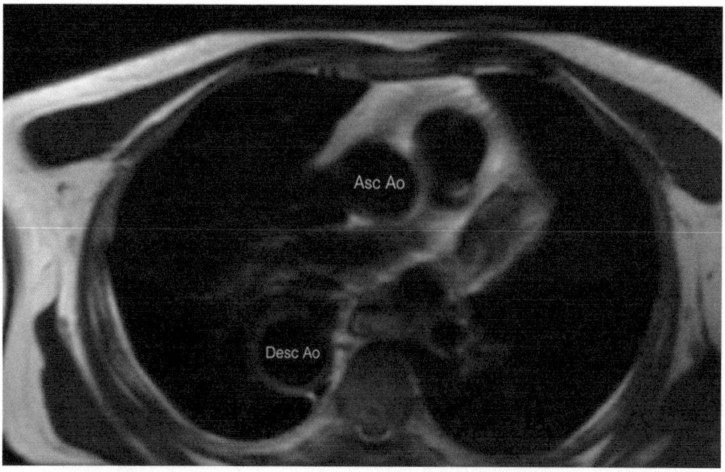

Fig. 6.21 Right aortic arch in a patient with repaired tetralogy of Fallot

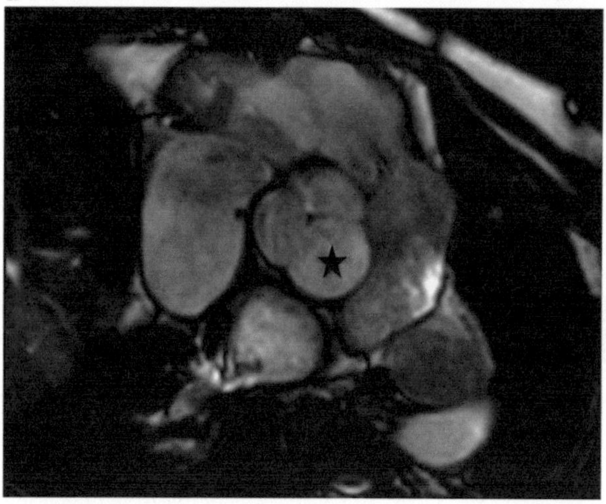

Fig. 6.22a Asymmetric dilatation of the left coronary aortic sinus (*) in a patient with repaired tetralogy of Fallot

6.3.5 Status Post-arterial Switch for d-Transposition of the Great Vessels

6.3.5.1 Echo

In post-arterial d-TGA switch patients, echo is commonly performed to assess for neo-pulmonary stenosis or regurgitation, supra-aortic stenosis, neo-aortic

b

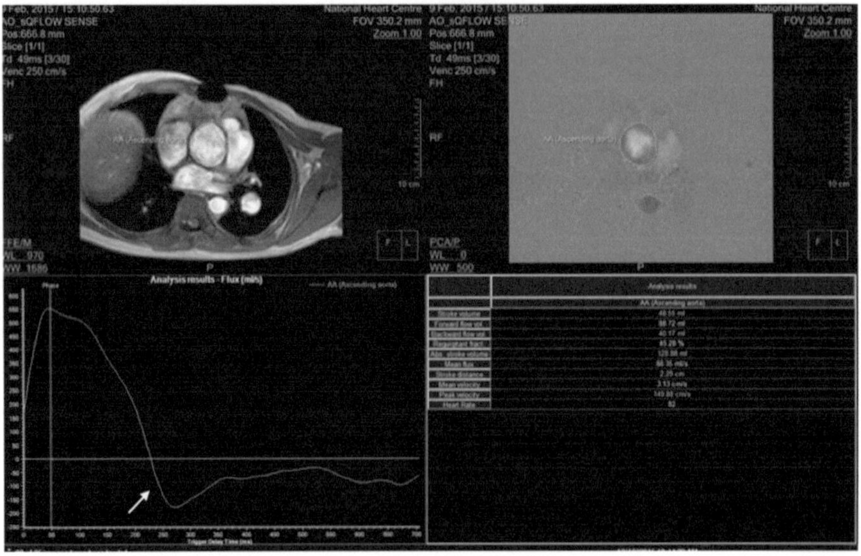

Fig. 6.22b Flow analysis showing severe aortic regurgitation (*white arrow*)

regurgitation, and neo-aortic root dilatation (Fig. 6.23a, b). Post Lecompte procedure and echo imaging of the anteriorly displaced neo-pulmonary valve and main and branch pulmonary arteries are often inadequate due to limited echo windows.

Neo-aortic root dilatation can occur as a result of the size discrepancy of the great arteries post-arterial switch (ASO). Risk factors for the development of neo-aortic root dilatation include older age at time of ASO, presence of VSD, bicuspid pulmonic valve, previous pulmonary artery banding, and higher neo-aortic root/ascending aorta ratio [28]. There is however no clear association with acute aortic dissection or increased mortality [29].

Co-Vu et al. reported neo-aortic root dilatation with z-scores of $\geq$2.5 in 66 % of ASO patients, and the root diameter z-score increased at an average rate of 0.08 per year after ASO. Freedom from neo-aortic root dilatation at 1, 5, 10, and 15 years after ASO was 84 %, 67 %, 47 %, and 32 %, respectively. At least moderate degree of neo-aortic valve regurgitation was present in 14 % of ASO patients, and neo-aortic root dilatation was a significant risk factor for this [30].

6.3.5.2 CT

Post-arterial switch relationship of the great vessels, dilatation of neo-aortic root (Fig. 6.24a, b), and presence of neo-aortic or neo-pulmonic stenosis are well demonstrated.

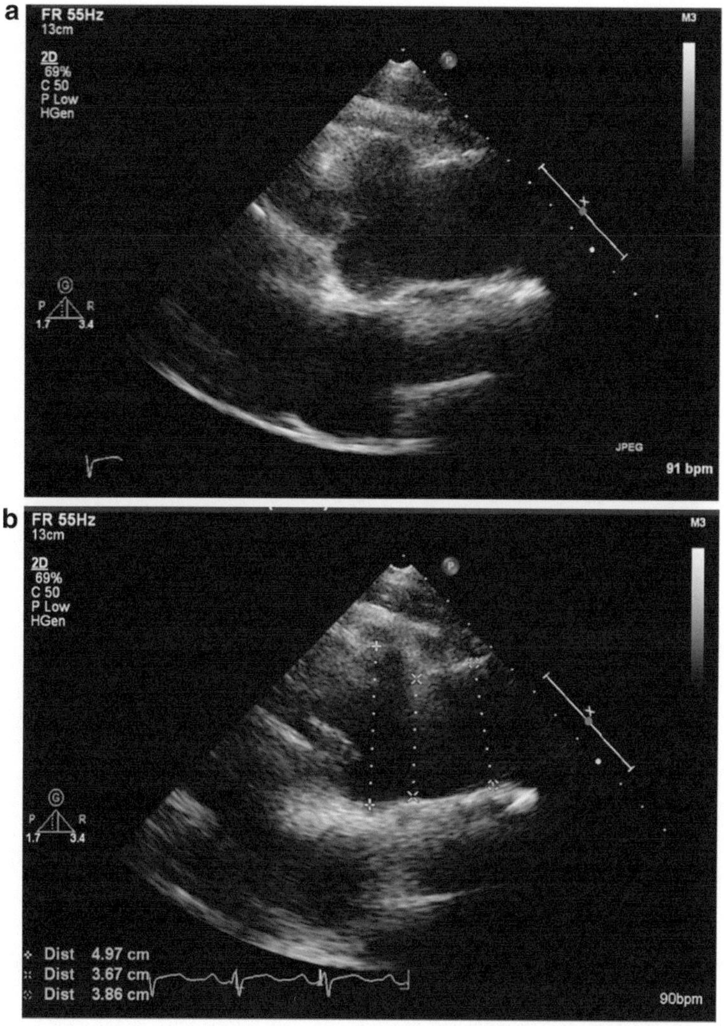

Fig. 6.23 (**a**, **b**) Patient with dilated aortic root (**a**) and ascending aorta (**b**) post-arterial switch operation

6.3.5.3 Cardiac MRI

The relationship of the great vessels can be better appreciated through cardiac MRI (see Fig. 6.25). It allows identification of dilatation of the ascending aorta (often at sites of coronary button transfer) and the presence of neo-aortic stenosis or supravalvular aortic stenosis.

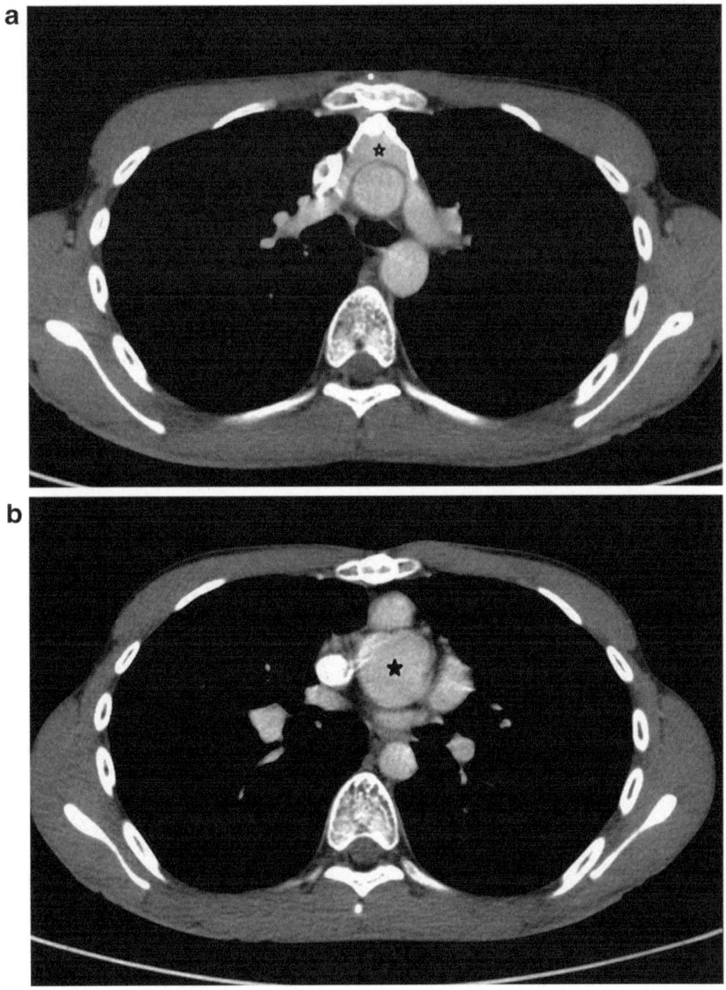

Fig. 6.24 (**a**, **b**) Axial images showing relationship of the great vessels and dilated SOV in a patient post-arterial switch operation for d-TGA

6.3.6 Miscellaneous

6.3.6.1 Status Post Fontan Palliation for Hypoplastic Heart Disease

Echo

Aortic dilatation in Fontan patients (Fig. 6.26a, b) may occur when the aortic valve is bicuspid or when Fontan completion is late resulting in prolong volume loading and hemodynamic stress through this single outlet trunk. In post Fontan patients born with hypoplastic left heart syndrome (HLHS), the native pulmonary valve

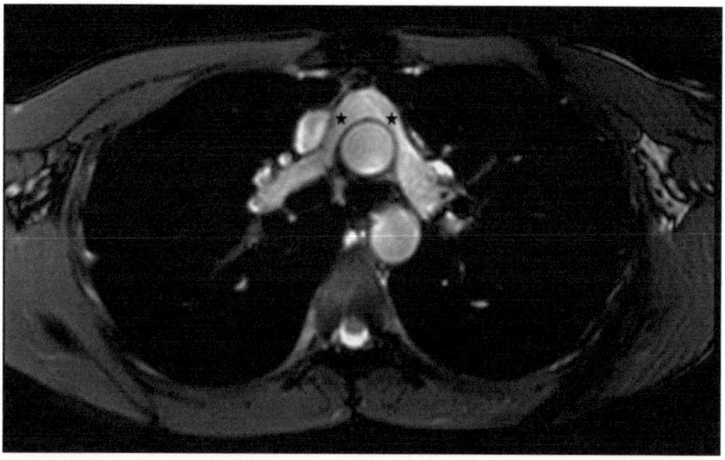

Fig. 6.25 Relationship of the great vessels post-arterial switch. Notice the kinking of the branch pulmonary arteries near the bifurcation (*)

would become the neo-aortic valve which had to withstand systemic pressure. Concomitant surgical intervention in HLHS such as patch augmentation of the ascending aorta may further increase the risk of aortic dilatation.

Cohen et al. reported that in a median 9-year follow-up of post Fontan HLHS patients, their neo-aortic root continued to dilate out of proportion to body size, with 98 % of patients having a root z-value of >2 [31].

Very few case reports of progressive neo-aortic root dilatation progress to requiring surgical intervention, but regular follow-up is required when aortic dilatation occurs [32, 33].

CT

CT provides adequate anatomical assessment for stenosis or thrombus formation in the Fontan pathways as well as aortic dilatation. When assessing Fontan pathway with contrast-enhanced CT, adequate opacification of both limbs of pathway may be tricky and will need either simultaneous injection of contrast through arm and leg veins or acquisition of images in early and delayed phases [34].

Cardiac MRI

Contrast-enhanced or 3D MRI allows for assessment of the arch reconstruction for residual obstruction. It also allows for characterization of the major aortopulmonary collateral arteries (MAPCAs).

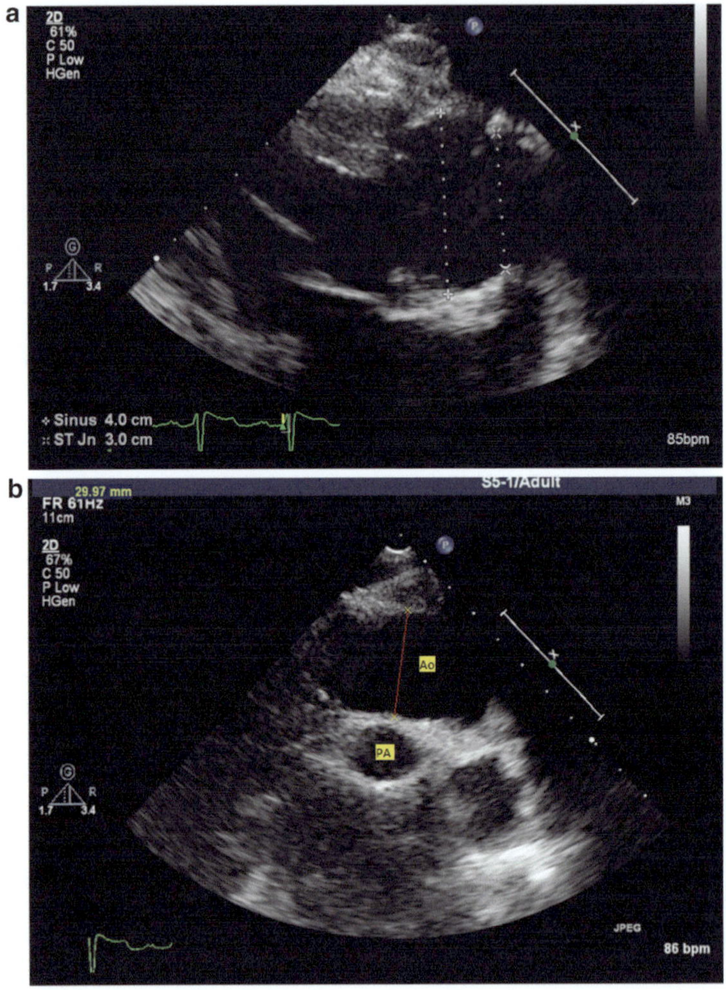

Fig. 6.26 (**a**, **b**) Dilated aortic root mainly involving the SOV (**a**) with relative sparing of the ascending aorta (**b**) in a patient with post-op Fontan. The great arteries are transposed with the aorta anterior to the pulmonary artery as shown in **b**

6.4 Summary

Due to easy accessibility and availability of expertise, echocardiography remains the key tool for initial assessment of the aorta in patients with congenital heart disease. However, as echo dropouts remain a challenge, additional information, vital to the decision-making in clinical care, have to be acquired through cardiac CT and MRI. Each modality carries its pros and cons, and the clinician will need to decide how best to utilize each modality to its fullest.

References

1. Goldstein SA, Evangelista A, Abbara S, Arai A, Asch FM, Badano LP, Bolen MA, Connolly HM, Cuellar-Calabria H, Czerny M, Devereux RB, Erbel RA, Fattori R, Isselbacher EM, Lindsay JM, McCulloch M, Michelena HI, Nienaber CA, Oh JK, Pepi M, Taylor AJ, Weinsaft JW, Zamorano JL, Dietz H, Eagle K, Elefteriades J, Jondeau G, Rousseau H, Schepens M (2015) Multimodality imaging of diseases of the thoracic aorta in adults: from the American Society of Echocardiography and the European Association of Cardiovascular Imaging: endorsed by the Society of Cardiovascular Computed Tomography and Society for Cardiovascular Magnetic Resonance. J Am Soc Echocardiogr 28(2):119–182
2. Roman MJ, Devereux RB, Kramer-Fox R, O'Loughlin J (1989) Two-dimensional echocardiographic aortic root dimensions in normal children and adults. Am J Cardiol 64(8):507–512
3. Vasan RS, Larson MG, Benjamin EJ, Levy D (1995) Echocardiographic reference values for aortic root size: the Framingham Heart Study. J Am Soc Echocardiogr 8(6):793–800
4. Hiratzka LF, Bakris GL, Beckman JA, Bersin RM, Carr VF, Casey DE Jr, Eagle KA, Hermann LK, Isselbacher EM, Kazerooni EA, Kouchoukos NT, Lytle BW, Milewicz DM, Reich DL, Sen S, Shinn JA, Svensson LG, Williams DM, American College of Cardiology F, American Heart Association Task Force on Practice G, American Association for Thoracic S, American College of R, American Stroke A, Society of Cardiovascular A, Society for Cardiovascular A, Interventions, Society of Interventional R, Society of Thoracic S, Society for Vascular M (2010) 2010 ACCF/AHA/AATS/ACR/ASA/SCA/SCAI/SIR/STS/SVM guidelines for the diagnosis and management of patients with thoracic aortic disease: executive summary. A report of the American College of Cardiology Foundation/American Heart Association Task Force on Practice Guidelines, American Association for Thoracic Surgery, American College of Radiology, American Stroke Association, Society of Cardiovascular Anesthesiologists, Society for Cardiovascular Angiography and Interventions, Society of Interventional Radiology, Society of Thoracic Surgeons, and Society for Vascular Medicine. Catheter Cardiovasc Interv 76(2):E43–E86
5. Burman ED, Keegan J, Kilner PJ (2008) Aortic root measurement by cardiovascular magnetic resonance: specification of planes and lines of measurement and corresponding normal values. Circ Cardiovasc Imaging 1(2):104–113. doi:10.1161/CIRCIMAGING.108.768911
6. Suh SY, Kim EJ, Choi CU, Na JO, Kim SH, Kim HJ, Han SW, Chung SM, Ryu KH, Park CG, Seo HS, Oh DJ (2009) Aortic upper wall tissue Doppler image velocity: relation to aortic elasticity and left ventricular diastolic function. Echocardiography 26(9):1069–1074. doi:10.1111/j.1540-8175.2009.00910.x
7. Gutstein A, Wolak A, Lee C, Dey D, Ohba M, Suzuki Y, Cheng V, Gransar H, Suzuki S, Friedman J, Thomson LE, Hayes S, Pimentel R, Paz W, Slomka P, Berman DS (2008) Predicting success of prospective and retrospective gating with dual-source coronary computed tomography angiography: development of selection criteria and initial experience. J Cardiovasc Comput Tomogr 2(2):81–90
8. Poll LW, Cohnen M, Brachten S, Ewen K, Modder U (2002) Dose reduction in multi-slice CT of the heart by use of ECG-controlled tube current modulation ("ECG pulsing"): phantom measurements. ROFO Fortschr Geb Rontgenstr Nuklearmed 174(12):1500–1505
9. Leschka S, Stolzmann P, Schmid FT, Scheffel H, Stinn B, Marincek B, Alkadhi H, Wildermuth S (2008) Low kilovoltage cardiac dual-source CT: attenuation, noise, and radiation dose. Eur Radiol 18(9):1809–1817. doi:10.1007/s00330-008-0966-1
10. Freeman LA, Young PM, Foley TA, Williamson EE, Bruce CJ, Greason KL (2013) CT and MRI assessment of the aortic root and ascending aorta. AJR Am J Roentgenol 200(6):W581–W592. doi:10.2214/AJR.12.9531
11. Lin FY, Devereux RB, Roman MJ, Meng J, Jow VM, Jacobs A, Weinsaft JW, Shaw LJ, Berman DS, Gilmore A, Callister TQ, Min JK (2008) Assessment of the thoracic aorta by multidetector computed tomography: age- and sex-specific reference values in adults without evident cardiovascular disease. J Cardiovasc Comput Tomogr 2(5):298–308

12. Holloway BJ, Rosewarne D, Jones RG (2011) Imaging of thoracic aortic disease. Br J Radiol 84(Spec No 3):S338–S354. doi:10.1259/bjr/30655825
13. Potthast S, Mitsumori L, Stanescu LA, Richardson ML, Branch K, Dubinsky TJ, Maki JH (2010) Measuring aortic diameter with different MR techniques: comparison of three-dimensional (3D) navigated steady-state free-precession (SSFP), 3D contrast-enhanced magnetic resonance angiography (CE-MRA), 2D T2 black blood, and 2D cine SSFP. J Magn Reson Imaging 31(1):177–184. doi:10.1002/jmri.22016
14. Loeys BL, Dietz HC, Braverman AC, Callewaert BL, De Backer J, Devereux RB, Hilhorst-Hofstee Y, Jondeau G, Faivre L, Milewicz DM, Pyeritz RE, Sponseller PD, Wordsworth P, De Paepe AM (2010) The revised Ghent nosology for the Marfan syndrome. J Med Genet 47 (7):476–485. doi:10.1136/jmg.2009.072785
15. Nollen GJ, van Schijndel KE, Timmermans J, Groenink M, Barentsz JO, van der Wall EE, Stoker J, Mulder BJ (2002) Pulmonary artery root dilatation in Marfan syndrome: quantitative assessment of an unknown criterion. Heart 87(5):470–471
16. Verma S, Siu SC (2014) Aortic dilatation in patients with bicuspid aortic valve. N Engl J Med 370(20):1920–1929. doi:10.1056/NEJMra1207059
17. Siu SC, Silversides CK (2010) Bicuspid aortic valve disease. J Am Coll Cardiol 55 (25):2789–2800. doi:10.1016/j.jacc.2009.12.068
18. Fazel SS, Mallidi HR, Lee RS, Sheehan MP, Liang D, Fleischman D, Herfkens R, Mitchell RS, Miller DC The aortopathy of bicuspid aortic valve disease has distinctive patterns and usually involves the transverse aortic arch. J Thorac Cardiovasc Surg 135(4):901–907
19. Malaisrie SC, Carr J, Mikati I, Rigolin V, Yip BK, Lapin B, McCarthy PM (2012) Cardiac magnetic resonance imaging is more diagnostic than 2-dimensional echocardiography in determining the presence of bicuspid aortic valve. J Thorac Cardiovasc Surg 144(2):370–376
20. Hope MD, Hope TA, Crook SE, Ordovas KG, Urbania TH, Alley MT, Higgins CB (2011) 4D flow CMR in assessment of valve-related ascending aortic disease. JACC Cardiovasc Imaging 4(7):781–787. doi:10.1016/j.jcmg.2011.05.004
21. Tan JL, Babu-Narayan SV, Henein MY, Mullen M, Li W (2005) Doppler echocardiographic profile and indexes in the evaluation of aortic coarctation in patients before and after stenting. J Am Coll Cardiol 46(6):1045–1053. doi:10.1016/j.jacc.2005.05.076
22. Underwood SR, Firmin DN, Klipstein RH, Rees RS, Longmore DB (1987) Magnetic resonance velocity mapping: clinical application of a new technique. Br Heart J 57(5):404–412
23. Varaprasathan GA, Araoz PA, Higgins CB, Reddy GP (2002) Quantification of flow dynamics in congenital heart disease: applications of velocity-encoded cine MR imaging. Radiographics 22 (4):895–905; discussion 905-896
24. Araoz PA, Reddy GP, Tarnoff H, Roge CL, Higgins CB (2003) MR findings of collateral circulation are more accurate measures of hemodynamic significance than arm-leg blood pressure gradient after repair of coarctation of the aorta. J Magn Reson Imaging 17(2):177–183
25. Julsrud PR, Breen JF, Felmlee JP, Warnes CA, Connolly HM, Schaff HV (1997) Coarctation of the aorta: collateral flow assessment with phase-contrast MR angiography. AJR Am J Roentgenol 169(6):1735–1742
26. Chong WY, Wong WH, Chiu CS, Cheung YF (2006) Aortic root dilation and aortic elastic properties in children after repair of tetralogy of Fallot. Am J Cardiol 97(6):905–909. doi:10.1016/j.amjcard.2005.09.141
27. Mongeon FP, Gurvitz MZ, Broberg CS, Aboulhosn J, Opotowsky AR, Kay JD, Valente AM, Earing MG, Lui GK, Fernandes SM, Gersony DR, Cook SC, Ting JG, Nickolaus MJ, Landzberg MJ, Khairy P, Alliance for Adult Research in Congenital C (2013) Aortic root dilatation in adults with surgically repaired tetralogy of fallot: a multicenter cross-sectional study. Circulation 127(2):172–179. doi:10.1161/CIRCULATIONAHA.112.129585
28. McMahon CJ, Ravekes WJ, Smith EO, Denfield SW, Pignatelli RH, Altman CA, Ayres NA (2004) Risk factors for neo-aortic root enlargement and aortic regurgitation following arterial switch operation. Pediatr Cardiol 25(4):329–335. doi:10.1007/s00246-003-0483-6

29. Schwartz ML, Gauvreau K, del Nido P, Mayer JE, Colan SD (2004) Long-term predictors of aortic root dilation and aortic regurgitation after arterial switch operation. Circulation 110 (11 Suppl 1):II128–II132. doi:10.1161/01.CIR.0000138392.68841.d3
30. Co-Vu JG, Ginde S, Bartz PJ, Frommelt PC, Tweddell JS, Earing MG (2013) Long-term outcomes of the neoaorta after arterial switch operation for transposition of the great arteries. Ann Thorac Surg 95(5):1654–1659. doi:10.1016/j.athoracsur.2012.10.081
31. Cohen MS, Marino BS, McElhinney DB, Robbers-Visser D, van der Woerd W, Gaynor JW, Spray TL, Wernovsky G (2003) Neo-aortic root dilation and valve regurgitation up to 21 years after staged reconstruction for hypoplastic left heart syndrome. J Am Coll Cardiol 42 (3):533–540
32. Erez E, Tam VK, Galliani C, Lashus A, Doublin NA, Peretti J (2012) Valve-sparing aortic root replacement for patients with a Fontan circulation. J Heart Valve Dis 21(2):175–180
33. Pizarro C, Baffa JM, Derby CD, Krieger PA (2011) Valve-sparing neo-aortic root replacement after Fontan completion for hypoplastic left heart syndrome. J Thorac Cardiovasc Surg 141 (4):1083–1084. doi:10.1016/j.jtcvs.2010.07.076
34. Goo HW, Park IS, Ko JK, Kim YH, Seo DM, Park JJ (2005) Computed tomography for the diagnosis of congenital heart disease in pediatric and adult patients. Int J Card Imaging 21 (2–3):347–365; discussion 367

Chapter 7
Pulse Wave Velocity and Augmentation Index

Tomoaki Murakami

Abstract Pulse wave velocity is obtained from the transit time of pulse wave and the distance between two measuring sites. It is considered the "gold standard" for assessment of arterial elastance and recognized as one of the most important risk factors for cardiovascular diseases.

Augmentation index is the index of aortic pressure wave reflection and defined as the ratio of augmented ascending aortic pressure and pulse pressure (Ps – Pi) / (Ps – Pd) where Ps is the peak systolic pressure, Pi is the pressure at the reflection point, and Pd the is minimum diastolic pressure. The reflected pressure wave enhances the coronary perfusion in young people (slow pulse wave velocity). However, it interferes with the systemic ventricular ejection and increases workload of the systemic ventricle in elderly people (fast pulse wave velocity). In patients after aortic surgery, the augmentation index is high because the surgical procedure would make a new reflection point on the aorta.

Keywords Pulse wave velocity • Pressure wave reflection • Augmentation index

7.1 Pulse Wave Velocity

Pulse wave velocity (PWV) is obtained from the transit time of pulse wave and distance between two measuring sites (Fig. 7.1). PWV is considered the "gold standard" for assessment of arterial elastance and recognized as one of the most important risk factors for cardiovascular diseases. The PWV is proportional to the stiffness and the thickness of the arterial wall and inversely proportional to the diameter of the vessels and the viscosity of the blood. It is also influenced by the blood pressure and the heart rate. In European countries, carotid-femoral PWV is often used for the noninvasive evaluation of the arterial stiffness. On the other hand, brachial-ankle PWV is used in Japan. The PWV becomes high with aging (Fig. 7.2) [1].

T. Murakami, M.D., Ph.D. (✉)
Department of Cardiology, Chiba Children's Hospital, 579-1 Heta-cho, Midori-ku, Chiba 266-0007, Japan
e-mail: murat@seagreen.ocn.ne.jp

K. Niwa, H. Kaemmerer (eds.), *Aortopathy*, DOI 10.1007/978-4-431-56071-5_7

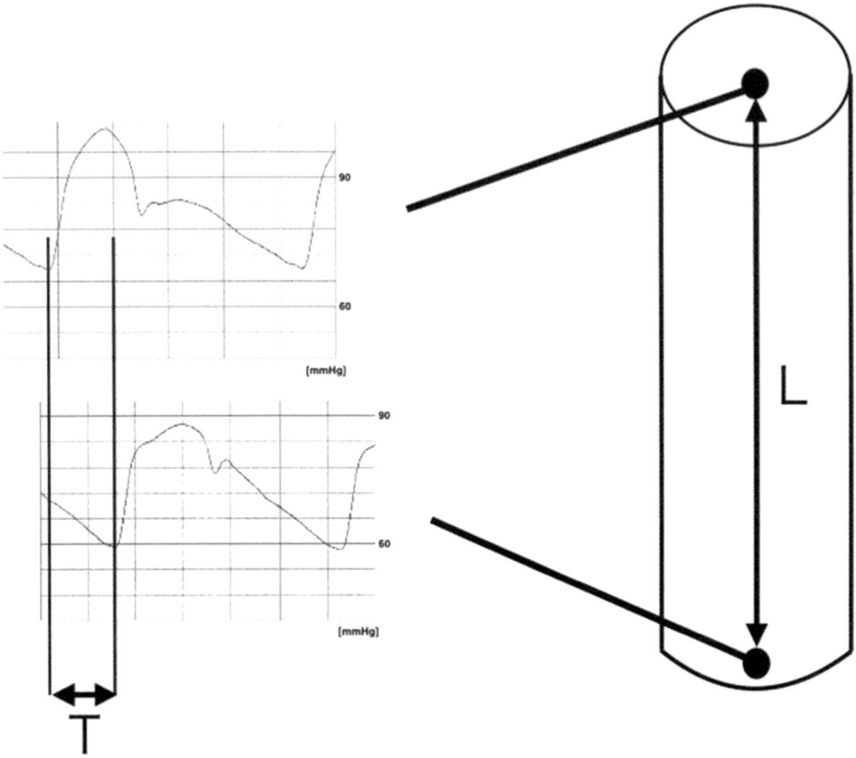

Fig. 7.1 Measurement of pulse wave velocity. The delay time between the two pressures is the transmission time (T), and the distance (L) between the two pressure recording sites divided by T is the pulse wave velocity

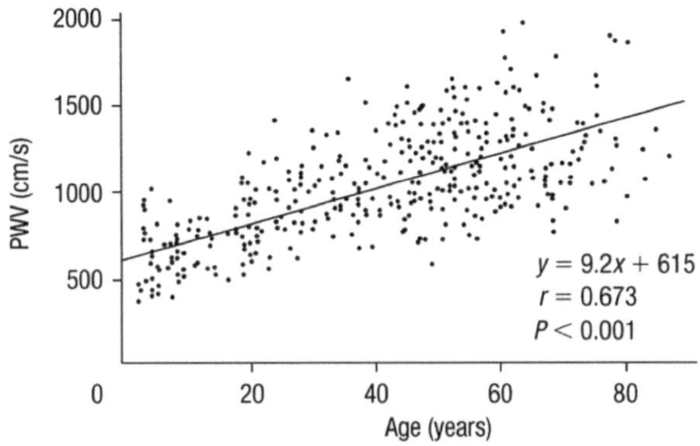

Fig. 7.2 Pulse wave velocity elevates with aging (Avolio et al. [1])

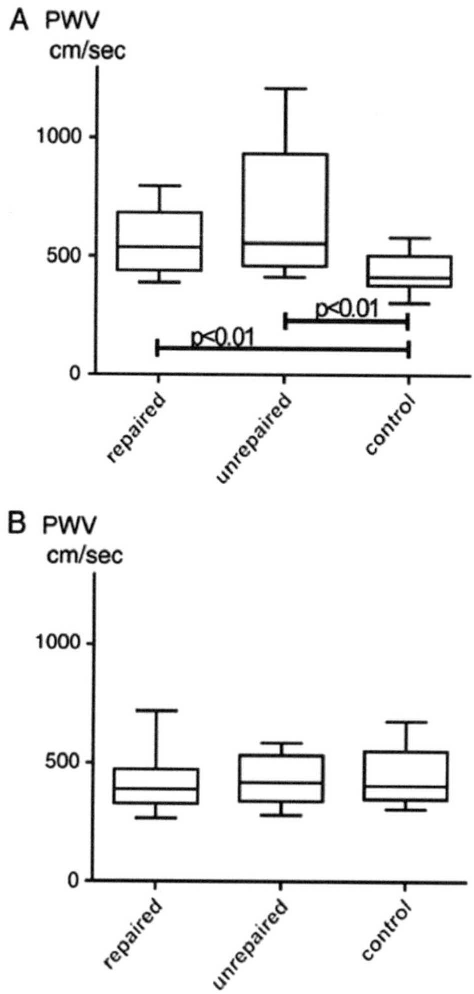

Fig. 7.3 Pulse wave velocity on the ascending aorta in repaired and unrepaired patients with tetralogy of Fallot increases in comparison with that in control (**a**). There is no difference on the pulse wave velocity on the descending aorta between the groups (**b**). PWV, pulse wave velocity (Saiki et al. [2])

Intriguingly, it is reported that the PWV in aneurysmal aorta in patients with tetralogy of Fallot is elevated [2], although the PWV is inversely proportional to the diameter of the vessel. This phenomenon could imply that the damage of the aortic wall precede the dilatation (Fig. 7.3).

7.2 Augmentation Index

Augmentation index (AI) is the index of the aortic pressure wave reflection. Aortic pressure waveform is composed of two pressure waveforms: the forward pressure wave and the reflected pressure wave (Fig. 7.4). The forward pressure wave is generated by the systemic ventricular ejection, and the backward pressure is the sum of the pressure wave reflections. The pressure wave reflections arise from any discontinuity in the elastic properties along the arterial tree in which there is a change (or mismatch) in impedance [3]. In normal aortic tree, the reflecting point that represents the integrated pressure wave reflections exists in the region of the aortic bifurcation [4]. Because of the slow PWV, the reflected pressure wave returns to the heart during diastole in young people, it means the timing after closure of aortic valve (Fig. 7.4b). Therefore, it enhances the coronary perfusion by pushing

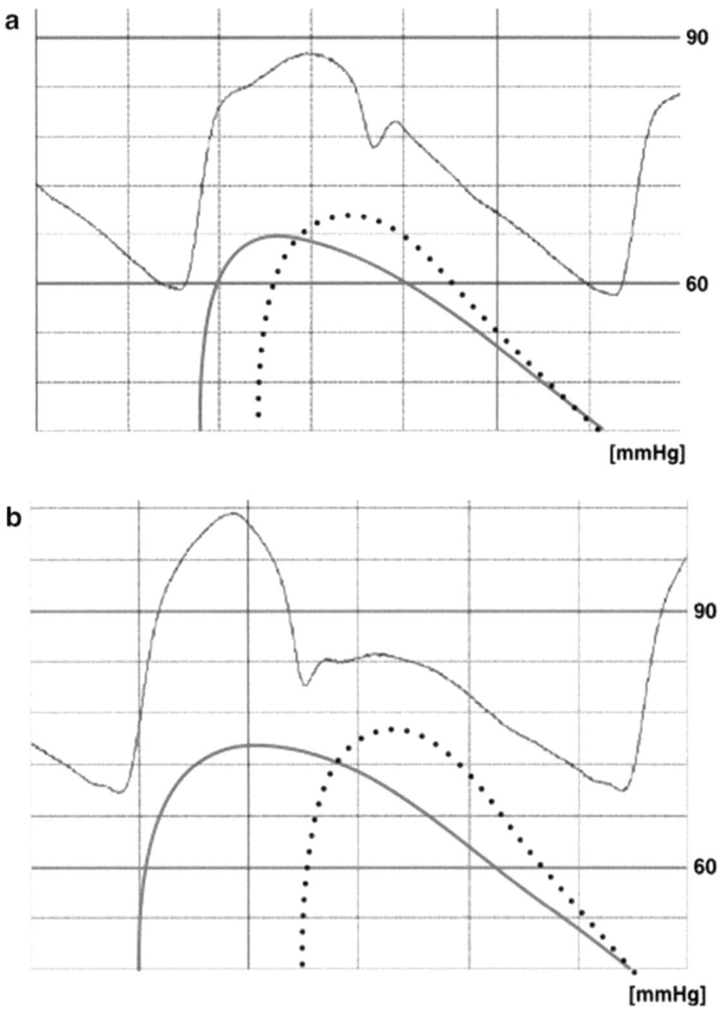

Fig. 7.4 Aortic pressure waveforms. A *solid line* means the forward pressure wave and *dotted line* stands for the reflected pressure wave. Early return of reflected pressure wave (**a**), namely, returns before closure of aortic valve, applies load to the systemic ventricle. On the other hand, late return of reflected pressure wave (**b**) can enhance coronary perfusion

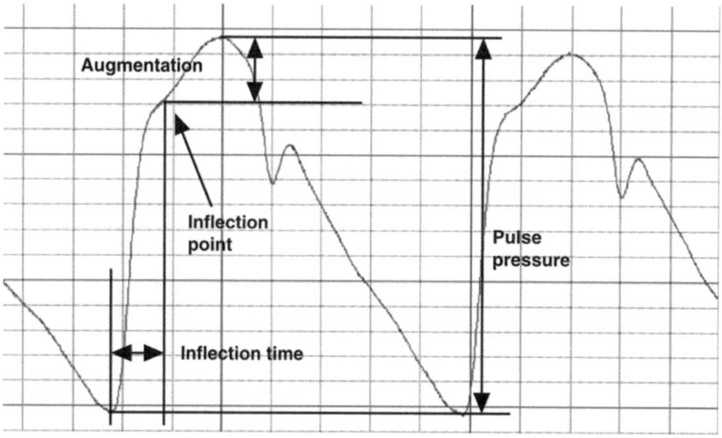

Fig. 7.5 Schematic representation of augmentation index. The augmentation index is the ratio of the augmentation pressure to the pulse pressure (Murakami et al. [5])

the aortic blood stored during systole. With aging, the PWV gradually increases. It means the early return of the reflected pressure wave (in systole) which impairs the arterial and ventricular functions. The opposite directional reflected pressure wave that returns to the heart during systole interferes with the systemic ventricular ejection and increases the workload of the systemic ventricle (Fig. 7.4a). To evaluate the degree of the pressure wave reflection, AI is calculated. The AI is defined as the ratio of the augmentation pressure to the pulse pressure (Fig. 7.5) (5). The inflection point is defined as the timing with the peak flow velocity or obtained by the fourth derivative of the original pressure waveform (Fig. 7.6) (6).

As the PWV increases with aging, the AI also rises (Fig. 7.7) (7). Moreover, it is well known that other factors could influence on the aortic pressure wave reflection. The distance from the heart to the inflection point is one of the important determinants of AI. It is reasonable that the short distance means early return of the reflected pressure wave. Practically, it is reported that the AI is high and inversely related to the body height in children (Fig. 7.8) [5], although their PWV is low (Fig. 7.2). When there is a strong inflection point nearer to the heart than the normal inflection point (aortic bifurcation), the AI could elevate. In patients after repair of aortic coarctation, the repaired site generates a new pressure wave reflection resulting in the elevation of the AI (Fig. 7.9) [8].

In adults with congenital heart disease, the history of the aortic surgery is one of the risk factors for the elevation of the AI [9]. Murakami et al. [9] proposed two possible mechanisms why aortic surgery enhances the pressure wave reflection. One is that direct aortic surgery can change the local vascular characteristics. For example, the repair of aortic coarctation makes the new plane generating the new pressure wave reflection at the anastomosis site [8]. Another mechanism is the

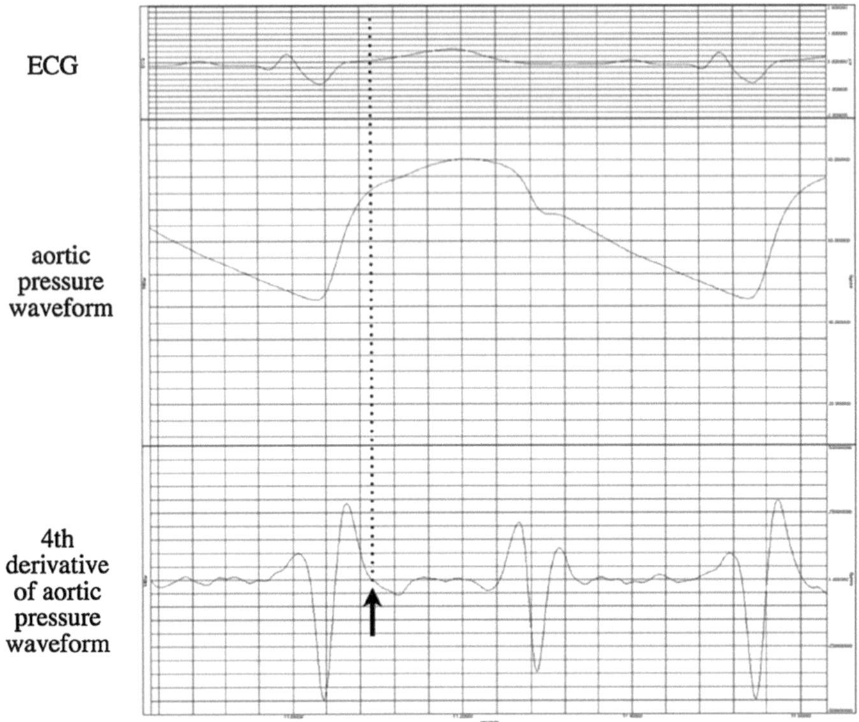

Fig. 7.6 Determination of the inflection point. The inflection point is obtained by the fourth derivatives of the original pressure waveform (Murakami et al. [6])

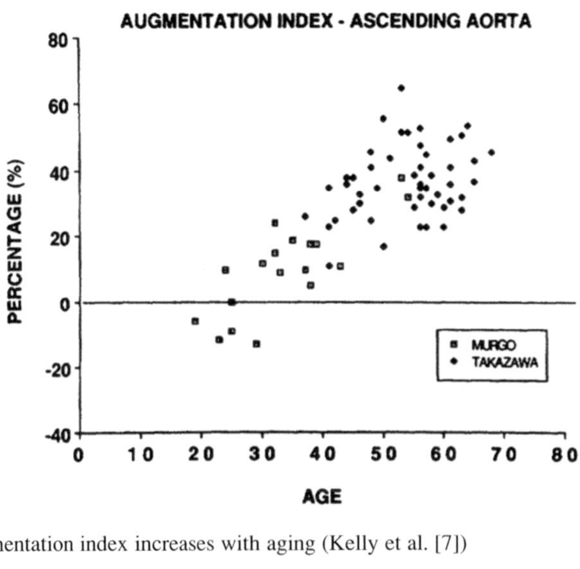

Fig. 7.7 Augmentation index increases with aging (Kelly et al. [7])

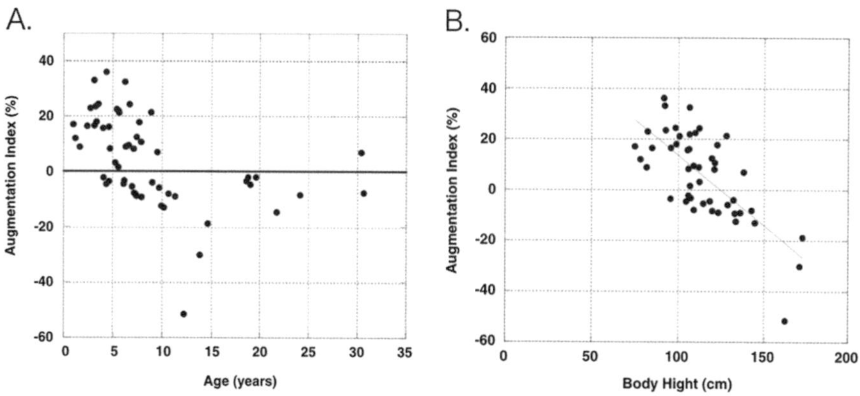

Fig. 7.8 Augmentation index in children. The augmentation index is high in youth (**a**), and it is inversely correlated to the age under 15 years old (**b**) (Murakami et al. [5])

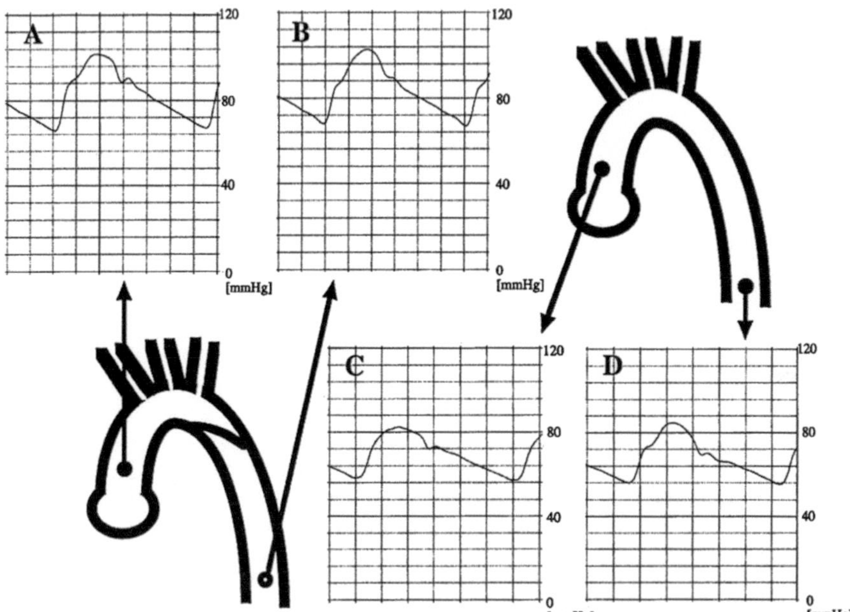

Fig. 7.9 Ascending (**a**) and descending (**b**) aortic pressure waveform in a 6-year-old patient after extended end-to-end anastomosis of the aortic arch. Ascending (**c**) and descending (**d**) aortic pressure waveform in a 6-year-old patient with normal aortic arch. The waveform **a** resembles **d** rather than **c** (Murakami and Takeda [8])

volume load of the partial aorta. For example, an aortopulmonary shunt produces volume overload of the ascending aorta. There could be the plane of the pressure wave reflection between the ascending and descending aorta. Practically, it has been reported that the aortopulmonary shunt is one of the risk factors of aortic root

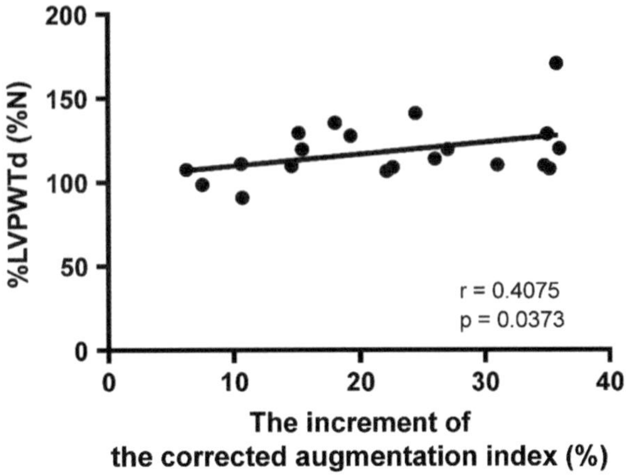

Fig. 7.10 The relationship between the increment of the corrected augmentation index and the percentage of the end-diastolic left ventricular posterior wall thickness in patients after the repair of aortic arch. The posterior wall thickness had a weak positive correlation with the increment of the corrected augmentation index. %LVPWTS, percentage of the end-diastolic left ventricular posterior wall thickness (Murakami et al. [13])

dilatation [10]. Namely, the heterogeneity or discontinuity of the aortic wall property could generate a new pressure wave reflection and elevate the AI [11, 12]. After repair or aortic coarctation, the elevation of the AI results in hypertrophy of the systemic ventricle (Fig. 7.10) [13].

References

1. Avolio AP, Chen SG, Wang RP et al (1983) Effects of aging on changing arterial compliance and left ventricular load in a northern Chinese urban community. Circulation 68:50–58
2. Saiki H, Kojima T, Seki M et al (2012) Marked disparity in mechanical wall properties between ascending and descending aorta in patients with tetralogy of Fallot. Eur J Cardio-thorac Surg 41:570–573
3. Nichols WW, O'Rourke MF, Vlachopoulos C (2011) McDonald's blood flow in arteries, 6th edn. Hodder Arnold, London
4. O'Rourke MF (1990) Arterial stiffness, systolic blood pressure, and logical treatment of arterial hypertension. Hypertension 15:339–347
5. Murakami T, Takeda A, Takei K et al (2010) Aortic pressure wave reflection in children. Hypertens Res 33:225–228
6. Murakami T, Takeda A, Takei K et al (2015) The cardiac blood supply-workload balance in children. Heart Vessel 30:626–631
7. Kelly R, Hayward C, Avolio A et al (1989) Noninvasive determination of age-related changes in the human arterial pulse. Circulation 80:1652–1659
8. Murakami T, Takeda A (2005) Enhanced aortic pressure wave reflection in patients after repair of aortic coarctation. Ann Thorac Surg 80:995–1000

9. Murakami T, Tateno S, Kawasoe Y et al (2014) Aortic surgery is one of the risk factors for enhancement of pressure wave reflection in adult patients with congenital heart disease. Int J Cardiol 175:451–454
10. Niwa K (2005) Aortic root dilatation in tetralogy of Fallot long-term after repair – histology of the aorta in tetralogy of Fallot: evidence of intrinsic aortopathy. Int J Cardiol 103:117–119
11. Murakami T, Niwa K (2015) Elastin fracture localized in ascending aorta could be one of the mechanisms of enhanced aortic pressure wave reflection in adult patients with congenital heart disease. Int J Cardiol 194:66–67
12. Murakami T, Shiina Y, Niwa K (2016) Final common pathway of aortic dilation?: heterogeneity of aortic wall property causes the aneurysmal change. J Am Coll Cardiol 67(6):735
13. Murakami T, Takeda A, Yamazawa H et al (2013) Aortic pressure wave reflection in patients after successful aortic arch repair in early infancy. Hypertens Res 36:603–607

Chapter 8
Comprehensive Assessment of Aortopathy Using Catheterization

Hirofumi Saiki and Hideaki Senzaki

Abstract Aortopathy is represented by aortic wall histological alterations, which are translated into alterations of mechanical property of the aortic wall. Because aortic pressure waveform in itself contains comprehensive information about aortic wall mechanical property, analysis of aortic pressure waveform either alone or coupled with aortic flow provides important diagnostic and therapeutic information about aortopathy. Catheter examination is the only way to precisely obtain the aortic waveform and thus plays an independent role compared to numerous noninvasive imaging modalities, such as echocardiogram, computed tomography, and magnetic resonance imaging. In this chapter, we summarize our knowledge about the aortic wall mechanical properties in several forms of aortopathy elegantly assessed by catheter examination.

Keywords Mechanical property • Pulse wave velocity • Impedance • Wave intensity • Wave reflection • Pressure–volume relationship

8.1 Introduction

Although the advancement of imaging technology has greatly contributed to the better understanding of hemodynamics in a variety of cardiac diseases, cardiovascular pressure waveform is still a fundamental factor that well characterizes cardiovascular properties. Invasive catheter insertion is the only method for obtaining actual pressure waveform in a specific location of the cardiovascular system, and the utility of alternative methods, such as applanation tonometry or MRI, has not yet been fully validated to estimate actual pressure waveform for patients with cardiovascular diseases [1, 2]. Pathology of the tunica media of the aortic wall is reportedly responsible for the onset of aortopathy in congenital or acquired cardiovascular diseases [3, 4], and hemodynamic stress as well as genetic backgrounds can induce it by activating inflammatory cascade and tissue permeability, which is

H. Saiki, M.D. • H. Senzaki, M.D. (✉)
Department of Pediatric Cardiology, Saitama Medical Center, Saitama Medical University, Room 415, Staff Office Building, 1981 Kamoda, Kawagoe, Saitama 350-8550, Japan
e-mail: hsenzaki@saitama-med.ac.jp

K. Niwa, H. Kaemmerer (eds.), *Aortopathy*, DOI 10.1007/978-4-431-56071-5_8

called mechanotransduction [5–11]. Accumulating evidence elucidated that intravascular blood pressure flow dynamics are closely related to the molecular mechanisms of the evolving aortopathy, particularly in patients with structural heart diseases [7, 10, 12, 13]. Accordingly, a precise understanding of cardiovascular mechanical properties and their interaction with aortic hemodynamics may allow us to identify optimal hemodynamic management that may ameliorate the clinical course of aortopathy, even under the significant influence of genetic factors. Thus, catheter examination has advantages over noninvasive assessments in terms of understanding the pathophysiology of aortopathy. This further understanding will contribute to the improvement of current hemodynamic management.

8.2 Aortic Hemodynamics and Pathology (Fig. 8.1, Details in Chaps. 2 and 3)

Elastic fiber disruption and fatigue of aortic tunica media are fundamental pathologies of the aortic dilatation in aortopathy. Although the elastic fibers in the aorta are considered to tolerate pulsatile stress by an intermittent ventricular ejection for more than decades [14], early disruption can be induced by inflammation or

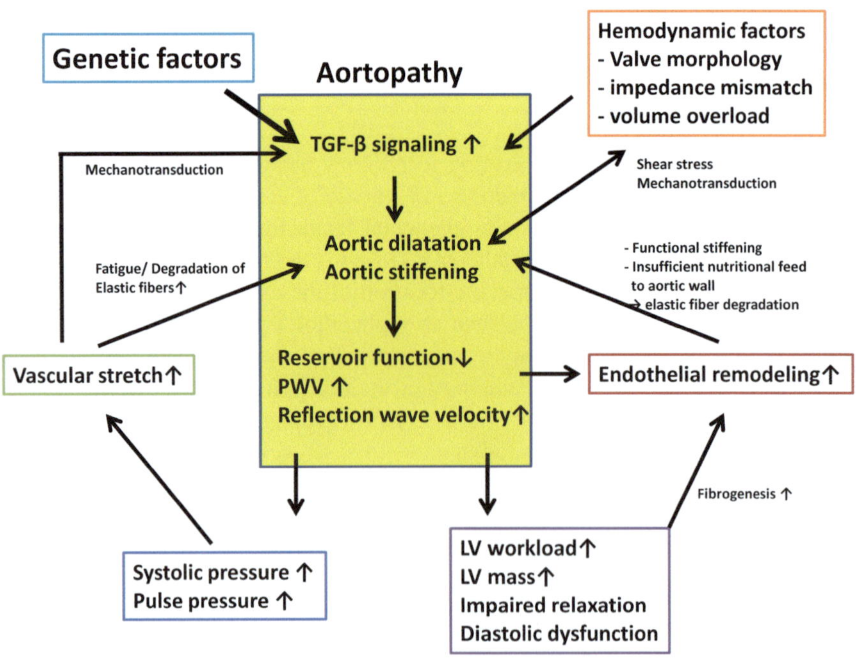

Fig. 8.1 Mechanisms for developing aortic dilatation

perturbation of the protein maintenance system, which is regulated by local gene expression [15, 16]. Although Marfan syndrome is the typical systemic disease that causes accelerated degradation of the aortic elastic fibers, mainly due to gene mutation encoding microfibril protein, fibrillin-1 [15, 17], similar pathology of the tunica media is also observed in patients with congenital heart disease, including bicuspid aortic valve, tetralogy of Fallot (TOF), and others [4]. Not limited to genetic factors or direct surgical vascular insults, characteristic hemodynamics such as excessive volume overload, augmented pressure load, or accelerated blood velocity induce vascular stress that activates inflammatory gene expression via mechanotransduction [10]. Mounting evidence has suggested a significant contribution of hemodynamics to the development of aortopathy [5, 7, 12]. Vascular mechanical stress, which can affect the aortic structure, mainly consists of normal stress and shear stress. Normal stress, which represents excessive vascular stretch, induces alteration of myosin–actin interaction and conformational changes of its linker proteins. Interaction with integrin, which connects the endothelial myosin–actin complex and extracellular matrix, ultimately stimulates TGF-β production, its release, and cellular growth [10]. When vascular endothelium senses an increase in shear stress, which is determined by both blood viscosity and blood flow velocity, relaxation of medial smooth muscle compensates to decrease it. Although shear stress regulates vascular dilatation in conductance arteries [18, 19], it also promotes endothelial permeability [20], proliferation of endothelial cells, and aortic remodeling [12]. A stiffened arterial system due to remodeling increases pulse pressure and ventricular afterload [21]. In addition, aortic remodeling decreases nutritional feed to the aortic wall from the aortic cavity, making it more dependent on the vasa vasorum, resulting in malnutrition of the tunica media. As reported by Stefanadis, the decrease of the aortic wall blood feed by removal of the vasa vasorum resulted in acute tunica media degradation and increased stiffness [22], suggesting a fundamental role of blood feeding for the maintenance of the tunica media. This is also supported by the fact that improper perfusion of the vasa vasorum relates to aortic wall stiffness [23]. Thus, degradation of the aortic tunica media is initiated by combined effects from inflammatory responses, pressure augmentation, and insufficient aortic wall blood supply; then, the aortic wall starts to dilate by a loss of elastic fibers. Eventually, the aortic wall becomes predominantly supported by the collagens, which are much stiffer than elastic fibers, and the characteristic features of aortopathy, including aortic dilatation and stiffness, are constructed. Accordingly, management of hemodynamics might be fundamentally important in preventing the development of aortopathy, because aortic mechanical stress is determined by blood pressure, velocity, and viscosity, which are factors of cardiac output, vascular resistance, and oxygen saturation.

8.3 Impedance Mismatch

Characteristic features of aortopathy, including augmented stiffness, aortic dilatation, and subsequent distal narrowing, result in heterogeneity of aortic properties, both in histological feature and aortic diameter. Although energy transmission between two locations of the vessel is maximized if the vascular property is uniform (known as impedance match), part of the blood energy can reflect at any part of the vessel and increase proximal input impedance if a vascular property difference exists [24–26]. In normal circulation, discontinuity of vascular properties in the peripheral arterial system, including relative narrowing and higher stiffness of the peripheral artery compared to that of the aorta, prevents end organs from exposure to high systolic blood energy by reflecting part of the energy. At the same time, it preserves redundant energy in the aortic wall as potential energy so that blood can be delivered to peripheral organs evenly during diastole [27]. In contrast, if central aortic stiffness becomes close to the level of that in peripheral arteries, then more pulsatile energy is delivered to the end organs and can impair their function [28, 29]. This also decreases reserved energy of the aorta, leading to decreased diastolic blood flow. Such discontinuity of vascular properties is called "impedance mismatch," and this can also accelerate the onset as well as progress of aortopathy by improper augmentation of proximal aortic waveform (Fig. 8.2). In addition to affecting the aorta and systemic circulation, an arising reflection wave in the proximal part of the aorta can be an additional ventricular afterload [21] and can impair ventricular function as well as myocardial energetic efficiency by affecting ventricular–arterial (VA) coupling [30, 31].

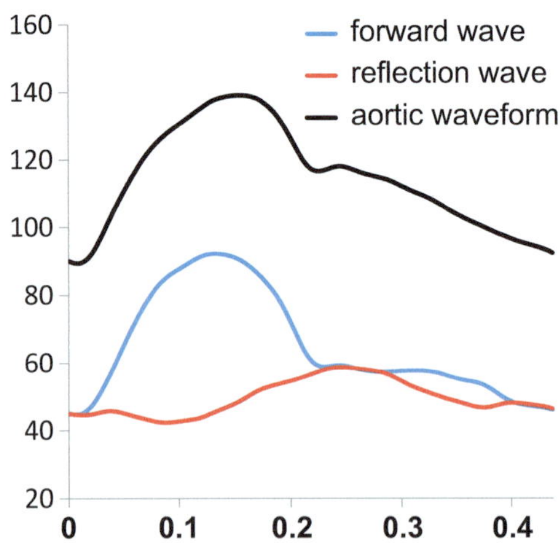

Fig. 8.2 Aortic pressure waveform consists of forward and backward pressure flows. The aortic pressure waveform can be factorized into forward-traveling flow and backward flow [44, 45]

8.4 Practical Utility of the Catheter Examination in Aortopathy

Although the shapes of the aorta are easily recognized using MRI or other imaging modalities of three-dimensional images, cardiovascular contrast imaging during catheter examination is two-dimensional and angle dependent, so its utility for morphological assessment is considerably limited in the current era. Meanwhile, having actual pressure waveform is a significant advantage in the assessment of vascular properties in catheter assessment. Catheter examination is commonly performed in patients with congenital heart diseases, so being conversant with such methods would highly support logical decision-making in the clinical setting.

8.4.1 *Pulse Wave Velocity*

One simple but reliable index for arterial stiffness assessed by catheter examination is pulse wave velocity (PWV). The American Heart Association identified PWV as a noninvasive and reliable marker of aortic stiffness [32]. Although noninvasive PWV is widely used in the clinical setting, PWV is also available during cardiac catheterization. During catheter drawback in the aorta, wave traveling distance is easily obtained by measuring the catheter extraction distance. The time gaps from the ECG R wave to the upstroke of aortic pressure at the starting point and at the end point of extraction represent wave traveling time. Thus, PWV can be calculated as extraction distance divided by wave traveling time [33]. As represented by the Moens–Korteweg equation (Eq. 8.1), PWV increases with the stiffening of the vascular wall, assuming that both vascular wall thickness and vessel area are almost the same.

$$\mathrm{PWV} = \left(\surd E^{*}\surd h\right)/\left(\surd \rho^{*}\surd D\right) \tag{8.1}$$

where E is Young's modules, h is vascular wall thickness, ρ is blood density, and D is vessel radius diameter. PWV is a predictor of cardiovascular events in heart failure or ischemic heart disease [34, 35]. Higher PWV is reported in patients with Marfan syndrome regardless of aortic dilatation [36], suggesting a possible relationship between PWV and histological change of the tunica media, as well as the predictive value for future aortopathy [37]. As represented in Eq. 8.1, PWV should theoretically decrease with the increase of aortic diameter. Accordingly, the increase of PWV in the dilated aorta further highlights significant stiffening of the aorta. In sharp contrast, PWV in bicuspid aortic valve patients without aortic dilatation was similar to that in tricuspid valve patients [38]. Even though PWV and arterial elastance were similar, aortic wall shear rate was significantly higher in bicuspid aortic valve patients than in tricuspid valve patients [38]. Although prospective observation is required, this result implies a significant contribution of hemodynamics.

We also reported increased aortic stiffness using catheter-based PWV in tetralogy of Fallot (TOF) both before and after anatomical repair compared to control patients [5, 39]. This trend was rather similar to that of Marfan syndrome, and it also implies the possible contribution of genetic factors for the development of aortopathy in TOF. Increased aortic stiffness was also observed in patients with a single ventricular heart, with close correlation with diameter of the ascending aorta [40]. Together, PWV can be a potential predictor for aortopathy, and it may also relate to aortic medial histology. Although those analyses might have been performed even with noninvasive methods [41, 42], catheter assessment allows the consideration of vascular morphological variety, which cannot be assessed with noninvasive methods. More importantly, aortic stiffness in a specific segment is also available if catheter-based PWV is utilized. In TOF patients, ascending aortic stiffness was significantly heightened, whereas that of descending aortic stiffness was not augmented, consistent with the reported distribution of tunica media degradation in similar patient cohorts [3, 43]. Because this method allows us to use PWV of the descending aorta as the internal control, catheter-based PWV is anticipated to be applied to a wide range of cardiovascular conditions.

8.4.2 Assessment of Blood Pressure Waveforms

The other advantage of invasive catheter examination is the availability of a blood pressure waveform at any site of the vessel. Pressure waveform consists of the sum of a forward-traveling pressure wave and a reflected wave (Fig. 8.2) [44, 45]. PWV increases with aortic stiffening, thus allowing the reflection wave to overlap earlier on the subsequent forward pressure wave in the proximal aorta. Because the local blood pressure waveform can be affected by any vascular property change (impedance mismatch) from the distal part of vessel, its morphology identifies how caliber change or stiffness change alters the actual blood pressure waveform. The augmentation index (AI), which is calculated as the augmentation pressure divided by pulse pressure, is the index of the vascular property found by observing the arrival of the wave reflex at a specific site (Fig. 8.3) [46]. Although AI can be affected by the length of the aorta (i.e., patient's height), heart rate, or cardiac output due to its innate nature, patients with a bicuspid aortic valve were reported to have increased aortic stiffness and high AI, both of which were correlated with aortic dilatation [8], suggesting aortopathy as the source of pressure augmentation. Lee et al. investigated AI using applanation tonometry in bicuspid aortic valve patients and revealed close correlation with E/e′ [47]. Because increased afterload can be a predisposing factor for ventricular stiffening [31], its finding endorses the impact of aortopathy to exert afterload that relates to the reflection wave. Together, the aortic pressure waveform might be a feasible index to determine VA interaction for patients with aortopathy.

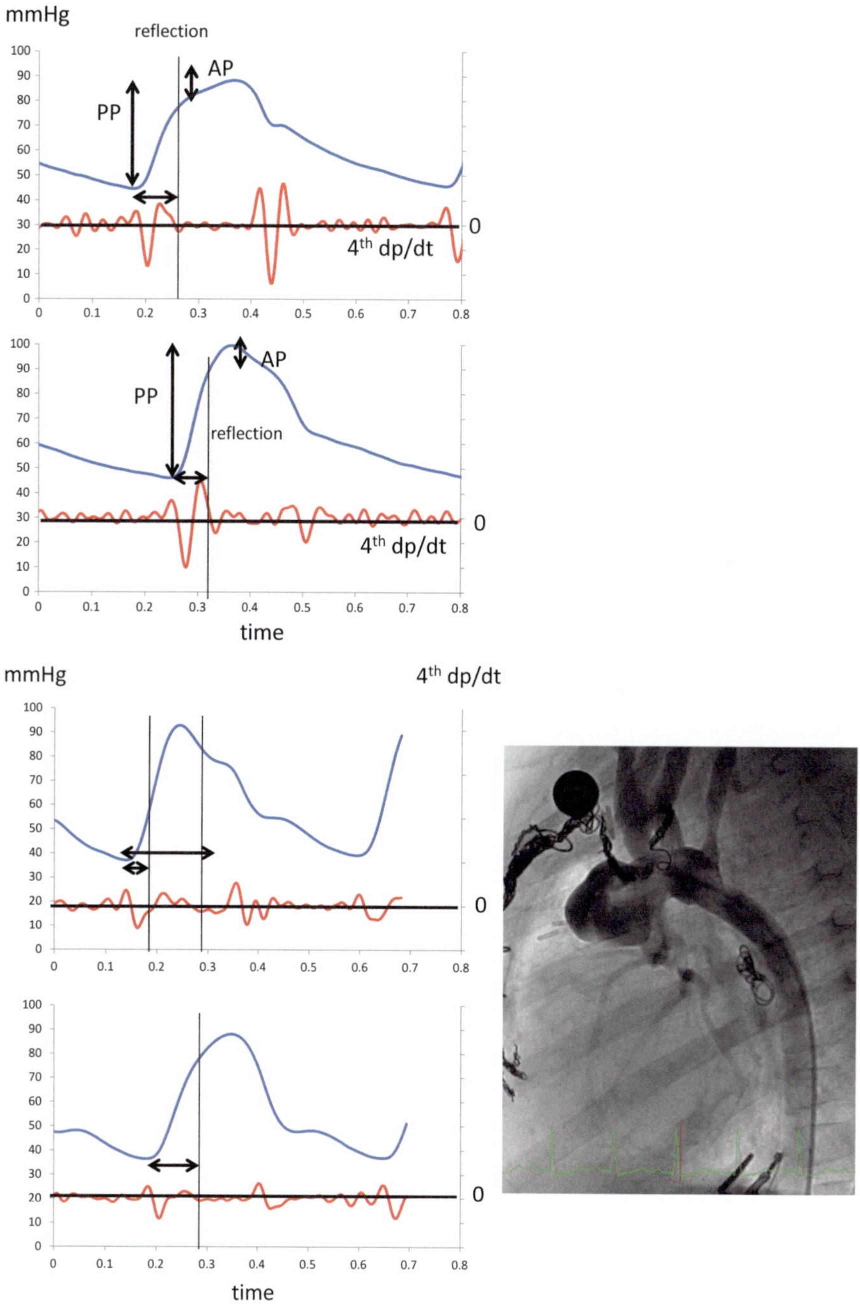

Fig. 8.3 Identification of pressure augmentation. *AP* augmentation pressure, *PP* pulse pressure. The onset of pressure augmentation by reflection (Ri) was identified by the fourth differentiate of the pressure waveform (Kelly et al.) [73]. (**a**) *Upper panel*: Ascending aortic pressure waveform in a patient with a normal aortic arch. The time interval between upstroke of pressure and Ri in the ascending aorta is relatively long, and peak aortic pressure is close to the time of dicrotic notch, allowing higher diastolic pressure. This is suitable for maximizing coronary driving pressure.

Pressure assessment using invasive catheterization is increasing its utility in the assessment of aortopathy. The case report published by Murakami et al. suggested aortopathy as a possible source of supra vena cava (SVC) stenosis [48]. Because SVC is a compliant vein and is considered to be durable against compression in general, we need to carefully interpret this case regarding whether surgical scars and postoperative adhesions associated with SVC/aortic cannulation contributed to functional stenosis of SVC pressure. Even with such limitations, catheter insertion is helpful for understanding whether morphological stenosis is hemodynamically problematic, particularly in a lesion where echocardiogram assessment can be inaccurate. Because SVC pressure can affect cerebral circulation [42, 49], assessment of SVC compression and its hemodynamic impact might be of further importance in preventing neurodevelopment or onset of dementia in patients with aortopathy.

8.4.3 Subendocardial Viability Ratio

Due to surgical scars or aortic caliber changes originating from specific operations (i.e., Norwood procedure or Damus–Kaye–Stansel procedure), aortic stiffness or aortic input impedance can be diverse in congenital heart diseases. A similar caliber change is observed in patients with aortopathy even without operation, and the bicuspid aortic valve is often complicated with complex heart diseases. Increased aortic stiffness is a burden for heart failure due to augmented afterload [50], and it also impairs coronary blood flow [51]. This is due to increased ventricular oxygen demand and decreased coronary arterial blood supply, as represented by augmented tension time index (TTI) and decreased diastolic time index (DTI), respectively [52]. Although the subendocardial viability ratio (SEVR) [53] is the simple result of the blood pressure waveform of the ascending aorta, its utility in clinical decision-making is sufficiently validated [52, 54, 55]. The SEVR is not limited to hearts with normal structures. We investigated SEVR in patients after the Norwood procedure, which reconstructs the ascending aorta using the pulmonary trunk and native aorta [54]. In our cohort without aortopulmonary shunts, SEVR was markedly lower than

---

Fig. 8.3 (continued) Lower panel: Descending aortic pressure waveform in a patient with a normal aortic arch. The interval between upstroke and Ri in the descending aorta is shorter than that of the ascending aorta, with systolic pressure higher than that of the ascending aorta. High pressure is suitable for preserving potential energy in the aortic elastic fiber to effectively deliver blood to the peripheral organ. (**b**) *Upper panel*: Ascending aortic pressure waveform in a patient who underwent the Norwood procedure. There were two possible inflection points. The first inflection represented the reflection from proximal impedance mismatch, which heightened early systolic pressure. The second reflection wave appeared to be derived from the distal part of the aorta. Lower panel: Descending aortic pressure waveform in a patient who underwent a Norwood procedure. In contrast to Fig. 8.3a, peak aortic pressure was biased to the late systolic phase, which resulted in less systolic pressure. This means impaired preservation of potential energy in the aorta that of control patients with neither significant heart disease nor aortopulmonary shunt in whom all pulmonary blood flow was supplied from the aorta (Fig. 8.4). Accordingly, we concluded that post-Norwood aortas predisposed patients to being more susceptible to coronary ischemia, even without significant coronary stenosis. In this study, aortic impedance mismatch, as was represented by descending aortic relative narrowing compared to that in the ascending aorta, was a significant determinant of SEVR. Furthermore, SEVR was negatively correlated with the renin–angiotensin–aldosterone system and natriuretic peptides (atrial natriuretic peptide [ANP] and brain natriuretic peptide [BNP]), suggesting a promising marker for fibrosis or heart failure. This was further supported by the fact that patient outcome was also associated with SEVR. Our novel finding regarding the role of SEVR emphasizes the importance of guiding proper aortic reconstruction in hypoplastic left heart syndrome, and this might be extrapolated to other congenital heart diseases. The aortic reservoir function in the TOF with aortopathy is expected to be decreased. Although impaired coronary perfusion reserve in patients with decreased aortic distensibility was identified using simultaneous measures of aortic and coronary pressure/flow [56], the possibility that SEVR might also detect similar myocardial blood flow demand–supply imbalances as well as late complications, such as arrhythmias, will be further investigated.

8.4.4 Estimation of Aortic Volume Flow

As mentioned, aortic blood flow velocity is closely related to shear stress. Guzzardi et al. investigated aortopathy patients using MR flow mapping and actual aortic

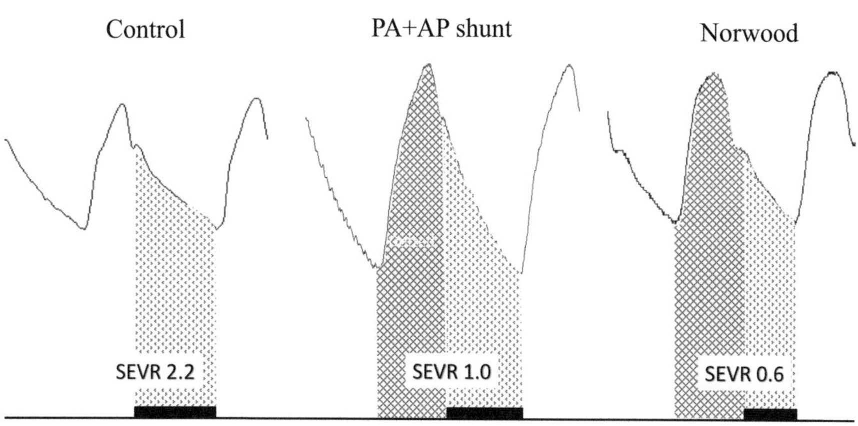

Fig. 8.4 Anatomical features of the subendocardial viability ratio. Mesh area, tension time index (TTI); dotted area, diastolic time index (DTI); filled area, pressure time integral of systemic ventricle. The ratio of DTI to TTI denotes the subendocardial viability ratio (SEVR). SEVR in a patient who underwent the Norwood procedure (RV-PA conduit) was significantly lower than that of controls and even lower than that of patients with pulmonary atresia plus aortopulmonary shunt

wall tissue sampled during surgery, and they elucidated that TGF-β1 and its downstream matrix metalloproteinases are upregulated in the aortic wall exposed to high shear stress but less so in the aortic wall, where less shear stress was observed [12]. Despite the advantages of MRI, which accurately assesses blood flow velocity at a specific location, heart rate variability due to room temperature, the small number of available beats for assessments, and existence of turbulence flow (i.e., pressure recovery in aortic stenosis) are limiting factors for obtaining clinically relevant aortic volume flow. Using cardiac catheterization, the Fick formula also allows us to estimate net aortic blood flow regardless of hemodynamic characteristics or existence of arrhythmias. Although available aortic flow, flow velocity, and shear stress itself cannot be directly estimated using the Fick method, they represent averaged volume loading to the aorta. Our previous data and those of others suggest the significant impact of aortic volume loading on the development of aortic dilatation [5, 6, 13].

The use of simultaneous Doppler flow and pressure wire further allow us to obtain actual blood flow velocity in a beat-by-beat manner with simultaneous measurements of the pressure waveform. Having both the pressure and flow waveforms allows us to factorize pressure/flow waveforms into forward (cardiac contribution) and backward (reflection) flow [44, 57]. The existence of backward flow that overlaps the systolic pressure is attributable to augmented ventricular pulsatile afterload. Accordingly, identifying backward flow and avoiding overlap of the upslope of forward pressure flow by pharmacological intervention will contribute to better management of aortopathy. Westerhof et al. reported the possibility of factorizing the pressure waveform into forward and backward pressure without measuring the flow waveform, but further validation is needed [45].

8.4.5 Cardiac Property

Progression of aortopathy implies afterload increase as well as coronary circulatory insufficiency [9, 21, 51]. Because both affect cardiac performance and geometry [9, 47], assessments of cardiac properties and ventricular–arterial coupling should be considered fundamental constituents of physiology in aortopathy. Venous congestion, which is often accompanied by heart failure, is known to predispose to fibrogenesis and inflammation [58]; therefore, coexistence of cardiac malfunction may accelerate aortic degradation. Using ventricular pressure and simultaneous ventricular volume measurements, the ventricular pressure–volume loop can be constructed either in structurally normal hearts or in those with congenital heart diseases (Fig. 8.5) [59–61]. Load-independent measurements for cardiac contractility (end-systolic pressure–volume relationship [ESPVR]) and diastolic passive stiffness (end-diastolic pressure–volume relationship [EDPVR]) can be determined, and those data allow us to determine therapeutic targets of hemodynamics to improve cardiac function or metabolism [62]. The ratio of end-systolic elastance (Ees) to arterial elastance (Ea) provides VA coupling (Ees/Ea), which is the

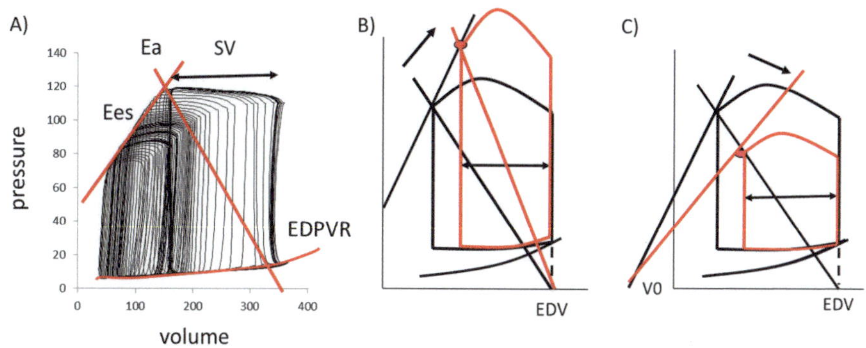

Fig. 8.5 Pressure–volume relationship of the ventricle. *Ea* effective arterial elastance, *Ees* end-systolic elastance, *EDPVR* end-diastolic pressure–volume relationship, *EDV* end-diastolic volume, *SV* stroke volume. (**a**) Pressure–volume relationship. Each loop represents the ventricular pressure–volume relationship during volume reduction (IVC occlusion), and the width of each loop represents stroke volume (SV). Ventricular pressure and volume at end systole construct a straight slope, and the end-systolic pressure–volume relationship (ESPVR) and its slope are called the end-systolic elastance (Ees), a load-independent measurement of ventricular contractility. Effective arterial elastance (Ea), a measurement of ventricular afterload, is calculated as the end-systolic pressure divided by the SV. The ventricular diastolic property is characterized by the slope of the pressure–volume relationship of the end diastole (end-diastolic pressure–volume relationship [EDPVR]). (**b**) Increase of afterload. Aortic stiffening augments the ventricular pulsatile load. Stroke volume declines with the increase of afterload (Red). Even without suppression of Ees, the increase of Ea reduces the Ees/Ea ratio; therefore, ventricular efficiency declines and cardiac energetic consumption increases (pressure–volume area↑). (**c**) Impaired cardiac contractility. Due to aortopathy and aortic stiffness, coronary perfusion can be suppressed; therefore, the decline of contractility (Ees↓) and the decline of SV can occur

measure of cardiac performance in relation to afterload [63]. Both ESPVR and coupling ratio (Ees/Ea) are associated with ventricular oxygen consumption in an experimental model [30]. As discussed in the previous section, myocardial circulation in the aortopathy might be impaired, so an energy-preserving strategy might be needed in cases in which unfavorable ventricular energetics is identified. Although aortopathy and ventricular stiffening appear to relate to ventricular diastolic properties, as was suggested by the close relationship between E/e′ and AI in the work by Lee et al. [47], they could not verify how relaxation or passive stiffness relates to arterial property. In addition, the utility of E/e′ was not fully validated in congenital heart diseases [64]; accordingly, more accurate and validated assessments of ventricular diastolic function further support the use of catheter assessment. Accumulating evidence suggests that the coronary microvasculature might be responsible for ventricular diastolic stiffness [65, 66]. In addition to innate cardiac function, external force derived from the pericardium or right ventricle can affect left ventricular preload and stroke volume, which can also be identified by the pressure–volume relationship during right ventricular unloading [67]. While high ventricular diastolic pressure derived from right ventricular dilatation or ventricular stiffening can hinder coronary circulation by decreasing the aorto-ventricular pressure gradient in the diastole, an increase of the RV load demands more coronary flow [68], causing a coronary supply–demand imbalance. Together, PV loops allow us to identify the issues predisposing to cardiac dysfunction coupled with aortopathy. Ventricular mechanics in patients with aortopathy is not well recognized, particularly when there is additional ventricular load. Further investigation is warranted in this field.

8.4.6 Possible Role of Impedance Analysis

Although PWV and aortic waveforms (AI) are simple but reliable indexes of aortic properties and impedance mismatch, they are relatively sensitive to blood pressure, aortic caliber change, and heart rate. Plenty of evidence that relates aortopathy to its fundamental constituents of focal aortic stiffening is available using PWV or AI; therefore, the additive role of relatively load-independent measurements of vascular properties, such as input impedance, may not be particularly needed in clinical practice. However, advances in noninvasive technology for measuring pressure and flow waveforms in the ascending aorta may expand the utility of input impedance for the management or better understanding of aortopathy.

Impedance denotes the sum of all types of opposition, which is confined to oscillatory motion (alternating current) to blood flow distal to the measurement site in the cardiovascular circuit. Whereas a few types of impedance (longitudinal impedance, input impedance, characteristic impedance, terminal impedance) are defined in the arterial system, input impedance, which defines the relationship between pulsatile flow and pulsatile pressure provided to the particular vascular system, is commonly used in cardiovascular research. Similar to the electrical circuit, it denotes the transfer function between blood flow and pressure waveforms. Impedance can be calculated using simultaneous measurements of blood flow and pressure waveforms at any site of the vessel. Advantages of having input impedance are the feature of comprehensive assessment in the entire vascular system distal to the measurement site (thus, resistance, characteristic impedance, and reflection coefficient can be evaluated at the same time) [27, 33] and relative independence of the caliber change or vascular wall thickness (includes segmental change of vascular property). Input impedance can be factorized into each harmonic property, where each harmonic represents a relatively specific vascular property, including proximal, distal, or pulsatile load. Taking advantage of this feature, the impedance of aortopathy can be evaluated regardless of stenosis or dilatation. In previous publications, aortic impedance in patients with Marfan syndrome was investigated in relation to aortic dilatation. Interestingly, most of the study concluded that the aortic characteristic impedance and reflection coefficient of Marfan syndrome were normal, even though aortic dilatation was significant [69, 70]. Assuming aortic dilatation is the result of compensation to maintain aortic impedance within a normal range under the condition of augmented aortic stiffness [10], analyses in these studies were cross-sectional; therefore, impedance analysis may still provide a predictive value for future development of aortopathy in Marfan syndrome and possibly other diseases susceptible to aortopathy. We evaluated pulmonary arterial properties in TOF patients utilizing input impedance and revealed that impedance at a fundamental frequency and pulmonary arterial compliance were significantly correlated with right ventricular eccentric hypertrophy [71]. We also found increased aortic input impedance in postoperative TOF patients. Increased impedance was associated with increased aortic diameter and reduced left ventricular ejection [72].

8.5 Conclusions

As reviewed in this chapter, catheter examination provides indispensable information regarding vascular properties of aortopathy even more so than advanced imaging modalities. Although the indication for catheter insertion in patients with a fragile aortic wall needs to be considered carefully, the assessments we introduced here are recommended for patients with congenital heart diseases who are at risk for aortopathy. Those patients require catheter examinations often for perioperative assessment and/or catheter interventions, so they have more opportunities for the insertion of catheters. In addition, hemodynamic assessments performed using catheters are the gold standard that is necessary to verify the appropriateness of noninvasive images, including echocardiograms or MRI scans. Extensive knowledge regarding hemodynamics is required for maximizing catheter examinations as the standard for hemodynamic assessments that contribute robust evidence regarding aortopathy. The goal of this chapter is to help others understand hemodynamics in aortopathy.

References

1. Cheng HM, Lang D, Tufanaru C, Pearson A (2013) Measurement accuracy of non-invasively obtained central blood pressure by applanation tonometry: a systematic review and meta-analysis. Int J Cardiol 167:1867–1876
2. Delles M, Rengier F, Jeong YJ, von Tengg-Kobligk H, Ley S, Kauczor HU, Dillmann R, Unterhinninghofen R (2013) Estimation of aortic pressure waveforms from 4d phase-contrast mri. Conf Proc IEEE Eng Med Biol Soc 2013:731–734
3. Tan JL, Davlouros PA, McCarthy KP, Gatzoulis MA, Ho SY (2005) Intrinsic histological abnormalities of aortic root and ascending aorta in tetralogy of fallot: evidence of causative mechanism for aortic dilatation and aortopathy. Circulation 112:961–968
4. Niwa K, Perloff JK, Bhuta SM, Laks H, Drinkwater DC, Child JS, Miner PD (2001) Structural abnormalities of great arterial walls in congenital heart disease: light and electron microscopic analyses. Circulation 103:393–400
5. Seki M, Kurishima C, Kawasaki H, Masutani S, Senzaki H (2012) Aortic stiffness and aortic dilation in infants and children with tetralogy of fallot before corrective surgery: evidence for intrinsically abnormal aortic mechanical property. Eur J cardiothorac Surg 41:277–282

6. de Simone G, Roman MJ, De Marco M, Bella JN, Izzo R, Lee ET, Devereux RB (2015) Hemodynamic correlates of abnormal aortic root dimension in an adult population: the strong heart study. J Am Heart Assoc 4
7. Girdauskas E, Borger MA, Secknus MA, Girdauskas G, Kuntze T (2011) Is aortopathy in bicuspid aortic valve disease a congenital defect or a result of abnormal hemodynamics? A critical reappraisal of a one-sided argument. Eur J cardiothorac Surg 39:809–814
8. Shim CY, Cho IJ, Yang WI, Kang MK, Park S, Ha JW, Jang Y, Chung N (2011) Central aortic stiffness and its association with ascending aorta dilation in subjects with a bicuspid aortic valve. J Am Soc Echocardiogr 24:847–852
9. Grotenhuis HB, Ottenkamp J, Westenberg JJ, Bax JJ, Kroft LJ, de Roos A (2007) Reduced aortic elasticity and dilatation are associated with aortic regurgitation and left ventricular hypertrophy in nonstenotic bicuspid aortic valve patients. J Am Coll Cardiol 49:1660–1665
10. Jeremy RW, Robertson E, Lu Y, Hambly BD (2013) Perturbations of mechanotransduction and aneurysm formation in heritable aortopathies. Int J Cardiol 169:7–16
11. Kim YG, Sun BJ, Park GM, Han S, Kim DH, Song JM, Kang DH, Song JK (2012) Aortopathy and bicuspid aortic valve: haemodynamic burden is main contributor to aortic dilatation. Heart 98:1822–1827
12. Guzzardi DG, Barker AJ, van Ooij P, Malaisrie SC, Puthumana JJ, Belke DD, Mewhort HE, Svystonyuk DA, Kang S, Verma S, Collins J, Carr J, Bonow RO, Markl M, Thomas JD, McCarthy PM, Fedak PW (2015) Valve-related hemodynamics mediate human bicuspid aortopathy: insights from wall shear stress mapping. J Am Coll Cardiol 66:892–900
13. Altit G, Sarquella-Brugada G, Dahdah N, Dallaire F, Carceller AM, Abadir S, Fournier A (2014) Effect of dual-chamber pacemaker implantation on aortic dilatation in patients with congenital heart block. Am J Cardiol 114:1573–1577
14. Sherratt MJ (2009) Tissue elasticity and the ageing elastic fibre. Age (Dordr) 31:305–325
15. Segura AM, Luna RE, Horiba K, Stetler-Stevenson WG, McAllister HA Jr, Willerson JT, Ferrans VJ (1998) Immunohistochemistry of matrix metalloproteinases and their inhibitors in thoracic aortic aneurysms and aortic valves of patients with marfan's syndrome. Circulation 98:II331–II337 discussion II337–338
16. Grewal N, Gittenberger-de Groot AC, DeRuiter MC, Klautz RJ, Poelmann RE, Duim S, Lindeman JH, Koenraadt WM, Jongbloed MR, Mohamed SA, Sievers HH, Bogers AJ, Goumans MJ (2014) Bicuspid aortic valve: phosphorylation of c-kit and downstream targets are prognostic for future aortopathy. Eur J cardiothorac Surg 46:831–839
17. Dietz HC, Pyeritz RE, (1995) Mutations in the human gene for fibrillin-1 (fbn 1) in the marfan syndrome and related disorders. Hum Mol Genet 4 Spec No: 1799–1809
18. Snow HM, Markos F, O'Regan D, Pollock K (2001) Characteristics of arterial wall shear stress which cause endothelium-dependent vasodilatation in the anaesthetized dog. J Physiol 531:843–848
19. Drexler H, Zeiher AM, Wollschlager H, Meinertz T, Just H, Bonzel T (1989) Flow-dependent coronary artery dilatation in humans. Circulation 80:466–474
20. Kang H, Cancel LM, Tarbell JM (2014) Effect of shear stress on water and ldl transport through cultured endothelial cell monolayers. Atherosclerosis 233:682–690
21. Senzaki H, Iwamoto Y, Ishido H, Matsunaga T, Taketazu M, Kobayashi T, Asano H, Katogi T, Kyo S (2008) Arterial haemodynamics in patients after repair of tetralogy of fallot: influence on left ventricular after load and aortic dilatation. Heart 94:70–74
22. Stefanadis C, Vlachopoulos C, Karayannacos P, Boudoulas H, Stratos C, Filippides T, Agapitos M, Toutouzas P (1995) Effect of vasa vasorum flow on structure and function of the aorta in experimental animals. Circulation 91:2669–2678
23. Angouras D, Sokolis DP, Dosios T, Kostomitsopoulos N, Boudoulas H, Skalkeas G, Karayannacos PE (2000) Effect of impaired vasa vasorum flow on the structure and mechanics of the thoracic aorta: implications for the pathogenesis of aortic dissection. Eur J cardiothorac Surg 17:468–473

24. Khono K, Tamai A, Kobayashi T, Senzaki H (2011) Effects of stent implantation for peripheral pulmonary artery stenosis on pulmonary vascular hemodynamics and right ventricular function in a patient with repaired tetralogy of fallot. Heart Vessel 26:672–676
25. Dobson G, Flewitt J, Tyberg JV, Moore R, Karamanoglu M (2006) Endografting of the descending thoracic aorta increases ascending aortic input impedance and attenuates pressure transmission in dogs. Eur J cardiothorac Surg 32:129–135
26. Senzaki H, Masutani S, Kobayashi J, Kobayashi T, Sasaki N, Asano H, Kyo S, Yokote Y, Ishizawa A (2002) Ventricular afterload and ventricular work in fontan circulation: comparison with normal two-ventricle circulation and single-ventricle circulation with blalock-taussig shunts. Circulation 105:2885–2892
27. Senzaki H, Chen CH, Ishido H, Masutani S, Matsunaga T, Taketazu M, Kobayashi T, Sasaki N, Kyo S, Yokote Y (2005) Arterial hemodynamics in patients after kawasaki disease. Circulation 111:2119–2125
28. Sedaghat S, Mattace-Raso FU, Hoorn EJ, Uitterlinden AG, Hofman A, Ikram MA, Franco OH, Dehghan A (2015) Arterial stiffness and decline in kidney function. Clin J Am Soc Nephrol 10 (12):2190–2197
29. Cooper LL, Woodard T, Sigurdsson S, van Buchem MA, Torjesen AA, Inker LA, Aspelund T, Eiriksdottir G, Harris TB, Gudnason V, Launer LJ, Mitchell GF (2015) Cerebrovascular damage mediates relations between aortic stiffness and memory. Hypertension 67(1):176–182
30. Burkhoff D, Sagawa K (1986) Ventricular efficiency predicted by an analytical model. Am J Phys 250:R1021–R1027
31. Senzaki H, Iwamoto Y, Ishido H, Masutani S, Taketazu M, Kobayashi T, Katogi T, Kyo S (2008) Ventricular-vascular stiffening in patients with repaired coarctation of aorta: integrated pathophysiology of hypertension. Circulation 118:S191–S198
32. Townsend RR, Wilkinson IB, Schiffrin EL, Avolio AP, Chirinos JA, Cockcroft JR, Heffernan KS, Lakatta EG, McEniery CM, Mitchell GF, Najjar SS, Nichols WW, Urbina EM, Weber T (2015) Recommendations for improving and standardizing vascular research on arterial stiffness: a scientific statement from the american heart association. Hypertension 66:698–722
33. Saiki H, Senzaki H (2015) Congenital heart disease: morphological and functional assessment chapter 6. Springer, Heidelberg
34. Kim J, Song TJ, Song D, Lee KJ, Kim EH, Lee HS, Nam CM, Nam HS, Kim YD, Heo JH (2014) Brachial-ankle pulse wave velocity is a strong predictor for mortality in patients with acute stroke. Hypertension 64:240–246
35. Regnault V, Lagrange J, Pizard A, Safar ME, Fay R, Pitt B, Challande P, Rossignol P, Zannad F, Lacolley P (2014) Opposite predictive value of pulse pressure and aortic pulse wave velocity on heart failure with reduced left ventricular ejection fraction: Insights from an eplerenone post-acute myocardial infarction heart failure efficacy and survival study (ephesus) substudy. Hypertension 63:105–111
36. Reed CM, Fox ME, Alpert BS (1993) Aortic biomechanical properties in pediatric patients with the marfan syndrome, and the effects of atenolol. Am J Cardiol 71:606–608
37. Nollen GJ, Groenink M, Tijssen JG, Van Der Wall EE, Mulder BJ (2004) Aortic stiffness and diameter predict progressive aortic dilatation in patients with marfan syndrome. Eur Heart J 25:1146–1152
38. Warner PJ, Al-Quthami A, Brooks EL, Kelley-Hedgepeth A, Patvardhan E, Kuvin JT, Heffernan KS, Huggins GS (2013) Augmentation index and aortic stiffness in bicuspid aortic valve patients with non-dilated proximal aortas. BMC Cardiovasc Disord 13:19
39. Seki M, Kurishima C, Saiki H, Masutani S, Arakawa H, Tamura M, Senzaki H (2014) Progressive aortic dilation and aortic stiffness in children with repaired tetralogy of fallot. Heart Vessel 29:83–87
40. Kojima T, Kuwata S, Kurishima C, Iwamoto Y, Saiki H, Ishido H, Masutani S, Senzaki H (2014) Aortic root dilatation and aortic stiffness in patients with single ventricular circulation. Circ J 78:2507–2511

41. Nakagawa R, Kuwata S, Kurishima C, Saiki H, Iwamoto Y, Sugimoto M, Ishido H, Masutani S, Senzaki H (2015) Arterial stiffness in patients after kawasaki disease without coronary artery involvement: Assessment by performing brachial ankle pulse wave velocity and cardio-ankle vascular index. J Cardiol 66:130–134
42. Saiki H, Kurishima C, Masutani S, Senzaki H (2014) Cerebral circulation in patients with fontan circulation: assessment by carotid arterial wave intensity and stiffness. Ann Thorac Surg 97:1394–1399
43. Saiki H, Kojima T, Seki M, Masutani S, Senzaki H (2012) Marked disparity in mechanical wall properties between ascending and descending aorta in patients with tetralogy of fallot. Eur J cardiothorac Surg 41:570–573
44. Westerhof N, Sipkema P, van den Bos GC, Elzinga G (1972) Forward and backward waves in the arterial system. Cardiovasc Res 6:648–656
45. Westerhof BE, Guelen I, Westerhof N, Karemaker JM, Avolio A (2006) Quantification of wave reflection in the human aorta from pressure alone: a proof of principle. Hypertension 48:595–601
46. Sakurai M, Yamakado T, Kurachi H, Kato T, Kuroda K, Ishisu R, Okamoto S, Isaka N, Nakano T, Ito M (2007) The relationship between aortic augmentation index and pulse wave velocity: an invasive study. J Hypertens 25:391–397
47. Lee SY, Shim CY, Hong GR, Seo J, Cho I, Cho IJ, Chang HJ, Ha JW, Chung N (2015) Association of aortic phenotypes and mechanical function with left ventricular diastolic function in subjects with normally functioning bicuspid aortic valves and comparison to subjects with tricuspid aortic valves. Am J Cardiol 116:1547–1554
48. Murakami T, Shirai T, Shiina Y, Niwa K (2015) Compression of superior caval vein - new clinical problem of aortopathy. Int J Cardiol 191:235–236
49. Saiki H, Sugimoto M, Kuwata S, Kurishima C, Iwamoto Y, Ishido H, Masutani S, Senzaki H (2015) Novel mechanisms for cerebral blood flow regulation in patients with congenital heart disease. Am Heart J 172:152–159
50. Tsao CW, Lyass A, Larson MG, Levy D, Hamburg NM, Vita JA, Benjamin EJ, Mitchell GF, Vasan RS (2015) Relation of central arterial stiffness to incident heart failure in the community. J Am Heart Assoc 4(11):e002189
51. Nobari S, Mongrain R, Gaillard E, Leask R, Cartier R (2012) Therapeutic vascular compliance change may cause significant variation in coronary perfusion: a numerical study. Comput Math Methods Med 2012:791686
52. Brazier J, Cooper N, Buckberg G (1974) The adequacy of subendocardial oxygen delivery: the interaction of determinants of flow, arterial oxygen content and myocardial oxygen need. Circulation 49:968–977
53. Buckberg GD, Fixler DE, Archie JP, Hoffman JI (1972) Experimental subendocardial ischemia in dogs with normal coronary arteries. Circ Res 30:67–81
54. Saiki H, Kuwata S, Kurishima C, Masutani S, Senzaki H (2016) Vulnerability of coronary circulation after norwood operation. Ann Thorac Surg 101(4):1544–1551
55. Tsiachris D, Tsioufis C, Syrseloudis D, Roussos D, Tatsis I, Dimitriadis K, Toutouzas K, Tsiamis E, Stefanadis C (2012) Subendocardial viability ratio as an index of impaired coronary flow reserve in hypertensives without significant coronary artery stenoses. J Hum Hypertens 26:64–70
56. Ohtsuka S, Kakihana M, Watanabe H, Sugishita Y (1994) Chronically decreased aortic distensibility causes deterioration of coronary perfusion during increased left ventricular contraction. J Am Coll Cardiol 24:1406–1414
57. Murgo JP, Westerhof N, Giolma JP, Altobelli SA (1981) Manipulation of ascending aortic pressure and flow wave reflections with the valsalva maneuver:relationship to input impedance. Circulation 63:122–132
58. Colombo PC, Onat D, Harxhi A, Demmer RT, Hayashi Y, Jelic S, LeJemtel TH, Bucciarelli L, Kebschull M, Papapanou P, Uriel N, Schmidt AM, Sabbah HN, Jorde UP (2014) Peripheral

venous congestion causes inflammation, neurohormonal, and endothelial cell activation. Eur Heart J 35:448–454
59. Senzaki H, Masutani S, Ishido H, Taketazu M, Kobayashi T, Sasaki N, Asano H, Katogi T, Kyo S, Yokote Y (2006) Cardiac rest and reserve function in patients with fontan circulation. J Am Coll Cardiol 47:2528–2535
60. Suga H, Sagawa K (1974) Instantaneous pressure-volume relationships and their ratio in the excised, supported canine left ventricle. Circ Res 35:117–126
61. Kass DA, Maughan WL (1988) From 'emax' to pressure-volume relations: a broader view. Circulation 77:1203–1212
62. Burkhoff D, Mirsky I, Suga H (2005) Assessment of systolic and diastolic ventricular properties via pressure-volume analysis: a guide for clinical, translational, and basic researchers. Am J Physiol Heart Circ Physiol 289:H501–H512
63. Senzaki H, Kyo S, Matsumoto K, Asano H, Masutani S, Ishido H, Matunaga T, Taketatu M, Kobayashi T, Sasaki N, Yokote Y (2004) Cardiac resynchronization therapy in a patient with single ventricle and intracardiac conduction delay. J Thorac Cardiovasc Surg 127:287–288
64. Masutani S, Saiki H, Kurishima C, Kuwata S, Tamura M, Senzaki H (2014) Assessment of ventricular relaxation and stiffness using early diastolic mitral annular and inflow velocities in pediatric patients with heart disease. Heart Vessel 29:825–833
65. Mohammed SF, Hussain S, Mirzoyev SA, Edwards WD, Maleszewski JJ, Redfield MM (2015) Coronary microvascular rarefaction and myocardial fibrosis in heart failure with preserved ejection fraction. Circulation 131:550–559
66. Paulus WJ, Tschope C (2013) A novel paradigm for heart failure with preserved ejection fraction: Comorbidities drive myocardial dysfunction and remodeling through coronary microvascular endothelial inflammation. J Am Coll Cardiol 62:263–271
67. Dauterman K, Pak PH, Maughan WL, Nussbacher A, Arie S, Liu CP, Kass DA (1995) Contribution of external forces to left ventricular diastolic pressure. Implications for the clinical use of the starling law. Ann Intern Med 122:737–742
68. Aburawi EH, Munkhammar P, Carlsson M, El-Sadig M, Pesonen E (2014) Coronary flow dynamics in children after repair of tetralogy of fallot. Int J Cardiol 172:122–126
69. Yin FC, Brin KP, Ting CT, Pyeritz RE (1989) Arterial hemodynamic indexes in marfan's syndrome. Circulation 79:854–862
70. Segers P, De Backer J, Devos D, Rabben SI, Gillebert TC, Van Bortel LM, De Sutter J, De Paepe A, Verdonck PR (2006) Aortic reflection coefficients and their association with global indexes of wave reflection in healthy controls and patients with marfan's syndrome. Am J Physiol Heart Circ Physiol 290:H2385–H2392
71. Inuzuka R, Seki M, Sugimoto M, Saiki H, Masutani S, Senzaki H (2013) Pulmonary arterial wall stiffness and its impact on right ventricular afterload in patients with repaired tetralogy of fallot. Ann Thorac Surg 96:1435–1441
72. Senzaki H, Iwamoto Y, Ishido H, Matsunaga T, Taketazu M, Kobayashi T, Asano H, Katogi T, Kyo S (2007) Arterial hemodynamics in patients after repair of tetralogy of fallot: Influence on left ventricular afterload and aortic dilation. Heart
73. Kelly R, Hayward C, Avolio A, O'Rourke M (1989) Noninvasive determination of age-related changes in the human arterial pulse. Circulation 80:1652–1659

Chapter 9
Pregnancy and Delivery

Shinji Katsuragi, Jun Yoshimatsu, Koichiro Niwa, and Tomoaki Ikeda

Abstract Exposure of estrogen and hemodynamic changes during pregnancy lead to the fragility of the elastic fiber of the aortic media. It elevates the risk for aortic dilatation and dissection. We observe cystic medial necrosis change in the aortic wall media during pregnancy, and the diameter of the aorta increases slightly. This phenomenon generally called aortopathy is especially important in the management of connective tissue diseases such as Marfan syndrome patients during pregnancy.

A large sinus of Valsalva, increased aortic size index, and rapid growth of the sinus of Valsalva are risk factors for aortic dilatation or dissection in pregnant women with Marfan syndrome.

Keywords Aortic dissection • Marfan syndrome • Pregnancy • Sinus of Valsalva • Aortic size index

9.1 Hemodynamic Changes During Pregnancy

During normal pregnancy, total blood volume increases by 40–50 % by the end of the second trimester. The heart rate increases about 20 % above baseline, and cardiac output approaches 30–50 % above baseline by the end of the second trimester. And peripheral resistance decreases by the 16 weeks of gestation to adopt the increased uterine blood flow, but it becomes higher than before conception by the increased level of renin and angiotensin II. These hemodynamic changes

---

S. Katsuragi, M.D. (✉)
Department of Obstetrics and Gynecology, Sakakibara Heart Institute, 3-16-1 Asahi-cho, Fuchu, Tokyo 183-0003, Japan
e-mail: skatsura12@yahoo.co.jp

J. Yoshimatsu
Department of Perinatology and Gynecology, National Cerebral and Cardiovascular Center, Osaka, Japan

K. Niwa
Department of Cardiology, St. Luke's International Hospital, Tokyo, Japan

T. Ikeda
Department of Obstetrics and Gynecology, Mie University, Tsu, Mie, Japan

K. Niwa, H. Kaemmerer (eds.), *Aortopathy*, DOI 10.1007/978-4-431-56071-5_9

may cause dilatation and dissection of the aorta for the mother especially with weak aortic media such as Marfan syndrome and Loeys-Dietz syndrome.

9.1.1 Estrogen Levels During Pregnancy and Aortopathy

During normal pregnancy estrogen level is high to support the growth development of the uterus, the fetus, and the mammary gland.

Exposure of estrogen during pregnancy leads to the fragility of the elastic fiber of the aortic media (elastic fiber fragmentation). This elevates the risk for aortic dilatation and dissection. Also it affects renin-angiotensin system and increases not only extracellular fluid and volume load but also the vulnerability of the aortic wall. We observe cystic medial necrosis change in the aortic wall media during pregnancy, and the diameter of the aorta increases slightly.

9.1.2 Marfan Syndrome and Incidence of Aortic Complications During Pregnancy

Marfan syndrome is an autosomal-dominant connective tissue disorder caused by mutations in the fibrillin-1 (FBN1) gene located on chromosome 15 [1]. These mutations result in weakness of the supportive tissue of the body and clinical characteristics including symptoms of the cardiovascular, skeletal, and ocular systems [2, 3]. Cardiovascular complications are the main cause of morbidity and mortality in patients with Marfan syndrome [4]. Before preventive surgical approaches to aortic diseases, the mean life expectancy for a patient with Marfan syndrome was below 40 years old, with aortic dissection, aortic rupture, and cardiac failure being the predominant causes of death [5]. However, beta-blocker therapy and elective surgical repair have increased life expectancy to near-normal values [6].

Pregnancy is strongly associated with life-threatening problems in Marfan patients. The risk of aortic dilatation or dissection increases during and after pregnancy in patients with Marfan syndrome due to superimposition of the hyperdynamic and hypervolemic circulatory state of pregnancy on the preexisting weakness of the aortic media [3]. Pacini describes that Marfan syndrome patients tend to experience dissection of the aorta during pregnancy than nonpregnant period (4.4 % vs. 0.9 %, $p < 0.05$) (Fig. 9.1). The rate of aortic dissection during pregnancy has been studied in previous reports. In 1981, Pyeritz reported no aortic complications during 105 pregnancies in 26 women affected by Marfan syndrome, based on phone interviews (Table 9.1.) [7]. Rossiter et al. prospectively followed 45 pregnancies in 21 women and found 2 cases complicated by dissection (Fig. 9.2) [8]; Lipscomb et al. reported 6 aortic events, including 4 aortic dissections, in

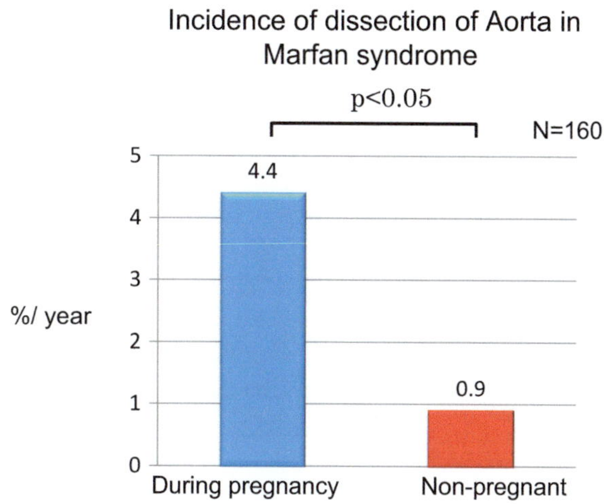

Fig. 9.1 Incidence of dissection of the aorta in Marfan syndrome. Marfan syndrome patients tend to experience dissection of the aorta during pregnancy than nonpregnant period (4.4 % vs. 0.9 %, $p < 0.05$)

91 pregnancies in 36 women [9]; Lind et al. found 5 aortic dissections in 117 pregnancies [10]; and Pacini et al. reported 7 aortic dissections in 160 pregnancies in 85 women [11]; and we reported 9 aortic dissections/dilatations in 29 pregnancies [12]. Combining all these data gives a risk of 5.3 % for aortic complication during pregnancy in women with Marfan syndrome who are not taking beta-blockers.

The basic aortic risks in pregnancy are an aortic diameter ≥4.0 cm [7–10, 12–14] and a steady increase in the aortic root dimension during pregnancy [9, 10, 12, 15]. Meijboom et al. reported that pregnancy in women with Marfan syndrome seems to be relatively safe up to an aortic root diameter of 45 mm [16]. However, most previous reports on Marfan syndrome in pregnancy have been from North America or Europe, and people in these areas have relatively larger number of physiques, or different physiques of patients might have been intermingled. Since normal aortic dimensions vary with age and body size [17], the same aortic dimension represents a proportionally greater diameter in smaller individuals, and proper interpretation of the aortic dimension requires that age and body size are accounted for. Therefore, the absolute aortic size cannot be directly used to evaluate risk in patients with a small physique [18], such as Japanese women.

The risk factors for aortic complications in pregnant patients affected with Marfan syndrome have not been examined with inclusion of a consideration of the body surface area. Therefore, to permit appropriate consultation and management of patients, we studied 29 consecutive pregnant patients with Marfan syndrome in one institution to determine the factors that influence maternal aortic complications.

Table 9.1. Aortic dissection/dilatation and Marfan syndrome complicated pregnancy

Number of pregnancy	Cardiac events (Dilatation/dissection) (%)	Report	Country
105	0	1981 Pyeritz	USA
45	2 (4.4)	1995 Rositter	USA
91	6 (6.6)	1997 Lipscomb	UK
117	5 (4.3)	2001 Lind	Holland
160	7 (4.4)	2009 Pacinni	France
29	9 (31)	2013 Katsuragi	Japan
547	29 (5.3)		

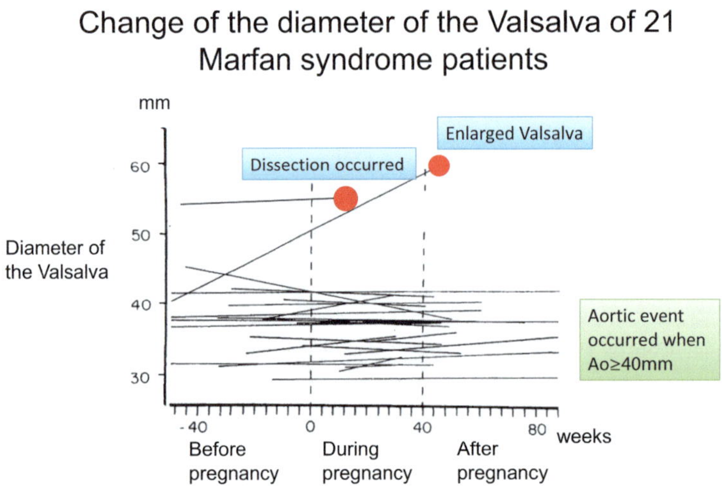

Fig. 9.2 Change of the diameter of the Valsalva of 21 Marfan syndrome patients. Aortic event occurred when Ao $\geq$ 40 mm

9.1.3 Monitoring for Dilatation and Dissection of the Aorta in Marfan Syndrome Patients During Pregnancy

9.1.3.1 Measurement of the Aortic Diameter and Indication for Surgery

Diameter of the sinus of Valsalva can be measured by echocardiography during pregnancy [17, 19]. MRI can be used during pregnancy, but CT is not usually examined due to radiation exposure. The Japanese Circulation Society recommends an operation for Marfan patients with a sinus of Valsalva over 5 cm [20]. Some surgeons also prefer an operation for patients with a sinus of Valsalva over 4.5 cm [21]. In our institution, surgical intervention is indicated according to the above criteria especially patients with a family history of dissection or sudden death. In general, surgical intervention is indicated for a sinus of Valsalva over 4.0 cm or in a case with steady aortic size growth [22, 23]. During pregnancy, surgical intervention is indicated if there is progressive aortic growth with a sinus of Valsalva of 4.0 cm (4.5 cm) or massive dissection. To standardize the measurement based on body size, the size of the sinus of Valsalva could be evaluated using the aortic size index (ASI), which is calculated as ASI = aortic diameter (mm)/body surface area (m^2) [18].

9.1.3.2 Cardiovascular Events Monitoring During Pregnancy

Echocardiographic follow-up including aortic diameter measurement and Holter electrocardiogram could be necessary at least once in each trimester during pregnancy and within 4 weeks after delivery. If the aortic root diameter is over $\geq$40 mm, echocardiography could be performed every 2 weeks in the second and the third trimester. Marfan syndrome is occasionally complicated with mitral valve prolapse and regurgitation. Regurgitation may be worsening from mild to severe during pregnancy, and it will develop arrhythmias. In these cases, Holter electrocardiogram is useful to decide whether it is better to introduce antiarrhythmic medication such as beta-blockade.

When surgical intervention is indicated, the operation should be performed after cesarean section when a fetus is already matured. But if the fetus is immature to live independently, the aortic operation could be performed with the fetus in the uterus.

9.1.4 Aortic Risks in Marfan Syndrome Patients During Pregnancy

9.1.4.1 Case Series of Aortic Dilatation or Dissection [12]

Eleven of 29 cases with Marfan women had aortic dilatation or dissection associated with pregnancy, including 7 that occurred during pregnancy and 4 within 1 year after pregnancy (group D). One case underwent hemiarch replacement and one underwent a David operation during pregnancy. Three underwent Bentall operations following delivery by cesarean section, and two received conservative therapy after cesarean section. The incidence of cesarean section was higher in patients with aortic dilatation/dissection. A family history of sudden death or aortic dissection was more frequent in patients with aortic dilatation/dissection.

9.1.4.2 Echocardiographic Data in Cases With and Without Aortic Dilatation or Dissection

By echocardiography, a sinus of Valsalva $\geq$40 mm in the first trimester was more frequent in patients with aortic dilatation/dissection (Fig. 9.3).

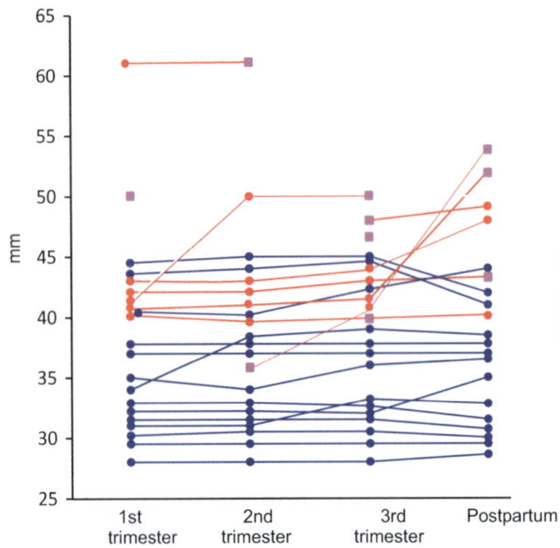

Fig. 9.3 Diameters of the sinus of Valsalva. D/D indicates aortic dilatation or dissection. Cases with and without aortic dilatation or dissection are shown by *red* and *blue circles*, respectively (group D and group ND, respectively). *Pink squares* indicate a cardiac event. In the first trimester, a larger sinus of Valsalva was found in group D compared to group ND (41.5±2.4 vs. 34.8±1.3, $P < 0.05$ by student t-test). The sinus of Valsalva was ≥40 mm in 6/7 cases in group D and 3/14 in group ND ($P < 0.05$ by chi-square test and Fisher exact test)

An aortic size index (ASI) (diameter of the sinus of Valsalva/body surface area) ≥25 mm/m^2 was more frequent in n patients with aortic dilatation/dissection (Fig. 9.4). Significantly faster growth of the sinus of Valsalva was also observed in patients with aortic dilatation/dissection (Fig. 9.5).

In the first trimester of pregnancy, patients with aortic dilatation/dissection showed more frequent moderate to severe aortic and mitral valve regurgitation.

9.1.5 Risk Factors for Aortic Dilatation/Dissection

The risk factors that differed significantly between groups D and ND were mostly consistent with those found in previous studies [7–10, 14]. The risk factors for pregnancy-associated dilatation or dissection are a large sinus of Valsalva, rapid growth of the sinus of Valsalva during pregnancy, moderate to severe aortic valve or mitral valve regurgitation, and family history of sudden death or aortic dissection [7–10, 15].

According to the relatively large prospective study of Meijboom et al. [16], pregnancy in women with Marfan syndrome seems to be relatively safe up to an aortic root diameter of 45 mm. Also, Canadian guidelines [23] recommend that women with an aortic root diameter beyond 44 mm should be strongly discouraged from becoming pregnant. In a case report of a patient who developed a massive retrograde type B aortic dissection 7 days after normal spontaneous vaginal

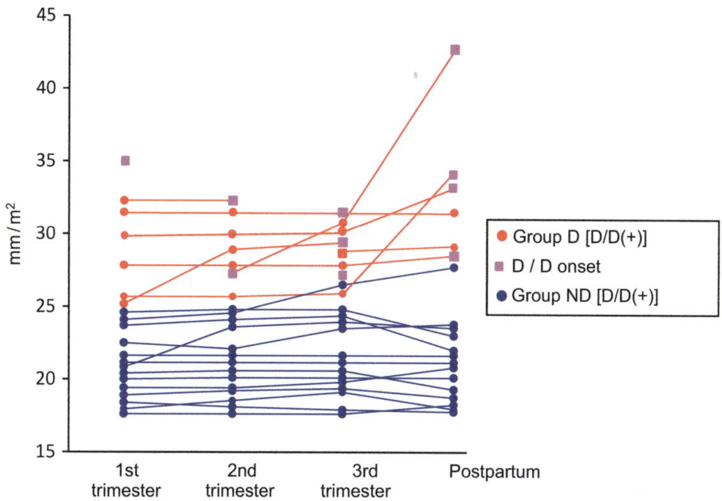

Fig. 9.4 Adjusted sizes of the sinus of Valsalva (size of the sinus of Valsalva/body surface area, mm/m^2). D/D indicates aortic dilatation or dissection. Cases with and without aortic dilatation or dissection are shown by *red* and *blue circles*, respectively (group D and group ND, respectively). In the first trimester, the adjusted size of the sinus of Valsalva was $\geq$25 mm/m^2 in 7/7 cases in group D and 0/14 in group ND ($P < 0.0001$ by chi-square test and Fisher exact test)

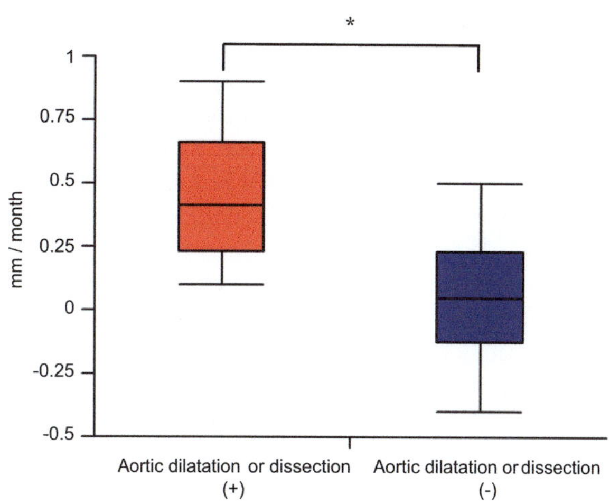

Fig. 9.5 Rate of growth of the sinus of Valsalva. Significantly faster growth of the sinus of Valsalva was observed in group D (*red box*) than in group ND (*blue box*). The middle bar indicates the 50th percentile; box edges are the 25th and 75th percentiles; and outer bars are the 10th and 90th percentiles. Data were analyzed by Wilcoxon test. $^*P < 0.05$

delivery, Gandhi et al. [24] described the patient as "petite" (body surface area, 1.69 m^2); however, in case of smaller physics such as Asian and Japanese woman, the cutoff value for regarding avoidance of pregnancy may be a sinus of Valsalva diameter $\geq$40 mm, rather than $\geq$45 mm.

9.1.6 Adjusted Aortic Size Index Is Applicable for Small Physics

The diameter of the sinus of Valsalva adjusted for body surface area (diameter of the Valsalva/body surface area, mm/m^2) may be more appropriate for selection of high-risk cases before pregnancy. The relative aortic size was first used to predict complications in patients with thoracic aortic aneurysms [18]. An aortic size index (ASI) $\geq$25 mm/m^2 in the first trimester is possibly a risk factor for aortic dilatation or dissection during pregnancy and postpartum. The ASI is a novel measurement of relative aortic size that predicts rupture of aortic aneurysm [18], and Davies et al. found that the ASI was more important than absolute aortic size in predicting aortic complications, especially in smaller women [18]. There was more rapid growth of the sinus of Valsalva in patients with Marfan syndrome with pregnancy-associated aortic dilatation or dissection, compared to those without these conditions. Therefore, even if the diameter of the sinus of the Valsalva is small, rapid growth carries a risk of aortic dissection or dilatation. The same phenomenon has been reported in nonpregnant cases of Marfan syndrome. Meijboom et al. [25] followed 108 women with Marfan syndrome and aortic root growth prospectively using serial echocardiograms and found that the patients could be divided into two normally distributed groups based on aortic growth rates: 90 % were slow growers and 10 % were fast growers. Higher incidence of dissections of the ascending aorta (25 % vs. 4 %, $P < 0.001$) is observed in the fast growers, and the average growth of the sinus of Valsalva in the fast group was 1.8 mm/year. The median growth in the five dissected cases was as high as 4.1 mm/year [12]. This larger increase relative to that in Meijboom et al. [16] is probably due to the influence of hemodynamic change including increased blood volume, heart rate, and stroke volume during pregnancy. Furthermore, hormonally mediated histological changes also occur in the aorta, including a decrease in mucopolysaccharides and loss of elastic fibers in the aortic wall [26–28]. Therefore, care is required in treating patients with a high growth rate of the sinus of Valsalva. The frequency and degree of aortic and mitral valve regurgitation were also higher in cases with aortic dilatation or dissection, and these valvular changes may have positive impact on dilatation or dissection.

An international expert panel established the revised Ghent criteria in 2010, which first put more weight on cardiovascular manifestations and in which aortic dilatation/dissection and ectopia lentis are the cardinal clinical features [29]. Second, in these revised criteria, a more prominent role is assigned to molecular genetic testing of FBN1 and other relevant genes in the diagnostic assessment. Third, some of the less specific manifestations of Marfan syndrome were either removed or made less influential in the diagnostic evaluation of patients. The new criteria also try to differentiate Marfan syndrome from Marfan-related syndromes such as Loeys-Dietz syndrome, Ehlers-Danlos syndrome, and familial thoracic aortic aneurysm syndrome, which are associated with a significantly greater risk of cardiovascular problems [29–31]. In the study of Katsuragi, patients with dilatation or dissection of the aorta less met major ocular criteria, more met the major cardiovascular criteria, and had a more frequent family history of dilatation or dissection [12, 32]. These findings indicate that the new nosology to diagnose Marfan syndrome facilitates to differentiate the high-risk patients for pregnancy-associated dilatation or dissection more accurately.

9.1.7 Loeys-Dietz Syndrome and Pregnancy

Loeys-Dietz syndrome (LDS), an autosomal-dominant connective tissue disorder first characterized by aortic aneurysms and generalized arterial tortuosity, hypertelorism, and bifid/broad uvula or cleft palate, was first described in 2005 [33,34]. Rapidly progressive aortic aneurysmal disease is a distinct feature of LDS, requiring close monitoring. Individuals with LDS 1/2 with severe craniofacial features are at particularly high risk, known to have ruptures at early ages and at smaller dimensions than those with other aneurysm syndromes [33, 34]. Aortic dissection has been reported in individuals as young as 3 months and cerebral hemorrhage as young as 3 years [35, 36]. Initial reports of LDS 1/2 cohorts described a mean age of death at 26.1 years, with aortic dissection and cerebral hemorrhages as major causes of death [33]. Better detection, surveillance, and early treatment are expected to extend the life span of affected individuals. Women with LDS can tolerate and have successful pregnancies and deliveries, although pregnancies should be considered high risk. In the absence of predictive characteristics of women who may have complications, counseling women about specific risks remains a challenge. In 21 pregnancies among 12 women with LDS 1/2, 6 women had a major complication either during pregnancy or immediately postpartum, comprised of 4 aortic dissections and 2 uterine ruptures [33]. These occurred in first, second, and third pregnancies. Two additional women experienced severe uterine hemorrhage independent of pregnancy. Arterial rupture may also be a pregnancy or postpartum complication. Cardiovascular medications should be addressed, with safe down-titration and discontinuation of angiotensin receptor blockers prior to pursuing a pregnancy. β-Blocker usage is recommended throughout pregnancy. Other pain, anticoagulation, and/or other medical therapy should be thoroughly discussed prior to pregnancy to reduce teratogenic effects on the fetus. Early delivery and the avoidance of high intra-abdominal pressure by means of cesarean section may reduce the risk of obstetric complications. No specific recommendations can be made, however, due to the absence of studies comparing the efficacy of cesarean and vaginal deliveries.

9.1.8 Ehlers-Danlos Syndrome and Pregnancy

Ehlers-Danlos syndrome is a multifaceted condition that has a number of different types, and within those types, each patient is affected in a different way. The most serious is type 4 or vascular EDS. If you are a female and diagnosed with this type, you will no doubt already understand that pregnancy is very risky and potentially life-threatening as it can increase the possibility of a catastrophic arterial or organ rupture. A study published in 2014 found that pregnancy-related deaths in women with vascular EDS occurred in 30 of 565 deliveries (5.3 %) [37]. Interviews with 39 women indicated that 46 % had uncomplicated pregnancies, while the most common pregnancy-related complications were third-/fourth-degree lacerations (20 %) and preterm delivery (19 %). Life-threatening complications occurred in 14.5 % of deliveries and included arterial dissection/rupture (9.2 %), uterine rupture (2.6 %), and surgical complications (2.6 %).

9.1.9 Turner's Syndrome and Pregnancy [38]

Ovarian failure is a typical feature in Turner's syndrome. Therefore, hormone replacement therapy (HRT) is necessary to achieve the development of normal female sexual characteristics and to prevent cardiovascular complications and osteoporosis. Spontaneous puberty occurs in 5–10 % of women with Turner's syndrome, and 2–5 % of them become pregnant spontaneously. Sexually active young women with Turner's syndrome need contraception. It can be administered as contraceptive pills, which also serve as HRT. Oocyte donation is now a treatment option for infertility of these women. Excellent results have been obtained with 46 % of embryo transfers resulting in pregnancy. The pregnancies carry high risks and have to be followed up carefully. The children born following oocyte donation have no additional risks. Risks can be reduced by transferring only one embryo at a time to the uterus, thus avoiding twin pregnancies. Ovarian tissue from young girls with Turner's syndrome could be cryopreserved for infertility treatment in the future, but the optimal age of ovarian biopsy has to be studied, and methods of replantation and maturation of oocytes in vitro have still to be developed. Fertility counseling has become important in the treatment of girls with Turner's syndrome.

9.1.10 Noonan Syndrome and Pregnancy

Noonan syndrome is a genetic disorder characterized by short stature, distinctive facial features, heart defects, bleeding problems, and skeletal abnormalities [39]. Earlier diagnosis will improve clinical management and genetic counseling. Most individuals with Noonan syndrome have normal intelligence, but some may have special educational needs or intellectual disability. Noonan syndrome occurs in about 1 in 2500 births. As this is an autosomal-dominant condition, the inheritance rate is 50 %. In molecular prenatal genetic testing, DNA is isolated from the cells of the developing baby through one of two procedures (chorionic villus sampling or amniocentesis) and is analyzed for the disease-causing mutation.

With appropriate counseling, a parent can then decide whether to carry the pregnancy to term or to end the pregnancy.

9.1.11 Genetics and Preconceptional Counseling

Differential diagnosis of Marfan syndrome includes Loeys-Dietz syndrome, familial thoracic aortic aneurysms, and Ehlers-Danlos syndromes. These are autosomal-dominant connective tissue disorders and responsible genes are discovered. Preconception genetic counseling is indicated to address recurrence risk and diagnostic testing options. The recurrence risk is 50 %. Prenatal diagnoses through amniocentesis or chorionic villus sampling are available options for autosomal-dominant connective tissue disorders. These information should be precisely informed to the mother and the husband by clinical geneticist before conception. Details of genetics, phenotype, and genotype are described in Chap. 5.

9.1.12 Drugs During Pregnancy

Angiotensin-converting enzyme inhibitor and angiotensin II-converting enzyme inhibitor should not be used during pregnancy because they have toxicity against fetal kidney, teratogenicity of congenital heart disease, and decrease of amniotic fluid volume. In the retrospective survey of pregnancies with cardiovascular diseases, fetal growth restriction is reported to be 7, 26, and 3 % in alpha-/beta-adrenergic blocker group, beta-adrenergic blocker group, and control group, respectively ($p < 0.05$) (submitting data, Tanaka Kayo et al.). And we admitted different ratio of fetal growth restriction in each beta-blockade: atenolol, propranolol > metoprolol, and bisoprolol.

9.1.13 Multidisciplinary Team Approach

For the management for Marfan syndrome during pregnancy, multidisciplinary team approach is important. Medical geneticist does the accurate diagnosis of Marfan syndrome including the genetic test and preconceptional counseling is necessary. In our institution, surgical intervention is indicated according to the criteria [29] and for patients with a family history of dissection or sudden death. In general, valve-sparing aortic root replacement is indicated for a sinus of Valsalva over 4.0 cm or in a case with steady aortic size growth [22, 23]. Vaginal delivery with epidural anesthesia is recommended.

9.1.14 Summary

Exposure of estrogen and hemodynamic changes during pregnancy lead to the fragility of the elastic fiber of the aortic media. An increased size of the sinus of Valsalva (≥40–45 mm) was found in patients with Marfan syndrome who experienced aortic dilatation or dissection during or after pregnancy. The aortic size index is a better indicator of the risk for aortic dilatation or dissection during pregnancy and postpartum, compared to the absolute size of the sinus of Valsalva. Until a molecular-based approach is available to identify patients at high cardiovascular risk, echocardiographic variables will remain as the most important prognostic factors. For the management of patients with aortopathy during pregnancy, multidisciplinary team approach is important.

References

1. Dietz HC, Cutting GR, Pyeritz RE, Maslen CL, Sakai LY, Corson GM et al (1991) Marfan syndrome caused by a recurrent de novo missense mutation in the fibrillin gene. Am J Hum Genet 49:662–667
2. Keane MG, Pyeritz RE (2008) Medical management of Marfan syndrome. Circulation 117:2802–2813
3. Ammash NM, Sundt TM, Connolly HM (2008) Marfan syndrome-diagnosis and management. Curr Probl Cardiol 31:7–39
4. Judge DP, Diez HC (2005) Marfan's syndrome. Lancet 366:1965–1976
5. Murdoch JL, Walker BA, Halpern BL, Kuzma JW, McKusick VA (1972) Life expectancy and causes of death in the Marfan syndrome. N Engl J Med 286:804–808
6. Silverman DI, Burton KJ, Gray J, Bosner MS, Kouchoukos NT, Roman MJ et al (1995) Life expectancy in the Marfan syndrome. Am J Cardiol 75:157–160
7. Pyeritz RE (1981) Maternal and fetal complications of pregnancy in the Marfan syndrome. Am J Med 71:784–790
8. Rossiter JP, Repke JY, Morales AJ, Murphy EA, Pyeritz RE (1995) A prospective longitudinal evaluation of pregnancy in the Marfan syndrome. Am J Obstet Gynecol 173:1599–1606
9. Lipscomb KJ, Smith JC, Bernard C, Donnai P, Harris R (1997) Outcome of pregnancy in women with Marfan's syndrome. Br J Obstet Gynaecol 104:201–206
10. Lind J, Wallenburg HC (2001) The Marfan syndrome and pregnancy: a retrospective study in a Dutch population. J Obstet Gynecol Reprod Biol 98:28–35
11. Pacici L, Digne F, Boumendil A, Muti C, Detaint D, Boileau C et al (2009) Maternal complication of pregnancy in Marfan syndrome. Int J Cardiol 136:156–161
12. Katsuragi S, Yamanaka K, Neki R, Kamiya C, Sasaki Y, Osato K et al (2012) Cir J 76:469–476
13. Goland S, Elkayam U (2009) Cardiovascular problems in pregnant women with Marfan syndrome. Circulation 119:619–623
14. Task Force on the Management of Cardiovascular Diseases during Pregnancy of the European Society of Cardiology (2003) Expert consensus document on management of cardiovascular diseases during pregnancy. Eur Heart J 24:761–781
15. Immer FF, Bansi AG, Immer-Bansi AS, McDougall J, Zehr KJ, Schaff HV et al (2003) Aortic dissection in pregnancy: analysis of risk factors and outcome. Ann Thorac Surg 76:309–314
16. Meijboom LJ, Timmermans J, Zwinderman AH, Engelfriet PM, Mulder BJ (2005) Aortic root growth in men and women with the Marfan's syndrome. Am J Cardiol 96:1441–1444

17. Roman MJ, Devereux RB, Kramer-Fox R, O'Loughlin J (1989) Two dimensional echocardiographic aortic root dimensions in normal children and adults. Am J Cardiol 64:507–512
18. Davies RR, Gallo A, Coady MA, Tellides G, Botta DM, Burke B et al (2006) Novel measurement of relative aortic size predicts rupture of thoracic aortic aneurysms. Ann Thorac Surg 81:169–177
19. Roman MJ, Rosen SE, Kramer-Fox R, Devereux RB (1993) Prognostic significance of the pattern of aortic root dilatation in the Marfan syndrome. J Am Coll Cardiol 22:1470–1476
20. (2006) Guidelines for diagnosis and treatment of aortic aneurysm and aortic dissection. Circ J 70:1627
21. Matsuyama K, Usui A, Akita T, Yoshikawa M, Murayama M, Yano T et al (2005) Natural history of a dilated ascending aorta after aortic valve replacement. Circ J 69:392–396
22. Davies RR, Goldstein LJ, Coady MA, Tittle SL, Rizzo JA, Kopf GS et al (2002) Yearly rupture or dissection rates for thoracic aortic aneurysms: simple prediction based on size. Ann Thorac Surg 73:17–27
23. Milewicz DM, Dietz HC, Miller DC (2005) Treatment of aortic disease in patients with Marfan syndrome. Circulation 111:e150–e157
24. Silversides CK, Kiess M, Beauchesne L, Bradley T, Connelly M, Niwa K et al (2010) Canadian Cardiovascular Society 2009 Consensus Conference on the management of adults with congenital heart disease: outflow tract obstruction, coarctation of the aorta, tetralogy of Fallot, Ebstein anomaly and Marfan's syndrome. Can J Cardiol 26:e80–e97
25. Gandhi SD, Iqbal Z, Markan S, Almassi GH, Pagel PS (2008) Massive retrograde acute type B aortic dissection in a postpartum woman with a family history of Marfan syndrome. J Clin Anesth 20:50–53
26. Whittaker PG, MacPhail S, Lind T (1996) Serial hematologic changes and pregnancy outcome. Obstet Gynecol 88:33–39
27. Hashimoto M, Miyamoto Y, Iwai C, Matsuda Y, Hiraoka E, Kanazawa K et al (2009) Delivery may affect arterial elasticity in women. Circ J 73:750–754
28. Manalo-Esrrella P, Barker AE (1967) Histopathologic findings in human aortic media associated with pregnancy. Arch Pathol 83:336–341
29. Loeys BL, Dietz HC, Braverman AC, Callewaert BL, Backer JD, Devereux RC et al (2010) The revised Ghent nosology for the Marfan syndrome. J Med Genet 47:476–485
30. Akutsu K, Morisaki H, Takeshita S, Sakamoto S, Tamori Y, Yoshimuta T et al (2007) Phenotypic heterogeneity of Marfan-like connective tissue disorders associated with mutations in the transforming growth factor-beta receptor genes. Circ J 71:1305–1309
31. Akutsu K, Morisaki H, Okajima T, Yoshimuta T, Tsutsumi Y, Takeshita S et al (2010) Genetic analysis of young adult patients with aortic disease not fulfilling the diagnostic criteria for Marfan syndrome. Circ J 74:990–997
32. De Paepe A, Devereux RB, Dietz HC, Hennekam RC, Pyeritz RE (1996) Revised diagnostic criteria for the Marfan syndrome. Am J Med Genet 62:417–426
33. Loeys BL, Schwarze U, Holm T et al (2006) Aneurysm syndromes caused by mutations in the TGF-beta receptor. N Engl J Med 355:788–798
34. Loeys BL, Chen J, Neptune ER et al (2005) A syndrome of altered cardiovascular, craniofacial, neurocognitive and skeletal development caused by mutations in TGFBR1 or TGFBR2. Nat Genet 37:275–281
35. Malhotra A, Westesson PL (2009) Loeys-Dietz syndrome. Pediatr Radiol 39:1015
36. Williams JA, Loeys BL, Nwakanma LU et al (2007) Early surgical experience with Loeys-Dietz: a new syndrome of aggressive thoracic aortic aneurysm disease. Ann Thorac Surg 83: S757–S763 ; discussion S785–90
37. Murray ML, Pepin M, Peterson S, Byers PH (2014) Pregnancy-related deaths and complications in women with vascular Ehlers–Danlos syndrome. Genet Med 16:874–880
38. Hovatta O (1999) Pregnancies in women with Turner's syndrome. Ann Med 31:106–110
39. Turner AM (2014) Noonan syndrome. J Paediatr Child Health 50:E14–E20

Chapter 10
Medications

Hsin-Hui Chiu and Mei-Hwan Wu

Abstract In patients born with congenital heart defects or genetic syndromes with connective tissue disorders such as Marfan syndrome, aortic dilatation is one of the major late complications even after corrective surgery. The pathogenesis of aortic dilatation is complex and multifactorial. It could be related to an intrinsic aortic wall abnormalities, genetic alterations, and aortic or ventricular dysfunction, which is defined as "aortopathy." The major purpose of medical treatment for the aortopathy is to reduce the structural changes within the aortic wall and to slow down the progression of aortic dilatation to reduce the risk from life-threatening aortic events. Several medications have been studied for the purpose, which include β-blockers, angiotensin II type I (AT1) receptor blockers (ARBs), angiotensin-converting enzyme (ACE) inhibitors, Ca-antagonists, statins, and tetracyclines. But, the results, except those in patients with Marfan syndrome, are still very limited. The studies in Marfan syndrome, from mouse model to clinical trials, indicate an important role of β-blockers as well as a better protection from losartan add-on β-blockers.

Coexistent cardiovascular risk factors, such as systemic arterial hypertension, dyslipidemia, and diabetes, can accelerate the progress of the dilated aorta to aneurysm, dissection, or even rupture and should be treated aggressively. With the advances in understanding the molecular mechanisms of aortopathies, treatments target the underlying defect which may be the horizon of individualized medicine. The therapeutic approaches could hopefully be moved from current phenotype/syndrome-driven strategies to genotype/pathogenesis-driven strategies.

H.-H. Chiu
Department of Pediatrics, National Taiwan University Hospital and School of Medicine, College of Medicine, National Taiwan University, No. 7, Chung-Shen South Road, Zhongzheng Dist, Taipei 10002, Taiwan

Department of Pediatrics, Taipei Medical University Hospital and School of Medicine, College of Medicine, Taipei Medical University, Taipei, Taiwan

M.-H. Wu, M.D. (✉)
Department of Pediatrics, National Taiwan University Hospital and School of Medicine, College of Medicine, National Taiwan University, No. 7, Chung-Shen South Road, Zhongzheng Dist, Taipei 10002, Taiwan
e-mail: wumh@ntu.edu.tw

K. Niwa, H. Kaemmerer (eds.), *Aortopathy*, DOI 10.1007/978-4-431-56071-5_10

Keywords Angiotensin-converting enzyme inhibitors • Angiotensin receptor blockers • Beta-blockers

10.1 Introduction

Optimal medical management to prevent progressive aortic dilatation and dissection in normotensive patients with congenital heart disease or genetic syndrome-related aortopathy is still uncertain. Recent molecular, surgical, and clinical researches have yielded new insights into the disease pathogenesis and open new perspectives on the therapeutic approaches. However, most of clinical evidences are restricted to Marfan syndrome and remain limited in congenital heart disease groups. Because of the histopathological and functional similarities in the aorta between Marfan syndrome and congenital heart diseases, similar medication regimens are usually recommended for patients with aortopathy from congenital heart disease [1–6].

β-blockers have been the mainstay of medical treatment for many years [7–10]. Recently, losartan, an angiotensin II type I receptor blocker (ARB), has been shown to be very promising in a mouse model of Marfan syndrome and subsequently in patients [11–16]. Several clinical studies, focusing on the modulation of the angiotensin II pathway, proposed angiotensin-converting enzyme (ACE) inhibitors as other alternatives or adjuncts to the standard treatment with β-blockers [17–20]. In addition, other medications, such as calcium channel blockers, statins, and tetracyclines, have also been demonstrated with some potential benefits [21–32].

In addition, good control of the risk factors, such as systemic hypertension, dyslipidemia, and diabetes, smoking cessation, and healthy lifestyle modifications with suitable exercise are also important and warranted to delay the progression of aortic dilatation. The blood pressure should be controlled as low as the patients could tolerate and at least below 120–130 mmHg of systolic blood pressure at resting [1–6].

10.2 Medications

10.2.1 Beta-Blockers

Beta-blockers are often suggested as the first-line therapy for the treatment of a variety of cardiovascular problems, such as hypertension, aortic dissection, arrhythmia, and others [1–6]. Its negative inotropic and chronotropic effects can decrease proximal aortic shear stress or change in pressure over time (dP/dT). Thereby, β-blockers may slow the progression of aortic root dilatation and decrease the risk of cardiovascular events (aortic insufficiency, dissection, cardiovascular surgery, congestive heart failure, or death) [7–9]. This strategy was first proposed in 1971 by

Halpern et al. [10] and was advocated by subsequent small trials for patients with Marfan syndrome. From a mouse study, β-blockers were also noted to stimulate cross-linking of extracellular matrix components and to improve aortic elastic properties [33].

However, various studies reported heterogeneous responses and suggested that the β-blockers either had limited effect or even worsened the aortic stiffness, especially in patients with increased body weight or end-diastolic aortic root diameter of >40 mm [34, 35]. A meta-analysis did not show that β-blockers reduce mortality or the incidence of aortic dissection in patients with Marfan syndrome [36]. Although the effects are controversial, β-blockers are still regarded as first-line drug to slow down the progression of aortic dilatation in patients with syndromic connective tissue disorders or other congenital heart diseases and an aortic root diameter of >40 mm [1–6]. The recent AHA/ACC guidelines recommend the use of β-blockers for aortic dilatation in non-Marfan patients and keep blood pressure as low as well tolerated [5].

Salim MA et al. reported the changes of aortic root growth rate over a patient's lifetime, which reaches a peak between 6 and 14 years [9]. Therefore, in patients with connective tissue disorder such as Marfan syndrome or high risk for aortic dissection, β-blockers are recommended to use at the time of diagnosis especially before puberty and are maintained throughout life, even after aortic surgery [1–6]. The dose could be titrated to keep the heart rate around 60–70 bpm at rest and less than 100 bpm during submaximal exercise in older children or adults and less than 110 bpm in young children [2, 5, 6]. Up to now, widely used β-blockers in pediatric patients are propranolol or atenolol due to scanty safety evidences of other β-blockers. Atenolol is more beta-1 selective than propranolol and may be more effective in the treatment of aortic root dilation [1–6]. Recently, some ongoing studies used beta-1 selective blockades including bisoprolol, metoprolol, or nebivolol in the treatment of aortopathy to reduce the possible side effects. Among them, nebivolol is the highest selectively for β1 receptors and differs chemically, pharmacologically, and therapeutically from all other β-blockers which seems to directly target matrix metalloproteinases (MMPs) and/or transforming growth factor (TGF)-β cascade.

10.2.2 Angiotensin Receptor Blockers

Extracellular matrix homeostasis is controlled and balanced by matrix metalloproteinases (MMPs) and their specific tissue inhibitors (TIMPs). Increased MMPs activity will cause apoptosis and degeneration of the aortic wall and lead to aortic dilatation or aneurysm formation [3–5]. Studies in mice models of Marfan syndrome suggest that a fibrillin-1 gene mutation might lead to excessive transforming growth factor (TGF)-β signaling and activate MMPs [37, 38].

Losartan, an angiotensin II type I (AT1) receptor blocker, has been shown to be effective in preventing aortic root dilatation in a mouse model of Marfan syndrome through blocking the AT1 receptor and the subsequent TGF-β signal cascade

[11]. Several prospective clinical studies with different study designs had been conducted and shown the safety and the efficacy of losartan in operated or unoperated Marfan patients [12–16]. The efficacy of losartan correlates with treatment at earlier age and longer therapy duration, but not correlates with the type of phenotypes.

However, other studies did not confirm the results. The Pediatric Heart Network study, a large-scale, prospective randomized trial, which compared the efficacy of losartan and atenolol in children and young adult Marfan patients (608 patients, mean age 11 years, range 0.5–25.0 years) with dilated aortic roots failed to demonstrate superiority of losartan in reducing the rate of aortic dilatation (-0.107 vs. -0.139 z score/year; $P = 0.08$) over a 3-year period [39]. The Marfan Sartan study, a randomized, double-blind, placebo-controlled, add-on trial, which compared losartan vs. placebo in >10 years Marfan patients (303 patients, mean age 29.9 years, 86 % receiving β-blocker therapy) also reported no significant difference in limiting aortic dilatation between the losartan and placebo groups [40]. Forteza A et al. used magnetic resonance imaging to compare the benefits of losartan vs. atenolol as a monotherapy in Marfan patients (140 patients, mean age 25.2 ± 13.7 years, range 0.5–25.0 years) [41]. After 3 years of follow-up, aortic root diameter increased in both groups: 1.1 mm (95 % CI 0.6–1.6) in the losartan and 1.4 mm (95 % CI 0.9–1.9) in the atenolol group, with aortic dilatation progression being similar in both groups. The discrepancies between these studies may be due to different study design, inclusion criteria, drug doses, and endpoints. More methodologically rigorous studies currently in progress are needed to evaluate the impact of drug therapy on clinical outcomes.

The *FBN1* mutation might influence the drug response. In Marfan Sartan study, losartan tended to be more beneficial in patients with an *FBN1* mutation compared with those without (-0.04 vs. 0.00 z score/year and 0.40 vs. 0.51 mm/year; *P* value not reported) [40]. In COMPARE trial, patients with haploinsufficient *FBN1* mutations seem to be more responsive to losartan therapy in slowing the rate of aortic root dilatation compared with dominant negative patients (0.5 ± 0.8 mm/3 years vs. 0.8 ± 1.3 mm/3 years; *P* value not reported) [16].

In summary of current trials with different study design and results, losartan seems not to provide better protection against aortic dilatation than β-blockers. Therapy with a combination of β-blockers and losartan may be more effective than β-blockers alone in both children and adults with Marfan syndrome and should be considered at least if aortic dilatation is severe or progressive. Until the results of ongoing trials and meta-analyses are known, losartan can safely be administered as an alternative treatment to β-blockers or add-on β-blockers.

10.2.3 Angiotensin-Converting Enzyme Inhibitors

Inappropriate activation of the renin-angiotensin system in human aortic aneurysms had been described [17, 42, 43]. Angiotensin II signaling will be transduced via activation of two different receptors: type I and type II (AT1 and AT2) receptors. Signaling through AT1 receptor induces fibrosis and apoptosis by increasing TGF-β expression and MMPs activities. In contrast, the signaling through AT2 receptor is protective by decreasing cell proliferation, MMPs activities, and fibrosis [3].

ACE inhibitors are suggested to reduce large artery stiffness and slow the progression of aortic aneurysm in animal and human subjects [17, 42, 43]. The effects are not fully understood and may attribute to blood pressure control or inhibition of the extracellular signal-regulated kinases (ERK1/2) [17, 44]. ERKs were implicated to be involved in the progression of aortic aneurysm through stimulation of TGF-β and AT1 receptor-dependent signals [45, 46]. Some small retrospective or nonrandomized clinical studies have reported that ACE inhibitors reduced both aortic stiffness and aortic root diameter and improved aortic distensibility as compared with β-blockers in patients with Marfan syndrome or abdominal aortic aneurysm [17, 18]. However, Phomakay V et al. [19] retrospectively compared aortic growth rate in pediatric Marfan patients (67 patients, 13 ± 10 years, follow-up 7.6 ± 5.8 years) who received β-blockers, ACE inhibitors, or no therapy and showed that aortic growth rate was higher than normal in ACE inhibitor and untreated groups but nearly normal in β-blockers group. A small randomized, double-blind, crossover study (18 patients, 30.4 ± 11.7 years, follow-up 0.35 years) indicated limited effect of ACE inhibitors on aortic growth [20]. In addition, ACE inhibitors showed to be less effective in slowing aortic dilatation compared with losartan in a mouse model [44]. This may be due to simultaneous inhibition of AT1 and AT2 pathway of ACE inhibitors, leading to a less protective effect than AT1 receptor blockade alone. Larger, randomized clinical trials are needed to better evaluate the safety and potential benefits of ACE inhibitors on aortic growth.

10.2.4 Calcium Channel Blockers

Calcium channel blockers have been recognized as an important agent in vascular remodeling and are considered an alternative medication if β-blockers are not tolerated. In mice models of abdominal aortic aneurysm, calcium channel blockers reduced the progression of aortic aneurysm by an anti-inflammatory effect which was independent of its antihypertensive effect [21–23]. The levels of MMP-2, MMP-9, and tumor necrosis factor-α (TNF-α) were decreased in the aortic wall after calcium channel blocker treatment [21–23].

However, the evidence of efficacy and safety in patients with congenital heart disease or genetic syndrome-related aortopathy is very limited [20, 24]. In a Marfan mouse study, calcium channel blockers were even noted to accelerate aortic aneurysm growth, rupture, and premature lethality [25]. The mechanism may be through activation of AT1 receptor-mediated ERK1/2 pathway, followed by increased TGF-β signaling cascades. Therefore, calcium channel blockers should be used with caution in patients with congenital heart disease or genetic syndrome-related aortopathy [25].

10.2.5 Statins

Statins are primarily used in the treatment of atherosclerosis disease to reduce blood cholesterol levels. In small studies of abdominal aortic aneurysm, statins are noted to suppress the production of MMP-9, prevent progressive aortic dilatation, and decrease long-term mortality [26, 27]. Goel et al. reported that the dilatation of the ascending aortic size was less in patients with bicuspid aortic valve treated with statin (76 patients) than the control group (71 patients) [28]. Such protection with preserved elastin volume in the aortic wall was also reported in a Marfan mouse model [29]. Although statin is generally safe, some adverse effects should be cautioned such as hepatic dysfunction, myalgia, and rarely rhabdomyolysis. Large-scale clinical trials are needed for further efficacy evaluation.

10.2.6 Tetracyclines

Doxycycline, a tetracycline, was noted to delay rupture of aortic aneurysm in mice models of Marfan syndrome via inhibiting the expression of matrix metalloproteinases (MMP-2, MMP-9) [30, 31]. In a small human pilot study of abdominal aortic aneurysm, doxycycline decreased the growth rate of aneurysm [32]. However, the empirical evidences in patients with aortopathies are still very limited.

10.3 Conclusion

Patients with congenital heart diseases or genetic disorder-related aortopathies require multidisciplinary care which includes close monitoring of aortic dimension, strict control of cardiovascular risk factors, timely medical intervention, and prophylactic operation. At present, similar medical therapies have been recommended in patients with Marfan syndrome or congenital heart disease-related aortopathy, though limited evidences exist in the latter. Aggressive blood pressure control is important since hypertension will accelerate the aortic dilatation. β-Blockers are still recommended as first-line medication for these patients. However, angiotensin receptor blockade, losartan, can safely be considered as an alternative treatment to β-blockers. A combination therapy with losartan and β-blockers may offer more protection especially in those with severe or progressive aortic dilatation. Other medications influenced the angiotensin pathway or TGF-β mediated activation pathway, including ACE inhibitors, Ca-antagonists, statins, and tetracyclines, which have also been demonstrated with some potential benefits against aortic dilatation.

With the advances in understanding the molecular mechanisms of aortopathies, precision medicine shall target the underlying defect individually. We are waiting for the results from many ongoing trials which may help us to move the therapeutic approaches from current phenotype-/syndrome-driven strategies to genotype-/pathogenesis-driven strategies.

References

1. Francois K (2015) Aortopathy associated with congenital heart disease: a current literature review. Ann Pediatr Cardiol 8:25–36
2. Attenhofer Jost CH, Greutmann M, Connolly HM et al (2014) Medical treatment of aortic aneurysms in Marfan syndrome and other heritable conditions. Curr Cardiol Rev 10:161–171
3. Abdulkareem N, Smelt J, Jahangiri M (2013) Bicuspid aortic valve aortopathy: genetics, pathophysiology and medical therapy. Interact Cardiovasc Thorac Surg 17:554–559
4. Zanjani KS, Niwa K (2013) Aortic dilatation and aortopathy in congenital heart diseases. J Cardiol 61:16–21
5. Hiratzka LF, Bakris GL, Beckman JA et al (2010) 2010 ACCF/AHA/AATS/ACR/ASA/SCA/SCAI/SIR/STS/SVM guidelines for the diagnosis and management of patients with Thoracic Aortic Disease: a report of the American College of Cardiology Foundation/American Heart Association Task Force on Practice Guidelines, American Association for Thoracic Surgery, American College of Radiology, American Stroke Association, Society of Cardiovascular Anesthesiologists, Society for Cardiovascular Angiography and Interventions, Society of Interventional Radiology, Society of Thoracic Surgeons, and Society for Vascular Medicine. Circulation 121:e266–e369
6. Canadas V, Vilacosta I, Bruna I et al (2010) Marfan syndrome. Part 2: treatment and management of patients. Nat Rev Cardiol 7:266–276
7. Shores J, Berger KR, Murphy EA et al (1994) Progression of aortic dilatation and the benefit of long-term beta-adrenergic blockade in Marfan's syndrome. N Engl J Med 330:1335–1341
8. Ladouceur M, Fermanian C, Lupoglazoff JM et al (2007) Effect of beta-blockade on ascending aortic dilatation in children with the Marfan syndrome. Am J Cardiol 99:406–409
9. Salim MA, Alpert BS, Ward JC et al (1994) Effect of beta-adrenergic blockade on aortic root rate of dilation in the Marfan syndrome. Am J Cardiol 74:629–633
10. Halpern BL, Char F, Murdoch JL et al (1971) A prospectus on the prevention of aortic rupture in the Marfan syndrome with data on survivorship without treatment. Johns Hopkins Med J 129:123–129
11. Habashi JP, Judge DP, Holm TM et al (2006) Losartan, an AT1 antagonist, prevents aortic aneurysm in a mouse model of Marfan syndrome. Science 312:117–121
12. Brooke BS, Habashi JP, Judge DP et al (2008) Angiotensin II blockade and aortic-root dilation in Marfan's syndrome. N Engl J Med 358:2787–2795
13. Chiu HH, Wu MH, Wang JK et al (2013) Losartan added to β–blockade therapy for aortic root dilation in Marfan syndrome: a randomized, open-label pilot study. Mayo Clin Proc 88:271–276
14. Groenink M, den Hartog AW, Franken R et al (2013) Losartan reduces aortic dilatation rate in adults with Marfan syndrome: A randomized controlled trial. Eur Heart J 34:3491–3500

15. Pees C, Laccone F, Hagl M et al (2013) Usefulness of losartan on the size of the ascending aorta in an unselected cohort of children, adolescents, and young adults with Marfan syndrome. Am J Cardiol 112:1477–1483
16. Franken R, den Hartog AW, Radonic T et al (2015) Beneficial outcome of losartan therapy depends on type of *FBN1* mutation in Marfan syndrome. Circ. Cardiovasc. Genet 8:383–388
17. Hackam DG, Thiruchelvam D, Redelmeier DA (2006) Angiotensin-converting enzyme inhibitors and aortic rupture: a population-based case-control study. Lancet 368:659–665
18. Yetman AT, Bornemeier RA, McCrindle BW (2005) Usefulness of enalapril versus propranolol or atenolol for prevention of aortic dilation in patients with the Marfan syndrome. Am J Cardiol 95:1125–1127
19. Phomakay V, Huett WG, Gossett JM (2014) β-Blockers and Angiotensin Converting Enzyme Inhibitors: Comparison of Effects on Aortic Growth in Pediatric Patients with Marfan Syndrome. J Pediatr 165:951–955
20. Williams A, Kenny D, Wilson D et al (2012) Effects of atenolol, perindopril and verapamil on haemodynamic and vascular function in Marfan syndrome - a randomized, double-blind, crossover trial. Eur J Clin Invest 42:891–899
21. Yokokura H, Hiromatsu S, Akashi H et al (2007) Effects of calcium channel blocker azelnidipine on experimental abdominal aortic aneurysms. Surg Today 37:468–473
22. Mieth A, Revermann M, Babelova A et al (2013) L-type calcium channel inhibitor diltiazem prevents aneurysm formation by blood pressure-independent anti-inflammatory effects. Hypertension 62:1098–1104
23. Kurobe H, Matsuoka Y, Hirata Y et al (2013) Azelnidipine suppresses the progression of aortic aneurysm in wild mice model through anti-inflammatory effects. J Thorac Cardiovasc Surg 146:1501–1508
24. Rossi-Foulkes R, Roman MJ, Rosen SE et al (1999) Phenotypic features and impact of beta blocker or calcium antagonist therapy on aortic lumen size in the Marfan syndrome. Am J Cardiol 83:1364–1368
25. Doyle JJ, Doyle AJ, Wilson NK et al (2015) A deleterious gene-by-environment interaction imposed by calcium channel blockers in Marfan syndrome. Elife 27;4. doi:10.7554/eLife.08648
26. Nagashima H, Aoka Y, Sakomura Y et al (2002) A 3-hydroxy-3-methylglutaryl coenzyme a reductase inhibitor, cerivastatin, suppresses production of matrix metalloproteinase-9 in human abdominal aortic aneurysm wall. J Vasc Surg 36:158–163
27. Schouten O, van Laanen JH, Boersma E et al (2006) Statins are associated with a reduced infrarenal abdominal aortic aneurysm growth. Eur J Vasc Endovasc Surg 32:21–26
28. Goel SS, Tuzcu EM, Agarwal S et al (2011) Comparison of ascending aortic size in patients with severe bicuspid aortic valve stenosis treated with versus without a statin drug. Am J Cardiol 108:1458–1462
29. McLoughlin D, McGuinness J, Byrne J et al (2011) Pravastatin reduces Marfan aortic dilation. Circulation 124:S168–S173
30. Xiong W, Knispel RA, Dietz HC et al (2008) Doxycycline delays aneurysm rupture in a mouse model of Marfan syndrome. J Vasc Surg 47:166–172
31. Chung AW, Yang HH, Radomski MW et al (2008) Long-term doxycycline is more effective than atenolol to prevent thoracic aortic aneurysm in marfan syndrome through the inhibition of matrix metalloproteinase-2 and -9. Circ Res 102:e73–e85
32. Mosorin M, Juvonen J, Biancari F et al (2001) Use of doxycycline to decrease the growth rate of abdominal aortic aneurysms: A randomized, double-blind, placebo-controlled pilot study. J Vasc Surg 34:606–610
33. Brophy CM, Tilson JE, Eilson MD (1989) Propranolol stimulates the crosslinking of matrix components in skin from the aneurysm-prone blotchy mouse. J Surg Res 46:330–332
34. Haouzi A, Berglund H, Pelikan PC et al (1997) Heterogeneous aortic response to acute beta-adrenergic blockade in Marfan syndrome. Am Heart J 133:60–63

35. Selamet Tierney ES, Feingold B et al (2007) Beta-Blocker therapy does not alter the rate of aortic root dilation in pediatric patients with Marfan syndrome. J Pediatr 150:77–82
36. Gersony DR, McClaughlin MA, Jin Z (2007) The effect of b-blocker therapy on clinical outcome in patients with Marfan's syndrome: a meta-analysis. Int J Cardiol 114:303–308
37. Neptune ER, Frischmeyer PA, Arking DE et al (2003) Dysregulation of TGF-beta activation contributes to pathogenesis in Marfan syndrome. Nat Genet 33:407–411
38. Isogai Z, Ono RN, Ushiro S et al (2003) Latent transforming growth factor b-binding protein 1 interacts with fibrillin and is a microfibril-associated protein. J Biol Chem 278:2750–2757
39. Lacro RV, Dietz HC, Sleeper LA et al (2014) Atenolol versus losartan in children and young adults with Marfan's syndrome. N Engl J Med 371:2061–2071
40. Milleron O, Arnoult F, Ropers J et al (2015) Marfan Sartan: a randomized, double-blind, placebo-controlled trial. Eur Heart J 36:2160–2166
41. Forteza A, Evangelista A, Sanchez V et al (2016) Efficacy of losartan vs. atenolol for the prevention of aortic dilation in Marfan syndrome: a randomized clinical trial. Eur Heart J 37:978–985
42. Huang W, Alhenc GF, Osborne-Pellegrin MJ (1998) Protection of the arterial internal elastic lamina by inhibition of the renin-angiotensin system in the rat. Circulation Res 82:879–890
43. Lu H, Rateri DL, Cassis LA et al (2008) The role of the renin–angiotensin system in aortic aneurysmal diseases. Curr Hypertens Rep 10:99–106
44. Xiong W, Meisinger T, Knispel R et al (2012) MMP-2 regulates Erk1/2 phosphorylation and aortic dilatation in Marfan syndrome. Circ Res 110:e92–e101
45. Habashi JP, Doyle JJ, Holm TM et al (2011) Angiotensin II type 2 receptor signaling attenuates aortic aneurysm in mice through ERK antagonism. Science 332:361–365
46. Holm TM, Habashi JP, Doyle JJ et al (2011) Noncanonical TGF beta signaling contributes to aortic aneurysm progression in Marfan syndrome mice. Science 332:358–361

Chapter 11
Clinical Diagnosis and Surgical Therapy of the Ascending Aorta and the Aortic Arch

Christian Detter and Jens Brickwedel

Abstract Thoracic aortic aneurysms have an incidence of 5–10 per 100 000 patients per year with a peak in the sixth and seventh decade. Males are affected 2–4 times more than females. The majority of thoracic aortic aneurysms occur in the ascending aorta (51 %), followed by the descending aorta (38 %), and the aortic arch (11 %).

Aortic aneurysms occur due to arterial wall degeneration, most commonly caused by arteriosclerosis, often in combination with hypertension. However, arterial wall degeneration is also evident in patients with congenital connective tissue disorders, such as Marfan syndrome (MFS), Loeys-Dietz syndrome, and Ehlers-Danlos syndrome and in patients with bicuspid aortic valve (BAV) and aortic isthmus stenosis caused by turbulent aortic flow.

Thoracic aortic aneurysms are typically asymptomatic and are often detected during routine imaging investigations or during elective preoperative screening. Since the growth rate of thoracic aneurysms is relatively slow, it often reaches a significant size before the manifestation of clinical symptoms. The biggest risk of an aortic aneurysm is an aortic rupture or acute aortic dissection. The risk for an aortic rupture is dependent on the diameter, the etiology, and the localization of the aneurysm.

To avoid acute aortic dissection or rupture with high early mortality, prophylactic surgery of the ascending aorta should be performed when indicated according to the recommendation of the AHA and ESC guidelines.

The aortic diameter is a major criterion for recommendation for elective replacement of the ascending aorta. These recommendations are markedly influenced by the underlying etiology and histopathology of aortic disease as well as other specific risk factors.

This chapter describes the clinical diagnosis and indication for surgery as well as the different techniques of surgical therapy of the ascending aorta and the aortic arch.

C. Detter, M.D. (✉) • J. Brickwedel, M.D.
Department of Cardiovascular Surgery, University Heart Center Hamburg, Martinistraße 52, 20246 Hamburg, Germany
e-mail: detter@uke.de; https://www.uhz.de

K. Niwa, H. Kaemmerer (eds.), *Aortopathy*, DOI 10.1007/978-4-431-56071-5_11

Keywords Thoracic aortic disease • Aortic arch surgery • Aortic dissection • Circulatory arrest • Cardiopulmonary bypass

11.1 Aneurysm of the Thoracic Aorta

11.1.1 Definition and Etiology

By definition, aortic aneurysm refers to a permanent, localized dilatation of the aortic diameter of at least 50 % increase in diameter compared with the expected norm diameter [8, 19].

Thoracic aortic aneurysms are subdivided according to its anatomical location into aneurysms of the ascending aorta, the aortic arch, and the descending aorta. Simultaneous involvement of more than one segment is not uncommon.

An aneurysm of the ascending aorta is located between the aortic valve annulus and the aortic arch. Anatomically, the ascending aorta is divided into two sections: (1) the aortic root, which includes the aortic annulus, the aortic valve with its three sinuses, and the left and right coronary orifices, and (2) the tubular part of the ascending aorta. The complexity of the surgical treatment and the operative risk is greatly influenced by the location of the aneurysm, i.e., whether the aortic root (aortic root aneurysm) is involved or not.

An aneurysm of the aortic arch is located between the brachiocephalic trunk and the left subclavian artery, while descending thoracic aneurysms are located distal to the left subclavian artery.

Aortic aneurysms occur due to arterial wall degeneration. The most common cause for arterial wall degeneration is arteriosclerosis, often in combination with hypertension. However, arterial wall degeneration is also evident in patients with congenital connective tissue disorders such as Marfan syndrome, Loeys-Dietz syndrome, and Ehlers-Danlos syndrome. Marfan syndrome is the most frequent heritable connective tissue disorder that is inherited in an autosomal dominant fashion and is caused by mutations in the fibrillin-1 gene.

Aortic aneurysms can also occur posttraumatic, following a deceleration trauma, due to poststenotic dilatation of the aortic valve particularly in patients with bicuspid aortic valve (BAV), due to aortic isthmus stenosis which causes a turbulent flow in the aorta, due to pregnancy, and due to aortitis.

Aortitis can be commonly caused by viral or bacterial (evidently syphilis) infections; autoimmune vascular disease, e.g., giant cell arteritis, Takayasu's arteritis, rheumatoid arthritis, Kawasaki syndrome, and polyarteritis; and IgG4-related diseases. At present, bacterial aortitis is very uncommon in westernized countries due to the fact that people receive early antibiotic treatment for syphilis.

11.1.2 Epidemiology

The incidence of thoracic aortic aneurysm is 5–10 per 100 000 patients per annum with a peak in the sixth and seventh decade [19]. Females and males have similar incidences of thoracic aortic disease, but the age at diagnosis is a decade higher in females (70s) than in men (60s). The majority of thoracic aortic aneurysms occur in the ascending aorta (60 %), followed by the descending aorta (38 %) and, finally, the aortic arch (11 %) [9].

If a thoracic aortic aneurysm is diagnosed during the second to fifth decade, the most probable cause is an underlying genetic disease. Typically, aortic root dilatation is the predominant aortic manifestation in individuals with connective tissue disease such as Marfan syndrome and Loeys-Dietz syndrome. In contrast, supracommissural aneurysms without aortic root involvement are commonly seen in arteriosclerotic disease.

11.1.3 Symptoms and Clinical Findings

Thoracic aortic aneurysms are typically asymptomatic and are often detected by coincidence during routine investigations, such as thoracic X-ray, CT, or MRI, or during elective preoperative screening. Since the growth rate of thoracic aneurysms is relatively slow, it often reaches a significant size before the manifestation of clinical symptoms due to compression of neighboring and anatomical structures. Dyspnea, coughing, hemoptysis, and stridor occur in the presence of compression of the trachea or the main bronchus with a consecutive tracheal shift. Compression of the esophagus causes dysphasia, while compression of intrathoracic structures can cause thoracic and lower back pain. A typical symptom of aortic arch aneurysm is hoarseness due to stretching of the left recurrent nerve. In the presence of an aortic root dilatation which leads to a high-grade aortic valve regurgitation, patients might complain of unspecific retrosternal chest pain or reduced exercise tolerance.

Acute pain is often an indication of a sudden increase in size of a thoracic aneurysm. Ascending aortic aneurysms mostly cause thoracic pain; aortic arch aneurysms could refer pain to the neck and jaw, and descending aortic aneurysms cause localized shoulder blade pain.

Aortic rupture and an acute aortic dissection are the most dreadful complications, presenting as excruciating thoracic pain which typically refers to the back.

11.1.4 Imaging Techniques

The precise localization and the extension of the aneurysm play a vital role in determining the therapeutic management and surgical approach. It is of particular importance to clarify whether or not the ascending, the descending, and/or the aortic arch with its supra-aortic vessels are involved in the aneurysm. The gold standard for diagnostic imaging is the high-resolution multislice spiral computed tomography (CT) with the option for three-dimensional (3-D) reconstruction or an angio-magnetic resonance imaging (MRI). Due to the different cross sections, the angio-MRI optimally displays neighboring soft tissue structures. The 3-D reconstruction, in particular, is of great importance in determining the extent of the aneurysm and the choice of surgical approach and therapy. It has the added advantage of assisting in accurate planning of surgical aortic procedures such as hybrid or endovascular operations in complex aortic pathologies.

The transthoracic and transesophageal echocardiogram are both accurate and useful in investigating the aortic root with the proximal ascending and proximal descending aorta. Investigation of the aortic arch with ultrasound, however, is limited due to the presence of the trachea. Furthermore, valve and myocardial function can be evaluated.

11.1.5 Natural History and Risk of Rupture

The diameter plays a deciding role in the incremental growth of the aortic aneurysm. If the diameter is less than 5 cm, the growth rate is statistically estimated at 0.17 cm per annum. If the diameter is greater than 5 cm, the growth rate is estimated at 0.79 cm per annum [4]. The above mentioned findings directly influence the long-term survival of these patients. The 3-year survival with a diameter less than 5 cm is 93 %, with a diameter greater than 5 cm is 60 %, and with a diameter greater than 6 cm is only 38 % [4].

The biggest risk of an aortic aneurysm is an aortic rupture or dissection. The risk for an aortic rupture is dependent on the diameter, the etiology, and the localization of the aneurysm [15]. There is a rapid increase in the risk of dissection or rupture when the aortic diameter is 60 mm for the ascending aorta in degenerative disease. However, the risk for rupture is markedly increased in patients with connective tissue diseases (e.g., Marfan syndrome, Loeys-Dietz syndrome). In a study conducted by Perko et al., the risk for rupture with an aortic diameter of less than 5 cm was 14 %, between 5 and 6 cm was 23 %, and greater than 6 cm was 66 %. The cumulative risk in patients with an aortic dissection was twice as high as compared to patients without a dissection. The mortality of untreated aneurysms was 78 % after 8 years, of whom 59 % died of aortic rupture [17].

11.2 Surgical Therapy

11.2.1 Indication for Surgical Therapy

To avoid acute aortic dissection or rupture, prophylactic surgery of the ascending aorta should be performed when indicated according to the recommendation of the AHA and ESC guidelines [7, 8]. Furthermore, the operative risk of a planned procedure is low in aortic surgery affecting the ascending aorta. Compared to high early mortality in an acute setting, both early and late mortality improve significantly with prophylactic intervention.

The recommendations for asymptomatic patients with ascending aortic aneurysms are depicted in Table 11.1. The aortic diameter is a major criterion for recommendation for elective replacement of the ascending aorta. These recommendations are markedly influenced by the underlying etiology and histopathology of aortic disease, such as patients with bicuspid aortic valve (BAV), Marfan syndrome (MFS), or Loeys-Dietz syndrome, as well as other specific risk factors.

11.2.2 Surgical Therapy of the Ascending Aorta

Open aortic surgery is performed through a median sternotomy approach, if the ascending aorta is affected. In some cases, a minimal invasive approach such as a partial upper hemisternotomy can be performed. Potential advantages are reduced pain, shorter recovery time, and improved cosmetic result. Minimal invasive approaches are mainly performed in younger patients with low operative risk like in Marfan syndrome.

Surgery is performed using extracorporeal circulation and cardioplegia-induced cardiac arrest. The aim of aortic surgery is to totally resect and replace the aortic aneurysm using a polyester vascular prosthesis. In most situations, the ascending

Table 11.1 Recommendation for elective replacement of the ascending aorta (2014 ESC guidelines [7][a])

Etiology aortic disease	
Degenerative or patients without connective tissue disorder	≥55 mm
Patients with bicuspid aortic valve (BAV)	≥55 mm
Patients with bicuspid aortic valve (BAV) and risk factors[a]	≥50 mm
Patients with Marfan syndrome (MFS)	≥50 mm
Patients with Marfan syndrome (MFS) and risk factors[b]	≥45 mm
Patients with Loeys-Dietz syndrome	>42 mm

[a]Bicuspid aortic valve with risk factors (ESC): aortic coarctation, hypertension, family history for aortic dissection, progression of the aortic diameter of <0.3 cm/year

[b]MFS with risk factors (ESC): family history for aortic dissection, progression of the aortic diameter of <0.3 cm/year, severe aortic or mitral regurgitation, or desire for pregnancy

aorta can be clamped before the origin of the innominate artery avoiding circulatory arrest. If the proximal or even the total aortic arch is involved or the aorta is dissected, hypothermic circulatory arrest is necessary for a bloodless surgical field and for cerebral protection.

Depending on the extent of the aneurysm, with or without the aortic root, there are different techniques available (Fig. 11.1).

In ascending aortic aneurysms without involvement of the aortic root, a supracoronary replacement of the ascending aorta can be performed using a tubular vascular prosthesis with low operative risk between 1 and 3 % early mortality. If the aortic root is affected (aortic root aneurysm), the surgical procedure is more complicated, because the aortic valve and the coronary ostia originate from the root. Depending on aortic valve pathology, there are two different techniques of aortic root replacement:

- If the aortic valve is affected (e.g., aortic stenosis or complex severe aortic regurgitation), the entire aortic root and valve have to be replaced with a valved composite graft using a biologic or mechanical valve conduit (Bentall procedure). The choice of biological tissue or a mechanical valve depends on patient age and risk factors for long-term anticoagulation therapy with vitamin K antagonist, such as warfarin.
- If the aortic valve is unaffected and the valve cusps are normal (no aortic stenosis or severe aortic regurgitation with complex pathology), the aortic root is resected and replaced by a vascular graft, while the aortic valve can be preserved using valve-sparing root replacement techniques, such as the
- Reimplantation (David procedure) or the remodeling technique (Yacoub or David procedure) with reimplantation of the coronary buttons.

Using valve-sparing root replacement technique, the entire diseased aortic root including all three aortic sinuses is resected, while the native aortic valve is preserved. Both coronary ostia are removed for later reimplantation into a Dacron graft. There are two different valve-sparing techniques: the reimplantation procedure according to David and the remodeling technique according to Yacoub.

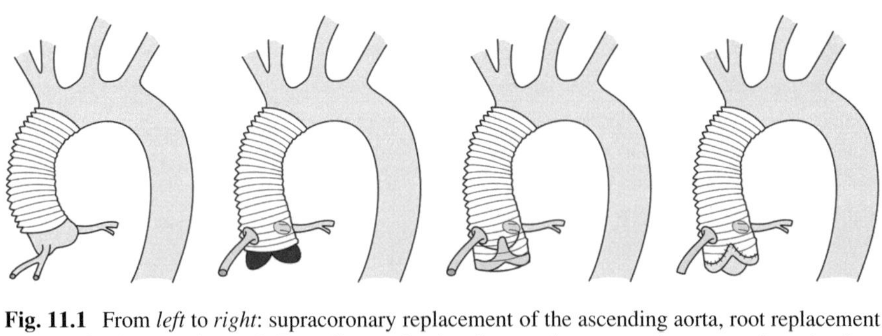

Fig. 11.1 From *left* to *right*: supracoronary replacement of the ascending aorta, root replacement with a valved composite graft (Bentall procedure), valve-sparing root replacement using reimplantation (David procedure), or remodeling technique (Yacoub procedure) with reimplantation of the coronary buttons

During the reimplantation procedure, a tubular or Valsalva graft is fixed by subvalvular sutures below the level of the aortic annulus. The aortic valve is then reimplanted into the graft using a continuous suture technique with respect to the valve anatomy (David technique, see Fig. 11.2). Using the remodeling technique, a tubular graft is incised at the base in three equal parts and tailored to the shape of the three aortic sinuses. The aortic valve with the three commissures is then sewn into the three incisions of the vascular graft to create neosinuses (Yacoub technique). Several studies showed excellent results for both valve-sparing root replacement techniques. David reported excellent freedom from reoperation at 15 to 18 years of 94.8 % [3]. Also both techniques show good long-term results, the David procedure demonstrated higher freedom from significant long-term aortic insufficiency in Marfan syndrome because the aortic root and annulus are better stabilized by the circular subannular fixation. Thus, current evidence is in favor of David rather than Yacoub technique in pathologies such as Marfan syndrome or other connective tissue disorders and in excessive annular dilatation.

If the aortic root and the aortic valve are diseased and have to be replaced, a combined replacement of the aortic root and valve with reimplantation of the coronary ostia is performed using a composite aortic valve graft (Bentall procedure, see Fig. 11.2). The choice of biological tissue or a mechanical valve depends on patient age and risk factors for anticoagulation therapy. Although mechanical valves have lifetime durability, there is need for lifelong anticoagulation, such as Coumadin with increased risk of bleeding complications. Using biological valves, lifelong antiplatelet therapy is sufficient for anticoagulation, and Coumadin is usually not necessary to prevent the development of blood clots. However, the durability compared to mechanical valves is poor with need of reoperation after 10–15 years in the majority of patients. In case of valve-sparing techniques, anticoagulation therapy is not required, and valve-related complications are rare. This is particularly important for younger women, who are planning to be pregnant. Furthermore, freedom from reoperation is excellent.

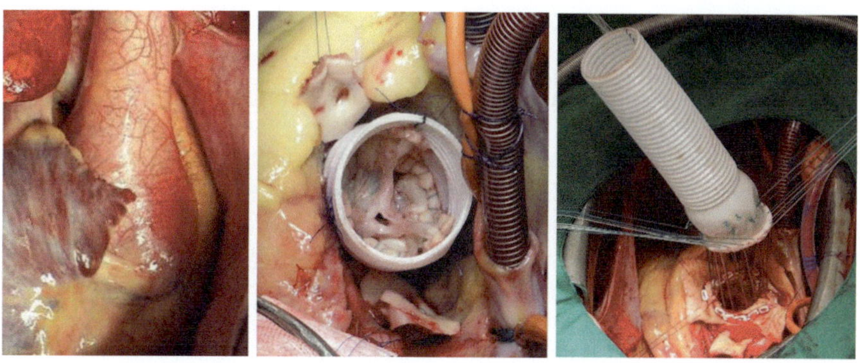

Fig. 11.2 From *left* to *right*: aortic root aneurysm, valve-sparing root replacement according to David with reimplantation of the native aortic valve into a Dacron graft, valved composite graft using a biologic valve conduit (Bentall procedure)

11.3 Surgical Therapy of the Aortic Arch

11.3.1 Indication for Operation

The surgical therapy of aortic arch aneurysms still remains a big challenge for the surgeon due to its topography. The introduction of deep hypothermic circulatory arrest for cerebral protection by Griepp and colleagues in 1975 made total aortic arch replacements by means of a vascular prosthesis possible.

The difficulty of the therapy can be attributed to the complex location of the aortic arch and the origin of the aortic arch vessels. The main intraoperative risk for the patient is that of cerebrovascular accident. Furthermore, the opening of the arch during surgery with interruption of the blood flow poses a particular risk for spinal cord ischemia with resultant paraplegia. Of utmost importance is also the sparing of the vagal and recurrent nerves. Patients must be informed preoperatively about the risk of postoperative stroke, paraplegia, and hoarseness.

Surgery for asymptomatic patients with isolated degenerative or atherosclerotic aortic arch aneurysm is indicated when a maximal diameter of ≥55 mm is reached or in patients who present symptoms or signs of local compression (2014 ESC guidelines [7]).

Earlier results published by Crawford reported a 30-day mortality between 9 and 26 %, depending on the extent of the aortic aneurysm. At present, this mortality during elective interventions has been reduced to 3.9–11.1 % [6, 21]. This can be primarily attributed to the improved techniques for cerebral protection (see Sect. 11.3.3). This justifies a prophylactic aortic arch replacement according to AHA and ESC guidelines. However, decision-making should weigh the perioperative risks, since aortic arch replacement is associated with higher rates of mortality and stroke than in surgery of the ascending and descending aorta (2014 ESC guidelines [7]).

11.3.2 Surgical Approach

The surgical approach in aortic arch pathology is determined by the extent of the aneurysm, as well as the local findings. If the ascending aorta is involved, a median sternotomy is the standard approach. However, if the arch aneurysm extends into the descending aorta, a lateral thoracotomy or bilateral anterior thoracotomy (clamshell approach) should be considered due to the technical difficulty via median sternotomy. An alternative surgical option for combined diseases of the aortic arch and the descending aorta is the "elephant trunk" (ET) technique (Borst 1983 [2]) during which the distal end of the prosthesis is positioned in the proximal descending aorta in preparation for the second surgical approach. A modified and more sophisticated method is the "frozen elephant trunk" (FET) technique, during which a hybrid stent graft prosthesis is used [12, 24]. The advantage of the FET is the possibility of a combined replacement of the ascending aorta, the aortic arch, and the proximal descending aorta in one stage. During this procedure the stented graft is placed in the proximal descending aorta in an antegrade fashion through the opened aortic arch via a median sternotomy.

11.3.3 Cerebral Protection and Extracorporeal Circulation

The complexity of aortic arch surgery is due to its awkward ventral to dorsal anatomical location and the unavoidable necessity to interrupt brain circulation during the opening of the aortic arch. This can result in irreversible brain cell damage. Therefore, aortic arch replacement is performed using extracorporeal circulation (ECC) and hypothermic circulatory arrest. During the last two decades, various techniques have been developed for cerebral protection in order to avoid neurological deficit. These well-established techniques primarily distinguish between the depth of the hypothermia and the technique of the selective cerebral perfusion [25]:

- Deep hypothermic circulatory arrest (<20 °C) without cerebral perfusion
- Deep hypothermic circulatory arrest (<20 °C) with retrograde cerebral perfusion via superior vena cava
- Moderate hypothermia and circulatory arrest (24–28 °C) with selective antegrade (uni- or bilateral) cerebral perfusion

11.3.3.1 Hypothermic Circulatory Arrest

Hypothermic circulatory arrest (HCA) alone was the standard technique in arch surgery during the last few decades and is still deemed to be secure technique for short circulatory arrest times. The risk for a permanent neurological dysfunction (PND) is estimated to be 1.9–9.6 % and for transient neurological deficit up to 20 % [14, 16]. The risk for neurological deficit is directly dependent on the time of circulatory arrest, increasing dramatically even after just 25 min of HCA [22]. The mortality rate also increases significantly after 1 h of HCA [22]. Furthermore, there is the added risk of clotting disorders due to the extended extracorporeal circulatory (ECC) time required for the long cooling and rewarming phase.

Various cerebral perfusion techniques in combination to HCA have been developed in order to reduce the high incidence of cerebral complications and, hence, mortality and morbidity.

11.3.3.2 Retrograde Cerebral Perfusion

Deep HCA (<20 °C) combined with retrograde cerebral perfusion via the superior vena cava was occasionally used for cerebral protection. Theoretical advantages are improved intracranial hypothermia, embolic washout, and the reduction of toxic metabolic products. Randomized controlled studies, however, have not reported an improved neurological or neuropsychological outcome using this method.

11.3.3.3 Selective Antegrade Cerebral Perfusion

At present, most centers in Europe adopt the combination of circulatory arrest and selective antegrade cerebral perfusion (SACP) at moderate hypothermia (24–28 °C) as a method of choice. The use of combining SACP and HCA in comparison to isolated HCA improves cerebral ischemic tolerance with significant reduction of CVAs [13].

Antegrade cerebral perfusion can be performed uni- or bilateral, as well as using different arterial cannulation techniques. One possibility is the cannulation of the right subclavian/axillary artery or the brachiocephalic trunk, with or without an 8 mm vascular prosthesis, and to supply the left carotid artery with arterial blood via an additional perfusion catheter. The left subclavian artery can either be perfused via another perfusion catheter or be occluded by clamping or insertion of an occlusion catheter. Alternatively, perfusion catheters can be inserted selectively in all supra-aortic vessels after aortic arch opening. The method of choice is dependent on the experience of the surgeon as well as the intraoperative anatomical findings.

Advantages of SACP include the continuous supply of the brain with oxygenated blood, improved de-airing of the aortic arch, reduction of clotting disorders through the avoidance of deep hypothermia, as well as a reduction of the extra circulatory perfusion time because of a reduced cooling and rewarming phase.

Current literature on selective cerebral perfusion supports the advantages of this technique. This technique leads to a reduced rate of cerebral complications and early mortality [1, 5, 13, 23].

11.3.4 Technical Aspects of Arch Surgery

The technique of arch surgery depends on the extent of the aortic arch aneurysm as is illustrated in Fig. 11.3.

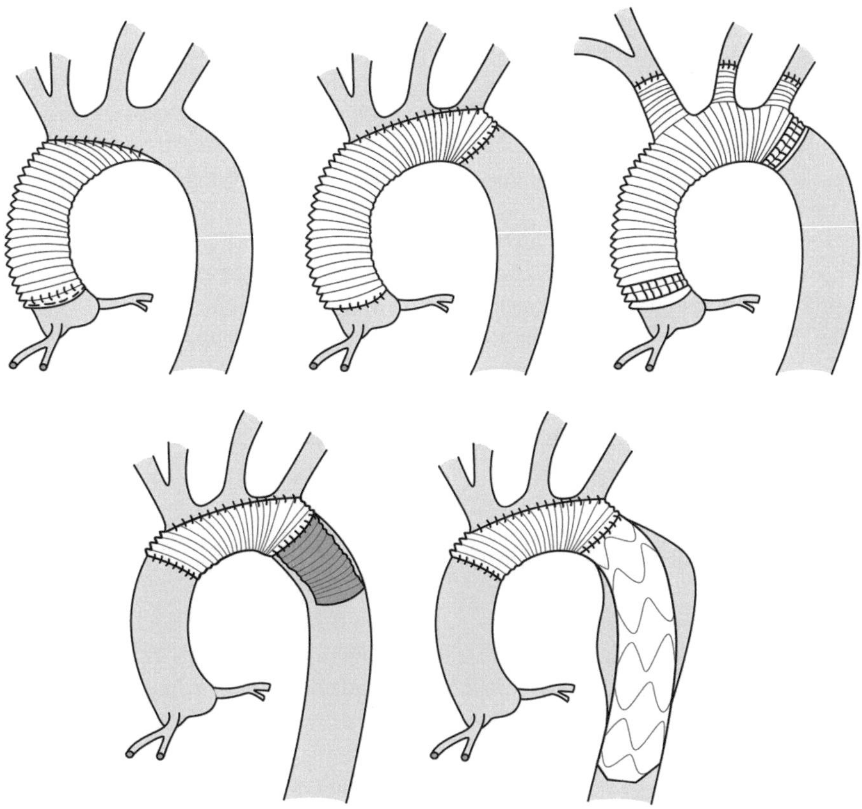

Fig. 11.3 From *left* to *right*: the technique of choice depends on the extent of the arch aneurysm
– Partial arch replacement (i.e., "hemi-arch") including the inner curvature while retaining the supra-aortic vessels
– Complete or total arch replacement, whereby the supra-aortic vessels of the big curvature are reimplanted as an island or cuff in the vascular prosthesis ("island" technique)
– Complete or total arch replacement including the replacement of the supra-aortic vessels using a branched prosthesis for the reimplantation of the arch vessels ("branched" technique)
– "Elephant trunk" technique in preparation for subsequent descending aortic replacement (two-stage procedure)
– "Frozen elephant trunk" technique for the combined replacement of the ascending aorta, the aortic arch, and the descending aorta with a combined hybrid stent graft prosthesis (one-stage procedure)

11.3.4.1 Partial Arch Replacement

Partial arch replacement is performed in addition to replacement of the ascending aorta when the aneurysm of the ascending aorta extends to the brachiocephalic trunk or also involves the proximal aortic arch. In this case, the distal anastomosis is done in a so-called open technique with circulatory arrest, i.e., without clamping the aorta. This allows a thorough visual examination of the aortic arch and the supra-aortic vessels and, hence, the complete resection of the aneurysm. The size of the implanted vascular prosthesis is chosen depending on the diameter of the remaining distal arch. Depending on the extent of the aneurysm, the smaller inner curvature is resected leaving the supra-aortic vessels in place, anastomosing the vascular prosthesis in an oblique fashion to the remaining native tissue. This has the advantage of significantly reducing the circulatory arrest time and simplifying the arch replacement because the supra-aortic vessels are not detached.

Partial aortic arch replacement is often indicated in aortic type A dissections since most aortic dissections extend beyond the brachiocephalic trunk (DeBakey type I), and clamping the dissected aortic wall is not recommended. As a general rule, the principles that apply to aortic arch aneurysms also apply to acute aortic type A aortic dissections. However, the fragile tissue of the dissected aortic wall imposes a clear surgical challenge. The dissected aortic wall is readapted, and the sutures are reinforced by using tissue glue and additional Teflon sutures to avoid further tearing of the aortic wall.

11.3.4.2 Complete Arch Replacement

Complete aortic arch replacement is indicated in the presence of aortic aneurysms that involve the entire arch with a maximal diameter $\geq$55 mm or who present symptoms or signs of local compression, in chronic dissections when a false lumen aneurysm is present, and in acute dissections when the arch is aneurysmal or there is extensive aortic arch destruction with further tears.

The aortic arch is resected and replaced with a vascular prosthesis while retaining the cuff with its supra-aortic vessels. This is followed by the reimplantation of the cuff with its vessels in the oval opening of the upper curvature of the vascular prosthesis ("island" technique). It is important to ensure a leak-proof suture line since postsurgical leakages are very difficult to repair due to its unfavorable anatomically position. If the aortic aneurysm involves the supra-aortic vessels or the vessels are dissected, a branched prosthesis is the choice of surgery ("branched" technique). Despite the improved techniques for cerebral protection and ECC systems, the mortality still remains between 4 and 15 % [6, 16, 18].

11.3.4.3 Elephant Trunk Technique

Borst et al. [2] introduced the "elephant trunk" (ET) technique for the treatment of complex diseases of the ascending aorta, aortic arch, and the descending aorta, which takes place in two stages. At the first stage, the ascending aorta as well as the aortic arch is replaced with a vascular prosthesis via a median sternotomy, and the distal end of the prosthesis is positioned in the proximal descending aorta to facilitate the second surgical stage. During ascending aortic and arch repair, the invaginated tubular graft material is positioned into the descending aorta resulting in the ET of the prosthesis floating freely in the descending aorta. Subsequently, the enveloped fold of the vascular prosthesis is anastomosed with the proximal descending aorta. Arch replacement is then performed when the invagination is withdrawn. The supra-aortic vessels are mostly implanted as a cuff in the convexity of the vascular prosthesis followed by the replacement of the ascending aorta.

At a subsequent date, the descending aorta is replaced via a lateral thoracotomy. The second approach has the advantage that the free floating ET can be used for anastomosis of an additional prosthesis. However, several complications have been reported using the ET technique, such as kinking or occlusion of the graft, spinal cord injury and malperfusion, thromboembolism, and aortic rupture during the interval between the two stages.

Ius summarized the results of several publications of conventional ET technique for the first and second stage [10]. The early mortality of the initial approach was reported as a mean of 8.9 % and the mortality of the subsequent treatment at 7.7 %, whereby only 46.3 % of the patients underwent the second operation. For this reason the ET technique has a higher overall risk [20]. Furthermore, the longtime interval between the two interventions results in a high mortality. Safi et al. reported an interval mortality of 16 % (7/45 patients). This is a clear limitation of this technique.

Alternatively, the possibility exists at subsequent treatment to implant a transfemoral aortic stent graft in the ET. This supplementary endovascular intervention following ET technique reduced the early mortality to 4.9 % [11] and, therefore, seemed a viable, low-risk subsequent approach.

11.3.4.4 Frozen Elephant Trunk Technique

The frozen elephant trunk (FET) procedure is a hybrid therapy combining conventional open surgical and endovascular techniques for a one-stage treatment of patients with extensive thoracic aortic disease. Classical indications are multifocal extensive thoracic aneurysms, acute extensive type A (DeBakey type I) dissections, and chronic dissections with false lumen aneurysms.

Since the first implant of a "custom-made" Chavan-Haverich hybrid stent graft (Curative GmbH, Dresden, Germany) in 2001, different prostheses have been developed including the commercially available JOTEC E-vita open plus prosthesis (JOTEC GmbH, Hechingen, Germany) and the Vascutek Thoraflex (Vascutek, Terumo, Inchinnan, Scotland, UK) hybrid stent graft (Fig. 11.4). Both hybrid prostheses consist of a proximal conventional gel-coated woven polyester graft and a distal self-expanding endoprosthesis constructed of polyester and nitinol ring stents. The difference between the two hybrid prostheses is that the woven vascular graft section of the E-vita hybrid prosthesis has no extra branches for the arch vessels and the supra-aortic vessels are reimplanted as an island into the vascular graft. The Thoraflex hybrid prosthesis consists of a proximal multi-branch aortic plexus graft with three arch branches for selective replacement of the supra-aortic vessels and one perfusion side branch for arterial cannulation to provide early antegrade lower body perfusion.

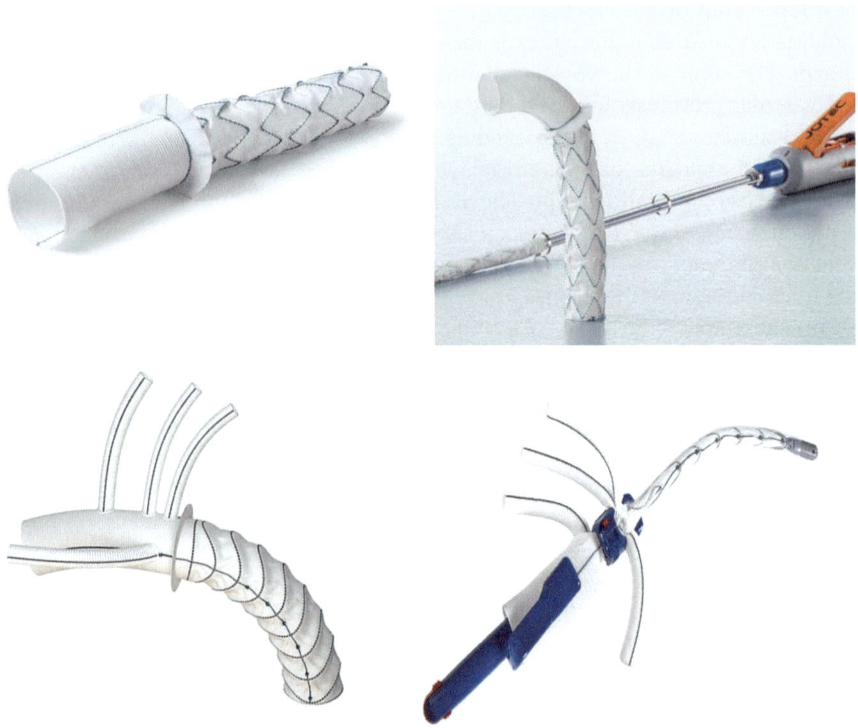

Fig. 11.4 JOTEC E-vita open plus (*above*) and Vascutek Thoraflex (*below*) hybrid stent graft prostheses with and without the delivery system. Both hybrid prostheses consist of a proximal conventional gel-coated woven polyester graft and a distal self-expanding endoprosthesis constructed of polyester and nitinol ring stents (Remark: both images are from JOTEC and Vascutek)

The hybrid stent graft prosthesis is implanted in a single-stage procedure through a median sternotomy approach during circulatory arrest with selective antegrade brain perfusion. The stent graft section is introduced in an antegrade fashion through the transected arch into the descending thoracic aorta and deployed using a delivery system. [12, 24]. After deployment of the stent graft, the incorporated vascular graft is sutured to the native aorta between the distal aortic arch and the proximal descending aorta using a circumferential running suture to provide fixation and proper hemostasis. An incorporated sewing collar between the graft segments facilitates the distal anastomosis. The hybrid stent graft comes in different stent sizes and lengths to match the individual anatomy of the patient. Thereafter, the aortic arch and the ascending aorta are replaced in conventional surgical technique using the woven polyester graft. Figure 11.5 is showing CT images of a patient with an acute type A aortic dissection preoperative and after implantation of a hybrid stent graft using the FET technique. The possible advantages of the FET technique for combined open and endovascular hybrid aortic repair are to treat

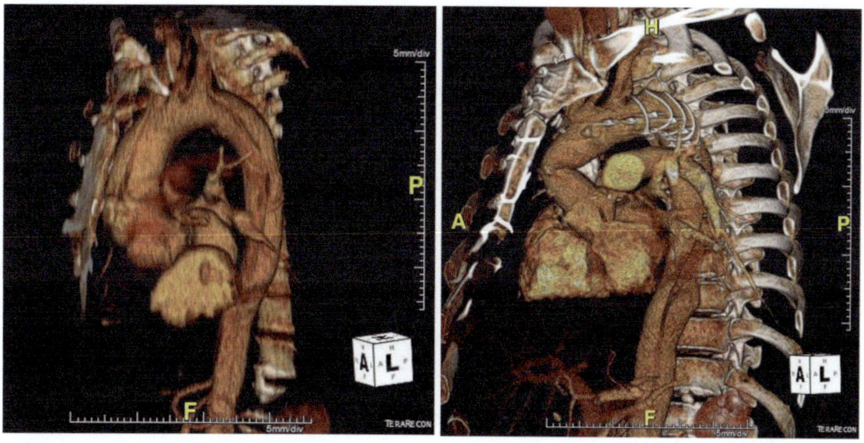

Fig. 11.5 CT image of a patient with an acute type A aortic dissection pre- and postoperative after implantation of a hybrid stent graft in frozen elephant trunk technique

patients with extensive diseases of the thoracic aorta in a single-stage procedure, to avoid the need for a second procedure to the downstream aorta, to reduce the surgical trauma, to promote remodeling in acute type A aortic dissection, or to produce an easy landing zone for secondary thoracic endovascular aortic repair (TEVAR) or open surgery if needed.

References

1. Bachet J (2010) What is the best method for brain protection in surgery of the aortic arch? Selective antegrade perfusion. Cardiol Clin 28:389–401
2. Borst HG, Walterbusch G, Schaps D (1983) Thorac Cardiovasc Surg 83:37–40
3. David TE, Feindel CM, David CM, Manlhiot C (2014) A quarter of a century of experience with aortic valve-sparing operations. J Thorac Cardiovasc Surg 148(3):872–879
4. Dapunt OE, Galla JD, Sadeghi AM, Lansman SL et al (1994) The natural history of thoracic aortic aneurysms. J Thorac Cardiovasc Surg 107:1323–1332
5. Di Bartolomeo R, Pilato E, Pacini D, Savini C, Di Eusanio M (2010) Cerebral protection during surgery of the aortic arch Multimed Manual Cardiothorac Surg. doi:10.1510/mmcts.2010.004457
6. Di Eusanio M, Berretta P, Cefarelli M, Castrovinci S, Folesani G, Alfonsi J, Pantaleo A, Murana G, Di Bartolomeo R (2015) Long-term outcomes after aortic arch surgery: results of a study involving 623 patients. Eur J Cardiothorac Surg 48:483–490
7. Erbel R, Aboyans V, Boileau C, Bossone E et al (2014) 2014 ESC guidelines on the diagnosis and treatment of aortic disease. Eur Heart J 35:2873–2926
8. Hiratzka LF, Bakris GL, Beckmann JA, Bersin RM et al (2010) 2010 ACCF/AHA/AATS/ACG/SCA/SCAI/SIR/STS/SVM guidelines for the diagnosis and management of patients with thoracic aortic disease. JACC 55(14):e27–e129
9. Isselbacher EM (2005) Thoracic and abdominal aortic aneurysm. Circulation 111:816–828
10. Ius F, Hagl C, Haverich A, Pichlmaier M (2011) Elephant trunk procedure 27 years after Borst: what remains and what is new? Eur J Cardiothorac Surg 40:1–12

11. Karck M, Kaamiya H (2008) Progress of the extended aortic aneurysms; is the frozen elephant trunk technique the next standard in the treatment of complex aortic disease including the arch? Eur J Cardiothorac Surg 33:1007–1013
12. Karck M, Hagl C, Kallenbach K, Haverich A (2003) The gut-first approach for repair of Crawford extent III thoracoabdominal aortic aneurysms. J Thorac Cardiovasc Surg 126: 602–604
13. Kazui T, Yamashita K, Washiyama N, Terada H, Bashar AHM, Suzuki K, Suzuki T (2007) Aortic arch replacement using selective cerebral perfusion. Ann Thorac Surg 83:796–798
14. Khaladj N, Shresta M, Meck S, Peterss S, Kamiya H, Kallenbach K, Winterhalter M, Hoy L, Haverich A, Hagl C (2008) Hypothermic circulatory arrest with selective antegrade cerebral perfusion in ascending aortic and aortic arch surgery: a risk factor analysis for adverse outcome in 501 patients. J Thorac Cardiovasc Surg 135(4):908–914
15. Kim JB, Spotnitz M, Lindsay ME, MacGillivray TH, Isselbacher EM, Sundt TM (2016) Risk of aortic dissection in the moderately dilated ascending aorta. JACC 68(11):1210–1219
16. Liu H, Chang Q, Zhang HT, Yu CT (2016) Predictors of adverse outcome and transient neurological dysfunction following aortic arch replacement in 626 consecutive patients in China. Heart Lung Circ xx:1–7
17. Perko MJ, Nørgaard M, Herzog TM, Olsen PS, Schroeder TV, Petterson G (1995) Ann Thorac Surg 59(5):1204–1209
18. Preventza O, Garcia A, Cooley DA, Hywood-Watson RJL et al (2015) Total aortic arch replacement: a comparative study of zone 0 hybrid arch exclusion versus traditional open repair. J Thorac Cardiovasc Surg 150:1591–1600
19. Saliba E, Sia Y (2015) The ascending aortic aneurysm: when to intervene? IJC Heart Vasculature 6:91–100
20. Safi HJ, Miller CCM, Estrera AL, Huynh TTT, Rubenstein FS, Subramaniam MH, Buja LM (2001) Staged repair of extensive aortic aneurysms: morbidity and mortality in the elephant trunk technique. Circulation 104:2938–2941
21. Settepani F, Cappai A, Basciu A, Barbone A, Tarelli G (2016) Outcome of open total arch replacement in the modern era. J Vasc Surg 63:537–545
22. Svensson LG, Kouchoukos NT, Miller DC, Bavaria JE, Coselli JS, Curi MA, Eggebrecht H, Elefteriades JA, Erbel R, Gleason TG, Lytle BW, Mitchell RS, Nienaber CA, Roselli EE, Safi HJ, Shemin RJ, Sicard GA, TM S 3rd, WY S, GH W (2008) Expert consensus document on the treatment of descending thoracic aortic disease using endovascular stent-grafts. Ann Thorac Surg 85(1 Suppl):S1–S41
23. Stamou SC, Rausch LA, Kouchoukos NT, Lobdell KW, Khabbaz K, Murphy E, Hagberg RC (2016) Comparison between antegrade and retrograde cerebral perfusion or profound hypothermia as brain protection strategies during repair of type A aortic dissection. Ann Cardiothorac Surg 5(4):328–335
24. Usui A, Fujimoto K, Ishiguchi T, Yoshikawa M, Akita T, Ueda Y (2002) Cerebrospinal dysfunction after endovascular stent-grafting via a median sternotomoy: the frozen elephant trunk procedure. Ann Thorac Surg 74(5):1825–1832
25. Yan DT, Bannon PG, Bavaria J, Coselli JS et al (2013) Consensus on hypothermia in aortic arch surgery. Ann Cardiothorac Surg 2(2):163–168

Chapter 12
Surgery (Bentall, Valve Sparing, Ross Procedure, Etc.)

Kozo Matsuo

Abstract Aortic dilatation is constantly observed in unrepaired or repaired congenital heart diseases (CHD). Aortic dilatation might cause aortic annular enlargement that will predispose to severe aortic regurgitation (AR). In such conditions, concomitant aortic valve plasty or replacement with aortic root replacement will be required. Bentall operation is root replacement with an aortic tube graft and a mechanical valve. Coronary ostia are reimplanted to the aortic graft. Remodeling method (Yacoub) and reimplantation method (David) had been developed in order to preserve the aortic valve with the same concept as the Bentall operation. These procedures are well known as valve-sparing operations. On the other hand, in Ross procedure a pulmonary autograft is used to replace the aortic root and aortic valve. RV outflow tract and pulmonary artery are reconstructed usually with homograft or other valved conduits. Superior hemodynamics, freedom from anticoagulation, and longevity of pulmonary autografts have been substantiated in many reports.

Keywords Aortic dilatation • Aortic root replacement • Bentall operation • Valve-sparing operation • Ross procedure

12.1 Introduction

In various congenital heart diseases (CHD), such as Marfan syndrome, Turner syndrome, bicuspid aortic valve (BAV) syndrome, single ventricle, and repaired or unrepaired tetralogy of Fallot (TOF), aortic dilatation is constantly observed.

Marfan syndrome is frequently associated with aortic dilatation or aortic dissection. Aortic dilatation might cause aortic annular enlargement that will in turn predispose to severe aortic regurgitation (AR). In such conditions, concomitant aortic valve plasty or replacement together with replacement of the aortic root or ascending aorta will be required. Sometimes arch replacement will also be necessary in the cases associated with arch dilation or dissection.

K. Matsuo (✉)
Chiba Cerebral and Cardiovascular Center, 575 Tsurumai, Ichihara, Chiba 290-0512, Japan
e-mail: mtso3@me.com

K. Niwa, H. Kaemmerer (eds.), *Aortopathy*, DOI 10.1007/978-4-431-56071-5_12

The Bentall operation [1] was introduced first as a root replacement for annulo-aortic ectasia (AAE) with a composite graft containing a mechanical valve.

The remodeling method [2] (Yacoub) and the reimplantation method [3] (David) had been developed with the same concept as the Bentall operation in order to preserve the aortic valve. Both procedures are well known as valve-sparing operations.

In contrast, in the Ross procedure [4], a pulmonary autograft is used to replace the aortic root and aortic valve. Enucleated RV outflow tract and the pulmonary artery are reconstructed usually with a homograft or other valved conduits. Superior hemodynamics, freedom from anticoagulation, and longevity of pulmonary autograft have been substantiated in many reports.

12.2 Aortic Root Replacement with Composite Graft – Bentall Operation

In 1968, Bentall and de Bono described the first successful complete replacement of the ascending aorta with a composite Teflon tube graft and a ball valve prosthesis (Starr valve) in a male associated with ascending aortic dilatation and aortic annular enlargement, which caused free AR. The arch vessels were not involved in the aortic dilatation.

The Bentall operation consists of aortic root and aortic valve replacement with an aortic valve conduit. The coronary arteries are reimplanted into the tube graft directly or interposing a small graft. In order to replace the ascending aorta as far distally as possible, cardiopulmonary bypass is usually established by retrograde arterial perfusion through the femoral artery. After cross-clamp of the ascending aorta, the aneurysmal ascending aorta is removed (Fig. 12.1a). The aortic valve is excised (Fig. 12.1b), and a composite tube graft prosthesis of appropriate size, including a prosthetic valve, is sutured to the aortic annulus. Usually a mechanical valve is used in this graft because of its longevity (Fig. 12.1c).

Two holes are made in the composite graft at the positions of the coronary ostia. Originally, coronary ostia were approximated to the graft and directly sutured to the

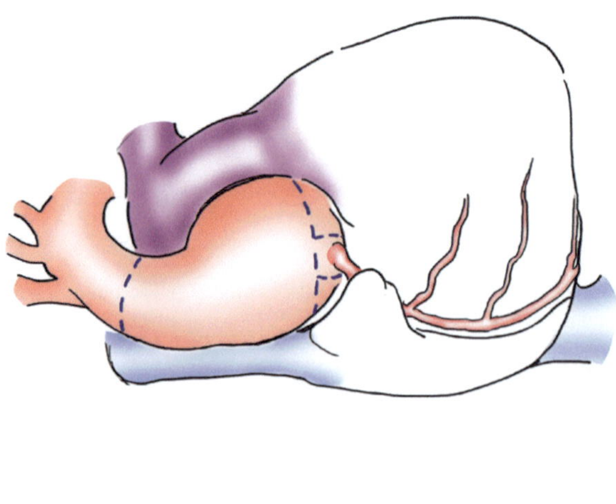

Fig. 12.1a The aneurysmal ascending aorta is removed from 10 mm above the coronary ostia to the normal distal ascending aorta

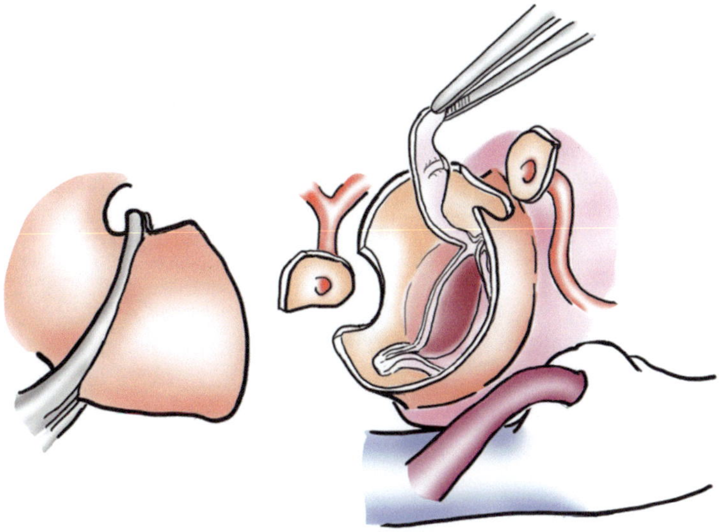

Fig. 12.1b Coronary ostia are detached as large buttons with the aortic wall. Aortic valve is removed

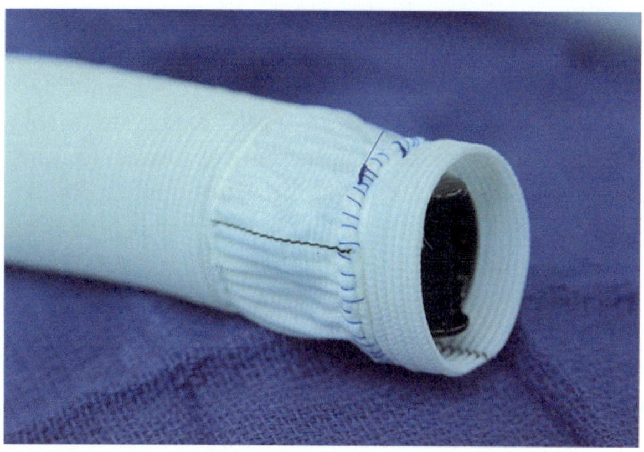

Fig. 12.1c Composite graft. A mechanical valve is fixed in the tube graft

holes of the graft. This method might cause significant tension to suture lines and bleeding, so that many modifications have been developed.

Nowadays, coronary ostia are detached as large buttons of the aortic wall and dissected free along their courses to ensure their mobility. The scalloped coronary buttons are sutured to the holes of the aortic graft directly (Carrel patch method) or interposing a small graft (Piehler method) (Fig. 12.1d).

The Bentall operation is usually indicated in AAE with a diseased aortic valve.

Aortic aneurysms in the patients with Marfan syndrome are also repaired with this technique. Marfan syndrome is frequently associated with aortic dissection.

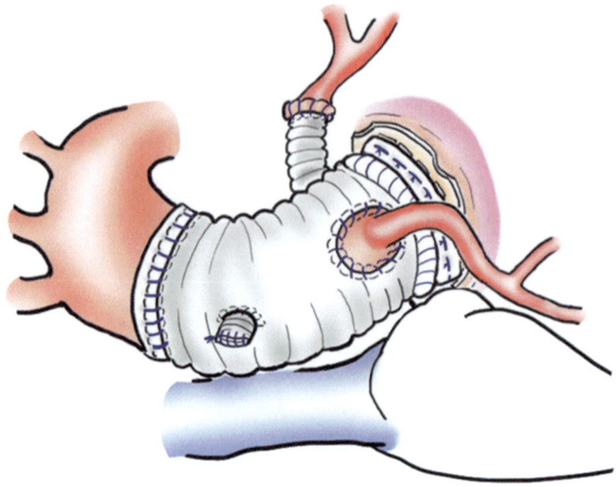

Fig. 12.1d Ascending aorta is replaced with a composite graft. Coronary ostium is reimplanted to the graft directly (Carrel patch method) or interposing a small graft (Piehler method)

Depending on the location and extent of the dissection, additional reconstruction or replacement of other parts of the aorta is necessary.

A large aorta is frequently observed in TOF, especially in the case of tetralogy of Fallot (TOF) with pulmonary atresia. Niwa [5] reported that 15 % of repaired adults with TOF had a dilated aortic root (Figs. 12.2a, 12.2b, and 12.2c).

Fortunately, only a small number of these patients seem to develop an aortic dissection [5]. For this reason, aortic replacement in TOF is indicated at a later stage compared to patients who developed an aortic aneurysm in other anomalies. However, when the diameter of the aortic root excesses 55 mm [6, 7], aortic replacement could be considered. If significant aortic regurgitation occurs due to annular dilatation, aortic valve replacement (AVR) combined with ascending aortic replacement or Bentall operation would be indicated.

12.2.1 Valve-Sparing Operation

Among patients with aortic dilatation, severe AR may occur only due to annular dilatation. When the aortic valve is not affected, it may be feasible to recover competence of the aortic valve by reducing the diameter of the aortic annulus and the suspension of cusps. Based on this concept, valve-sparing root replacement had been developed by Yacoub in 1979 (remodeling method [2]) and by David in 1992 (reimplantation method [3]).

12.2.1.1 Remodeling Method

Cardiopulmonary bypass is established in the same manner as in the Bentall operation. The aneurysmal ascending aorta is removed from the distal portion to the

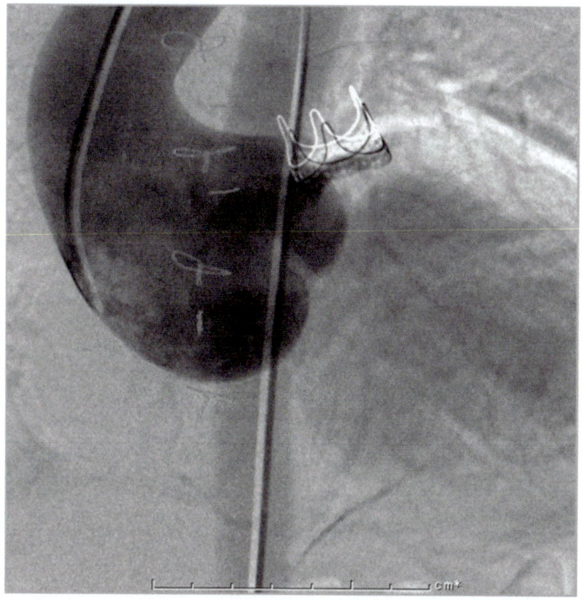

Fig. 12.2a Aortogram of a 46-year-old male who underwent TOF repair 41 years ago. Three years after pulmonary valve replacement at 43 year of age, aortic dilatation and aortic regurgitation were rapidly developed

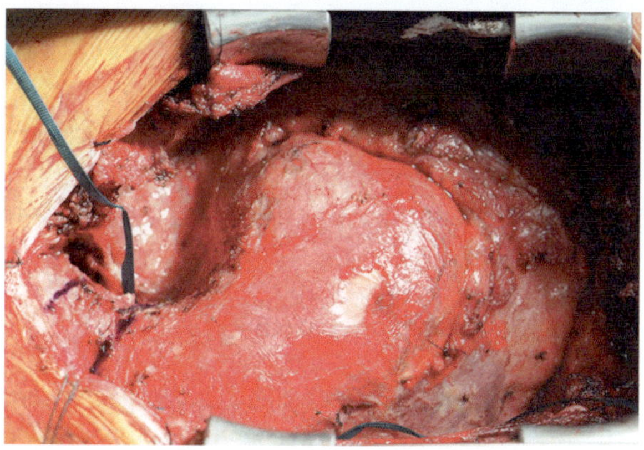

Fig. 12.2b Marked aortic dilation of the patient. Left is the cranial side

sinus of Valsalva. The coronary ostia are detached from the aortic wall as large buttons. The sinus of Valsalva is resected, whereas the aortic valve is preserved. A proper size tube graft, usually determined by the diameter of the sino-tubular junction at the time of competent approximation of the cusps, is prepared to fit the shape of the Valsalva sinuses and is sutured to the wall of the sinuses. As in the Bentall operation, two holes are made in the tube graft at the corresponding positions of the coronary ostia (Fig. 12.3). The coronary buttons are sutured to the tube graft in the same way as in the Bentall operation. Since the aortic annulus is untouched in the remodeling method, aortic root dilation may develop.

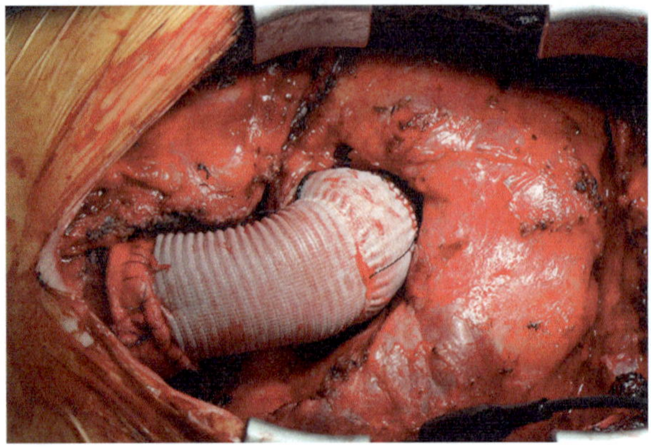

Fig. 12.2c Aneurysmal ascending aorta was replaced aortic a composite graft

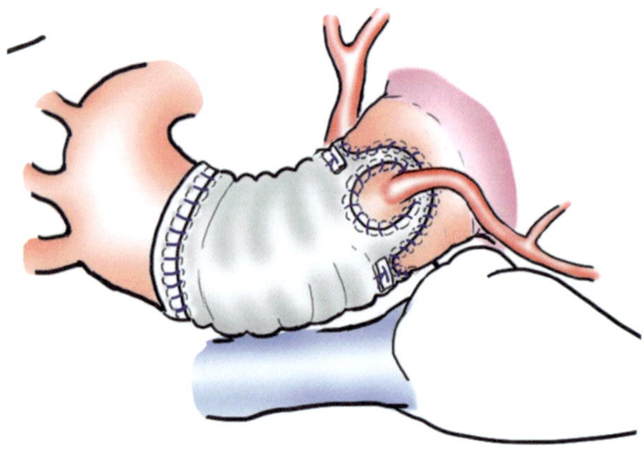

Fig. 12.3 Completion of remodeling method. Aneurysmal ascending aorta is removed to Valsalva sinuses. Coronary ostia are removed as large buttons. A proper size tube graft is trimmed to fit the figure of Valsalva sinuses. The ascending aorta is replaced with this graft. Coronary ostia are reimplanted to the tube graft

12.2.1.2 Reimplantation Method

Preservation of the aortic valve and enucleation of coronary buttons are performed in the same manner as in the remodeling method. A tube graft of 4-5 mm larger than the diameter of the aortic annulus is selected. The first row sutures are placed inside to outside just below the aortic cusps to fix the tube graft. Commissural walls are pulled into a tube graft (Fig. 12.4a), and then first row sutures are put in the edge of the graft and tied down. Each commissural wall is suspended to the inside of the tube graft arranging competence of the aortic valve. The free edge of the Valsalva sinuses is sutured continuously to the inside of the tube graft (second row sutures) (Fig. 12.4b). Two holes are made in the tube graft at the positions of the corresponding coronary ostia. The coronary buttons are sutured to the tube graft in the same fashion as in other forms of root replacement (Fig. 12.4c). This method is particularly indicated in young female with Marfan syndrome (Fig. 12.5). Although often a straight tube graft is used for root replacement, also a new type of grafts with a bulged midportion for improvement of valve movement is utilized.

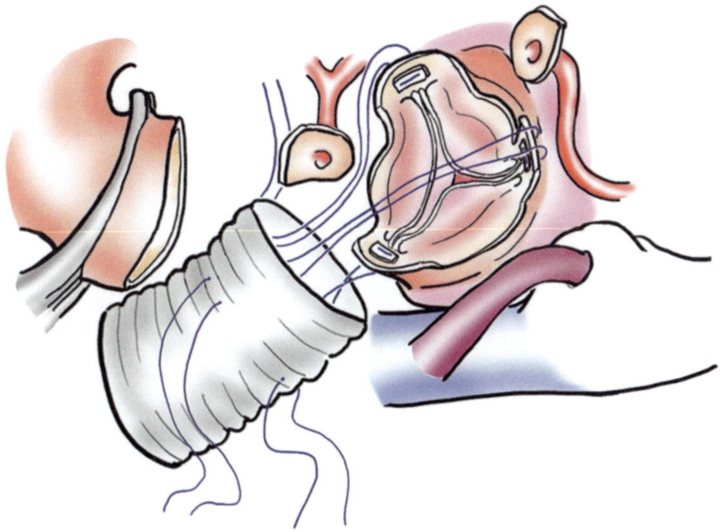

Fig. 12.4a The aneurysmal ascending aorta is removed from the distal portion to Valsalva sinuses. After the first row sutures are placed (not drawn in the figure), the commissural walls are pulled into the tube graft

12.2.1.3 Differences of Various Valve-Sparing Operations

As in the remodeling method, aortic annulus and aorto-ventricular junction are left untouched, the risk of root dilatation remains in the long term. However, in the remodeling method the function of the Valsalva sinuses is preserved. Leyh et al. [8] reported that aortic root elasticity and aortic valve motion are superior in the remodeling method compared to the reimplantation method. Richardt et al. [9] reported in Marfan syndrome excellent long-term results of the reimplantation method and a superiority of this method in the prevention of aortic root dilatation.

12.2.2 Ross Operation

In 1967, Donald Ross [4] developed the idea of using an autologous pulmonary valve to replace the aortic valve. At first the pulmonary valve was trimmed in scallop and reimplanted at subcoronary position. Inclusion cylinder method had also been performed to simplify the procedure. Nowadays full root replacement with pulmonary autograft is most prevailed.

After establishment of the cardiopulmonary bypass, the main pulmonary artery is transected just below its branches. The pulmonary valve is satisfactorily inspected if not diseased. Then the ascending aorta is cross-clamped and transected just above the sino-tubular junction. The aortic valve is removed. Both coronary

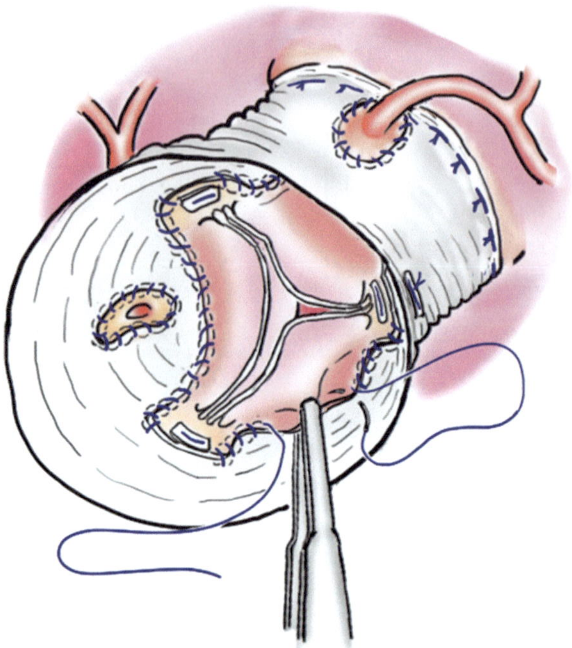

Fig. 12.4b After the first row sutures are placed, the commissural walls are pulled into the tube graft. The tube graft is fixed with the first row sutures, and then the commissural walls and the free edge of Valsalva sinuses are sutured inside of the tube graft

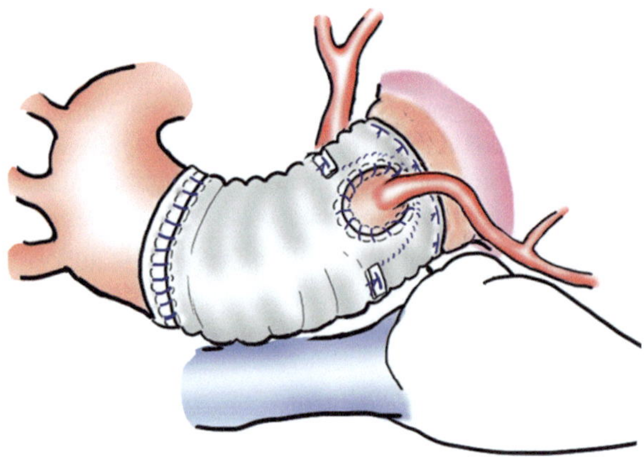

Fig. 12.4c The ascending aorta is replaced with the tube graft. Coronary ostia are reimplanted to the tube graft

ostia are removed with a large button of the aortic wall. The pulmonary artery is separated from the ascending aorta. The RV free wall is incised a few millimeters below the pulmonary annulus. After that, the incision is extended transversally and posteriorly. The endocardium on the posterior aspect of the RV is incised below the pulmonary valve, and the pulmonary artery is enucleated (Fig. 12.6a). Great care is necessary not to injure the first septal branch of the left anterior descending coronary artery.

The pulmonary autograft is sutured to the aortic annulus with many simple interrupted sutures or a mixture of continuous running and interrupted sutures.

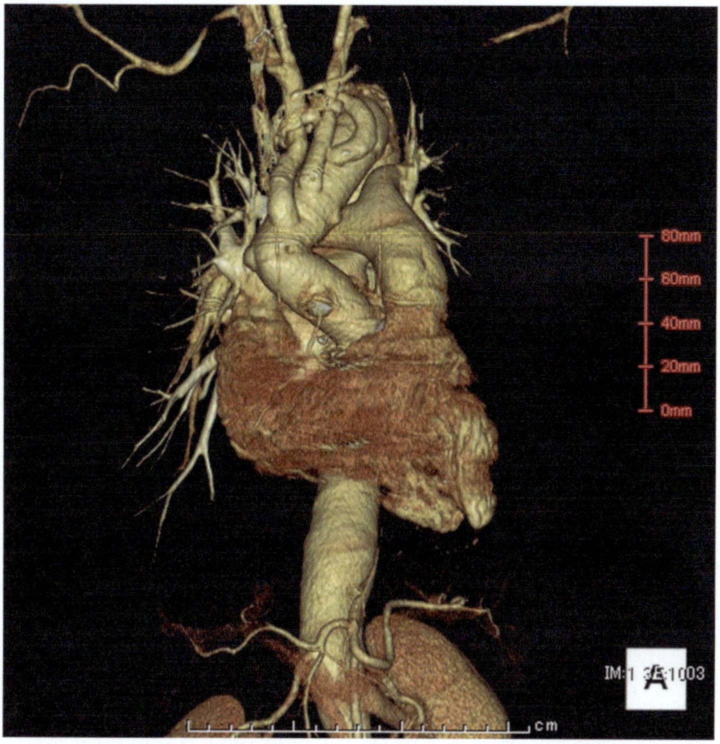

Fig. 12.5 CT image of a 29-year-old female associated with Marfan syndrome, who underwent the reimplantation method and arch replacement after attack of dissecting aneurysm

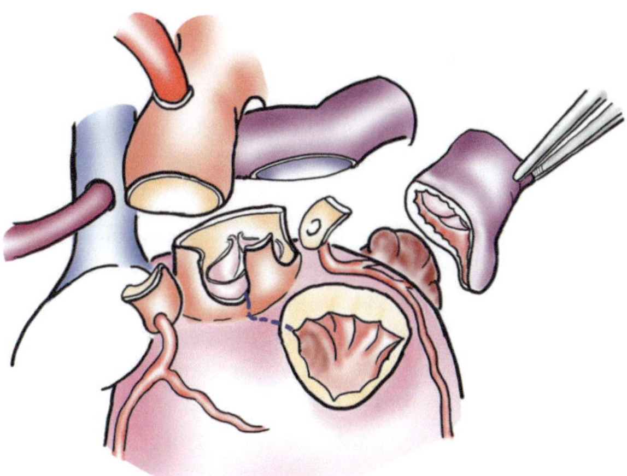

Fig. 12.6a Procedures of Ross-Konno operation. The pulmonary autograft is harvested. The ascending aorta is transected just above sino-tubular junction. Coronary ostia are removed as large buttons. The aortic valve is removed

Fig. 12.6b The pulmonary autograft is sutured to the aortic annulus. When the aortic annulus is too small for the autograft, a vertical incision is made to the ventricular septum

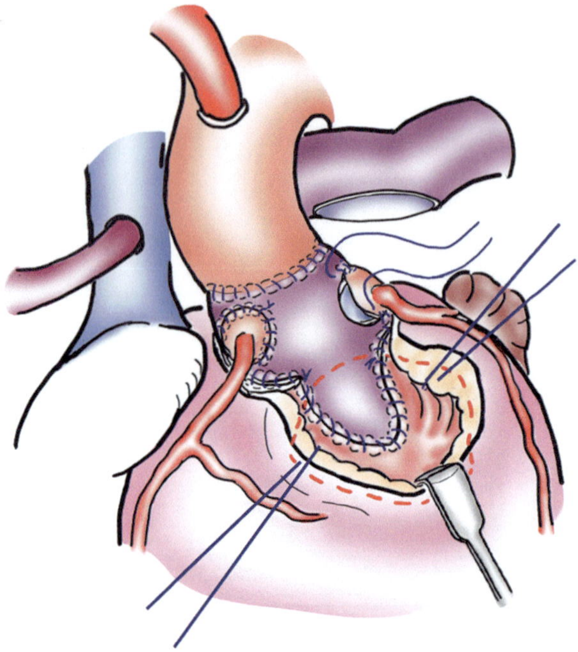

Usually autologous pericardial strip is used to reinforce the suture line. Then incisions are made in the corresponding area of the left and right coronary artery. Large enough holes are made, and both coronary buttons are sutured to the pulmonary autograft. The distal end of the pulmonary autograft is trimmed and sutured to the distal ascending aorta. The enucleated RV outflow tract and the pulmonary artery are reconstructed, usually with a homograft or other valved conduits (Fig. 12.6c) (Fig. 12.7).

The most prevalent indication for Ross operation is aortic stenosis or a combination of stenosis and insufficiency. When the aortic annulus is too small for the pulmonary autograft, Ross-Konno operation [10] can be performed (Figs. 12.6a, 12.6b, and 12.6c).

Superior hemodynamics, freedom from anticoagulation, and longevity of the pulmonary autograft have been substantiated. Growth potential with somatic growth or merely pathological dilatation of the autograft is also expected among young patients. Elkins RC et al. [11] reviewed 487 consecutive patients with the age from 2 days to 62 years (median 24 years), who underwent Ross procedure between 1986 and 2002. Actuarial survival was 82 ± 6 % at 16 years, freedom from autograft failure was 74±5 %, and freedom from allograft reoperation or reintervention was 82±4 %. Kieverik et al. reported their 146 patients of Ross procedure, aged 4 months to 52 years (mean 22 years). The survival at 13 years was excellent as much as 94±2 %; freedom from autograft and allograft reoperation were 69.7±7 % and 87.5±5 % at 13 years, respectively. Adult patients tended to be associated with higher risk of autograft reoperation, so that the Ross operation is

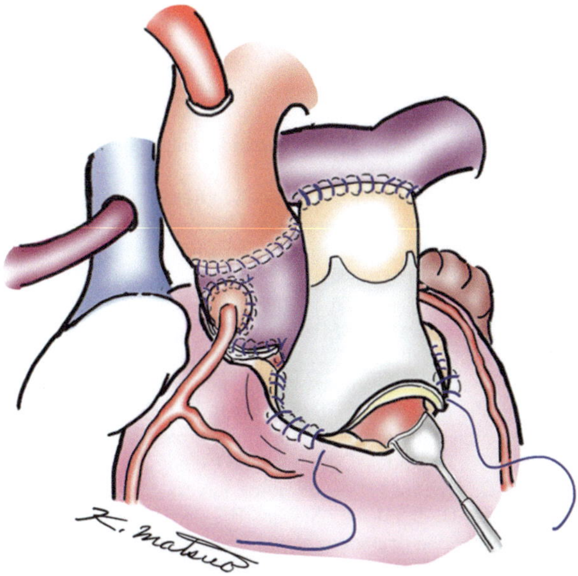

Fig. 12.6c Enucleated RV outflow tract and the pulmonary artery are reconstructed usually with homograft or other valved conduits

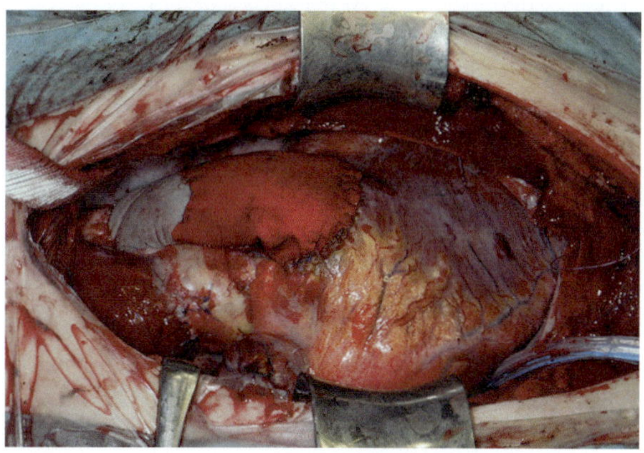

Fig. 12.7 A 15-year-old male with bicuspid valve and severe AS is repaired with Ross operation. RV-PA route is reconstructed with a handmade valved conduit

performed only in infants and children in their center [12]. In contrast to this study, Sievers et al. reviewed 1779 adult patients with the Ross procedure in eight centers in Germany, and the Ross procedure should be considered in young and active patients based on the excellent results in their study [13]. Since the Ross procedure requires considerable experience to obtain acceptable results, introduction of the Ross procedure to the adult patients is still controversial.

References

1. Bentall H, De Bono A (1968) A technique for complete replacement of the ascending aorta. Thorax 23(4):338–339
2. Sarsam MA, Yacoub M (1993) Remodeling of the aortic valve anulus. J Thorac Cardiovasc Surg 105(3):435–438
3. David TE, Feindel CM, Bos J. (1995) Repair of the aortic valve in patients with aortic insufficiency and aortic root aneurysm. J Thorac Cardiovasc Surg 109(2):345–351; discussion 51–2
4. Ross DN (1967) Replacement of aortic and mitral valves with a pulmonary autograft. Lancet 2(7523):956–958
5. Niwa K (2005) Aortic root dilatation in tetralogy of Fallot long-term after repair-histology of the aorta in tetralogy of Fallot: evidence of intrinsic aortopathy. Int J Cardiol 103:117–119
6. Wanes CA, William RG, Bashore TM et al (2008) ACC/AHA 2008 guidelines for the management of adults with congenital heart disease. Circulation 118:e714–e833
7. Gatzoulis MA, Webb GD, Daubeney PEF (2003) Diagnosis and management of adult congenital heart disease. Churchill Livingstone, Edinburgh, pp p315–p326
8. Leyh RG, Schmidtke C et al (1999) Opening and closing characteristics of the aortic valve after different types of valve-preserving surgery. Circulation 100(21):2153–2160
9. Richardt D, Stierle U, Sievers HH (2015) Long-term results after aortic valve-sparing-reimplantation operation (David) in bicuspid aortic valve. J Heart Valve Dis 24(1):4–9
10. Hraska V, Photiadis J, Poruban R, et al. (2008) Ross-Konno operation in children. Multimed Man Cardiothorac Surg 2008(915):mmcts 2008 003160
11. Elkins RC, Thompson DM, Lane MM, et al. (2008) Ross operation: 16-year experience. J Thorac Cardiovasc Surg 136(3):623–630, 30 e1–5
12. Klieverik LM, Takkenberg JJ, Bekkers JA et al (2007) The Ross operation: a trojan horse? Eur Heart J 28(16):1993–2000
13. Sievers HH, Stierle U, Charitos EI et al (2016) A multicentre evaluation of the autograft procedure for young patients undergoing aortic valve replacement: update on the German Ross Registry-dagger. Eur J Cardiothorac Surg 49(1):212–218

Chapter 13
Stenting in Aortopathies

Joanna Ghobrial and Jamil Aboulhosn

Abstract Transcatheter stent deployment within the aorta is generally used for two purposes: (1) relief of aortic obstruction as seen in aortic coarctation and (2) the use of covered stents to exclude an aneurysm or pseudoaneurysm of the aorta. For the purpose of relieving obstruction, balloon angioplasty alone is associated with reasonable short-term improvement in stenosis severity but limited by a high incidence of restenosis and aneurysm formation. Uncovered large diameter stent platforms are a more durable alternative for relief of stenosis but do not obviate the risk of aneurysm formation and do not protect the aorta in cases of rupture, dissection, or pseudoaneurysm formation. Covered balloon expandable stent platforms are ideal for relief of stenosis and reduce the risk of extravascular hemorrhage, dissection, and aneurysm formation. Transcatheter stent placement has become the treatment modality of choice for most children and adults with native coarctation or those with postsurgical sequelae or complications. The advent of large diameter self-expanding covered stent grafts allows for treatment of complex aneurysms, pseudoaneurysms, and dissections. Hybrid transcatheter and surgical techniques can also be utilized to treat hypoplasia and focal coarctations of the aortic arch. This chapter will review the role of transcatheter stenting for the treatment of aortopathies that are manifested by obstruction, aneurysm formation, or both.

Keywords Aortopathy • Coarctation • Stent • Angioplasty • Aneurysm

13.1 Aortopathy and Coarctation and Indications for Intervention

Aortopathy is defined as any disease of the aorta. This includes the inherited connective tissue disease syndromes with related aortic disease such as Marfan, Ehlers-Danlos, Loeys-Dietz, bicuspid aortic valve-associated aortopathy, and the

J. Ghobrial, M.D., M.S. (✉) • J. Aboulhosn, M.D.
Ahmanson/UCLA Adult Congenital Heart Disease Center, University of California, 100 Medical Plaza, Suite 630 East, Los Angeles, CA 90095, USA
e-mail: JGhobrial@mednet.ucla.edu

K. Niwa, H. Kaemmerer (eds.), *Aortopathy*, DOI 10.1007/978-4-431-56071-5_13

aortopathy associated with aortic coarctation. This section specifically considers aortopathies that can be intervened upon in the cardiac catheterization laboratory using stenting techniques, specifically native and postsurgical aortic coarctation, with or without aneurysm.

On histology, the aortic wall consists of three layers: the intima (the innermost layer with endothelial lining), the media (the muscular layer and contains smooth muscle cells, fibrillin, elastin, and collagen), and the adventitia (the outer lining) [1–3].

Aortopathies are related to abnormalities in the connective tissue of the aorta. On histologic examination, there is degeneration and disruption of smooth muscle cells, collagen, elastin, and fibrillin in the aortic media [3].

A coarctation of the aorta consists of a narrowing of a segment of the aortic arch that leads to varying degrees of obstruction, which causes hypertension proximal to the narrowing and lower pressure beyond. The most frequent location of a simple coarctation is just distal to the takeoff of the left subclavian artery at the area of the ductus/ligamentum arteriosum. Less common is a coarctation in the abdominal aorta or a diffusely narrowed aortic arch. Collateral vessels may arise proximal to the obstruction to help supply the distal organs, notably these collaterals can also mask the degree of obstruction on clinical examination or Doppler interrogation by allowing the distal aortic pressure to be adequately maintained. There are two possible underlying concepts explaining the development of coarctation. The first concept is related to blood flow limitation during development with outflow obstruction lesions such as aortic stenosis leading to the coarctation, the second is related to abnormal ductal tissue extending into the arch leading to constriction with ductal closure, supporting the latter concept is presence of abnormal smooth muscle and collagen in the aortic tissue surrounding the coarctation, and this also explains the predilection of the surrounding tissue to dissection and rupture [4–8].

Coarctation of the aorta is a common congenital heart lesion affecting 6–8 % of patients with congenital heart disease; it occurs up to two times more commonly in males than in females. While coarctation can present as the sole lesion, it can also present in association with other congenital conditions such as bicuspid aortic valve, ventricular septal defect, patent ductus arteriosus, aortic stenosis, subaortic stenosis, supravalvular aortic stenosis, and mitral valve abnormalities, as well as circle of Willis cerebral artery aneurysm and genetic conditions such as Turner syndrome [9–15].

Surgical repair of aortic coarctation was first described in 1944 by Crafoord et al. [16], and balloon dilation was first mentioned in 1979 [17], introduced in 1982 by Singer et al. [18], and performed in 1991 [19]. Medical therapy with beta-blockers, ACE-inhibitors, or angiotensin-receptor blockers is typically employed to control hypertension and to decrease shear stress in the abnormal aortic tissue. In adults, accepted indications for intervention to relieve native aortic coarctation include [20] (Fig. 13.1):

- Peak-to-peak coarctation gradient greater than or equal to 20 mmHg

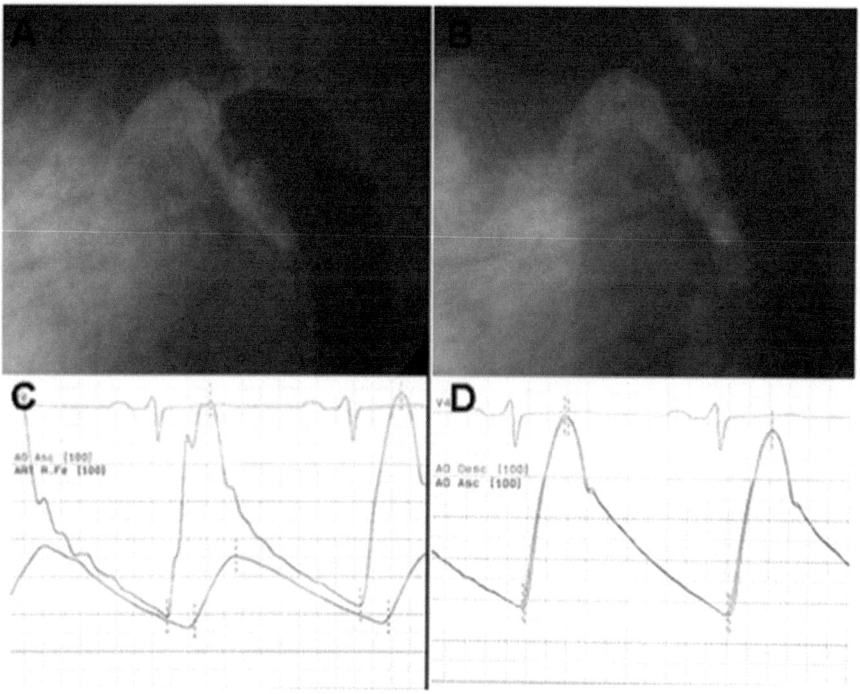

Fig. 13.1 (**a**) Aortic angiogram, lateral projection demonstrating near interruption of the distal aortic arch. (**b**) Angiogram following stent placement demonstrating a patent aorta without evidence of dissection or pseudoaneurysm. (**c**) Simultaneous ascending and descending aortic pressures. The ascending aortic systolic pressure is 80 mmHg higher than the descending aortic pressure distal to the coarctation. Also note that the ascending aortic diastolic pressure is also greater, and there is a delayed upstroke of the descending aortic systolic pressure; these findings are consistent with a severe fixed obstruction of the aorta. (**d**) Simultaneous pressure ascending and descending aortic pressures following successful stent deployment demonstrating no residual systolic or diastolic gradient and rapid systolic upstroke of both waveforms

- Imaging evidence of significant coarctation, with a peak-to-peak coarctation gradient less than 20 mmHg due to collateral flow (collaterals will decrease the gradient despite a hemodynamically significant coarctation)

Furthermore, for recoarctations, percutaneous stent placement is favored for discrete narrowing, whereas surgical intervention may be preferable for long-segment hypoplasia and aortic arch hypoplasia.

The European Society of Cardiology (ESC) [21] guidelines for the treatment of adult congenital heart disease list the following indications for intervention:

- Gradient >20 mmHg between upper and lower limbs.
- Upper limb hypertension.
- Pathological BP response to exercise.

- Aortic coarctation diameter <50 % of the diameter of the aorta at the level of the diaphragm.

In many ACHD centers presently, surgery is reserved for cases that are not amenable to percutaneous intervention, whether native coarctation or recoarctation, such as long tortuous segments, large aneurysms, and transverse aortic arch hypoplasia. There has been some experience in small series of patients with successful percutaneous stenting of transverse arch hypoplasia. Partial or complete coverage of the arch vessels with uncovered stents does not appear to cause significant obstruction to flow through these vessels but is nevertheless generally avoided due to concerns over thromboembolism [22–24]. The use of self-expanding covered stent grafts or covered stents within the aortic arch is accompanied by surgical bypass of occluded vessels (Fig. 13.2). In some cases where surgical aortic valve or ascending aortic repair or replacement is necessary in a patient with a coexistent coarctation of the aorta, transcatheter stenting of the coarctation can be performed at the time of or before surgical intervention. The complications of surgical repair in adults with coarctation, or recoarctation, are not negligible. Such complications include extensive bleeding from collaterals, severe rebound hypertension early after repair, recurrent laryngeal or phrenic nerve palsy, need for cardiopulmonary bypass, aneurysm or pseudoaneurysm formation especially with Dacron patch

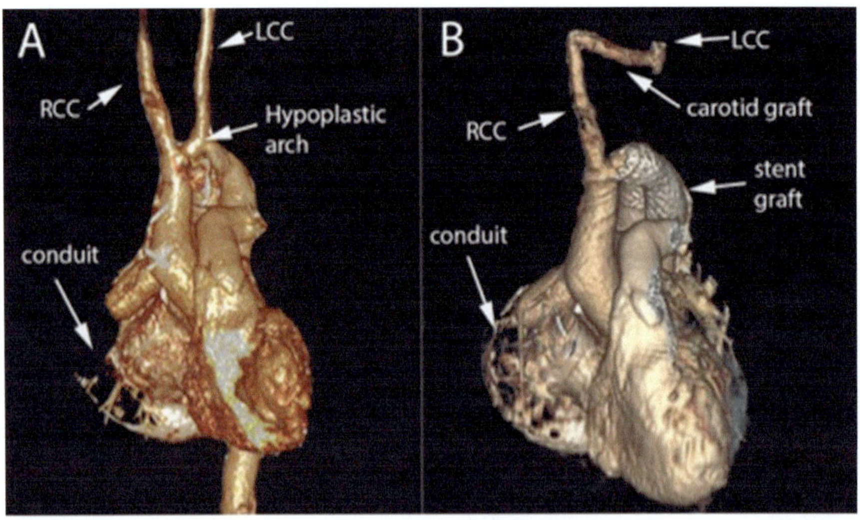

Fig. 13.2 (**a**) CT angiogram with 3-D volume rendering, shallow left anterior oblique view, demonstrating a hypoplastic aortic arch in a patient that had previously undergone surgical placement of an ascending to descending aortic conduit. The conduit had subsequently thrombosed. The right common carotid (RCC) and left common carotid (LCC) are labeled. The left subclavian artery is not visualized because it had previously been utilized to surgically augment the aorta as a subclavian flap. (**b**) Covered aortic stent graft placement within the aortic arch has increased the arch diameter. A surgically placed carotid bypass graft ensures flow from the patent RCC to the LCC

repair, subclavian steal syndrome, and rarely paraplegia due to spinal cord ischemia [25]. Complications of coarctation stenting include major aortic complications such as rupture, dissection or pseudoaneurysm formation in ~ 1 % of patients, [26] femoral arterial injury, bleeding, stent fracture, or stent embolization (Figs. 13.3 and 13.4).

Unlike stenting in aortic coarctation, which is oftentimes used as line treatment, stenting in other aortopathies due to underlying connective tissue disease, such as

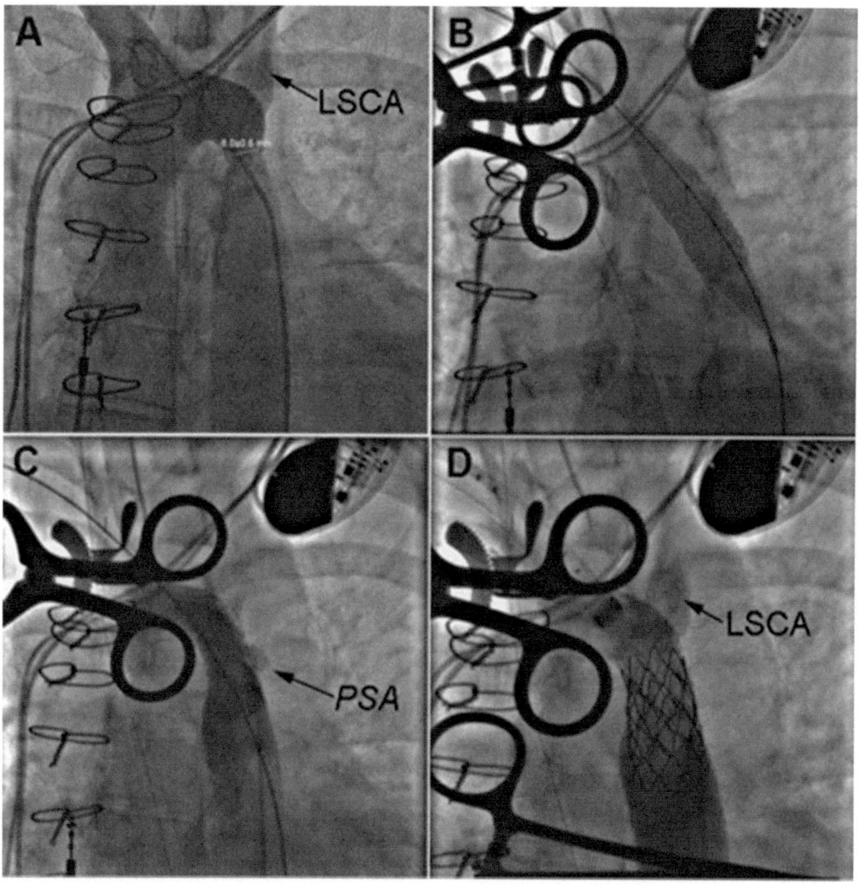

Fig. 13.3 (**a**) Aortic angiogram demonstrating a residual coarctation distal to the left subclavian artery in a patient that had undergone surgical end-to-end repair as a child yet developed upper extremity hypertension in adulthood. (**b**) High pressure balloon expansion of an uncovered stent with minimal residual waist. (**c**) Rotational angiography demonstrated an expanding pseudoaneurysm (PSA) at the site of stent deployment. (**d**) Angiogram following deployment of a covered stent with occlusion of the PSA. Note the left subclavian artery is not obstructed by the covered stent. Also note that arterial access for this case was via surgical cutdown of the right subclavian artery due to obstruction of both femoral arteries from prior catheterization procedures during childhood

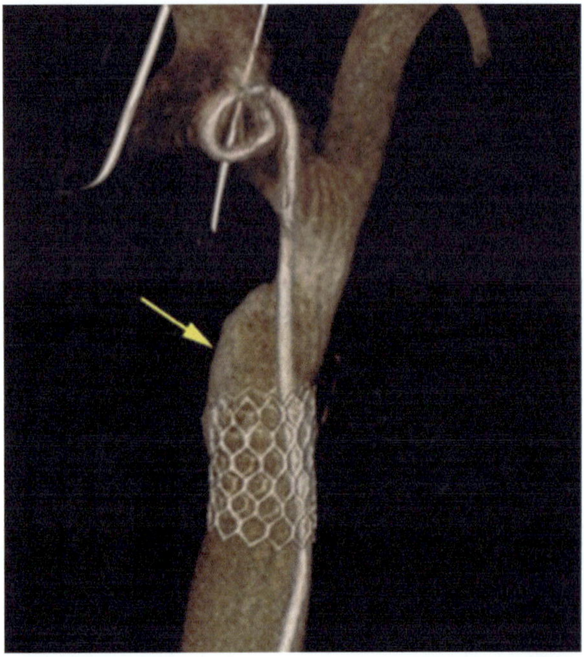

Fig. 13.4 Rotational aortic angiogram with 3-D volume rendering demonstrating an uncovered stent that embolized from its initial position just distal to the left subclavian artery to the mid-descending thoracic aorta. The *yellow arrow* points to an aneurysm or pseudoaneurysm

Marfan syndrome, is reserved for high-risk surgical patients. While endovascular repair of aneurysms and dissection due to underlying connective tissue disease has been shown to be feasible [27–30], it has also been associated with higher risk of dissection extension, endoleaks, stent graft migration, high re-intervention rates, and need for conversion to open surgical repair [31–34], and that is why expert consensus documents have recommended reserving stenting in patients with connective tissue disease-related aortopathies to only those with prohibitive surgical risk [35, 36].

13.2 Procedure Mechanism and Technique

Percutaneous intervention in aortic coarctation initially consisted of balloon dilation, but this technique has been supplanted by stent placement due to the decreased efficacy and increased risk of dissection or aneurysm formation with balloon angioplasty alone. Balloon dilation of narrowed segments in vessels involves the creation of small intimal and medial tears that heal with time. In fact, intravascular ultrasound study by Sohn et al. [37] confirmed the occurrence of such tears post angioplasty, with follow-up ultrasounds showing resolution and evidence of remodeling. However this very mechanism also can lead to aneurysm formation with a rate ranging from 2 % to as high as 20 % post-balloon angioplasty, especially in the setting of underlying aortopathy [19, 38–42].The advent of stenting of the coarctation has decreased this high rate of aneurysm formation and has now become the treatment of choice in older children and adult patients. The stent buttresses the aortic wall including the areas with intimal flaps or dissections [19, 43, 44], and this is also one of the main reasons why overdilation and oversizing are avoided.

Pre-procedural planning is essential, and the use of multiple imaging modalities aids in achieving a successful result. Echocardiography will evaluate for the presence of associated congenital lesions, such as left-sided outflow lesions or valvular abnormalities. Echocardiography also measures Doppler gradients across the coarctation, but such gradients are unreliable in the presence of collaterals. The echocardiogram can be limited however in assessing the size and dimensions of the coarctation, especially in relation to the aorta at the level of the diaphragm; that is where MRI or CT imaging is invaluable as it provides anatomic, and in the case of MRI also functional, evaluation of the aortic arch [45–47].

The procedure is typically performed under general anesthesia or deep sedation in adults; cross-matched blood should be available in the cardiac catheterization lab. The femoral artery is the preferred approach. Heparin is used as the procedural anticoagulant using 70–150 IU/Kg intravenously, with an activated clotting time (ACT) maintained >200 s. A femoral arterial sheath is inserted, an end-hole catheter is advanced over a soft-tip J wire in a retrograde fashion into the ascending aorta, and a pullback gradient is obtained. Alternatively, a separate radial artery line can be placed for continuous upper extremity pressure measurement. In cases where femoral arterial anatomy is prohibitive, a hybrid approach can be utilized with surgical cutdown and arterial access via the subclavian artery (Fig. 13.3).

After the hemodynamic assessment, the anatomy of the transverse arch and the coarctation is obtained with angiographic projections in the lateral and either left/right anterior oblique (20°) or anteroposterior views depending on right- or left-sided arch anatomy. Rotational angiography may be utilized if available and provides excellent three-dimensional assessment of the aorta (Figs. 13.4 and 13.5). Measurements made include the narrowest portion of the coarctation, the transverse arch, the ascending aorta, and the aorta distal to the coarctation and at the level of the diaphragm. The length of the narrowing is also measured to aid in stent sizing. The origins of the brachiocephalic, carotid, and subclavian arteries are noted, and presence of aneurysms is assessed.

The interventional portion of the procedure starts by introducing a stiff guidewire through the catheter into the ascending aorta or subclavian artery. If the coarctation is not more than 10 mm from the origin of the left subclavian artery, then positioning the wire there should be avoided as stent migration can cause "jailing" of this artery. The tip of the guidewire must be maintained at all times away from the coronary ostia, the carotid, and vertebral arteries.

Balloon angioplasty to "prepare" the lesion for stenting was previously widely utilized but has been generally abandoned due to concerns for aortic dissection, rupture, or aneurysm formation. If angioplasty is considered, it is imperative that the balloon size does not exceed that of the dimensions of the aorta at the level of the diaphragm and does not exceed two times the size of the minimal coarctation dimension [48–50]. The shortest balloons covering the length of the coarctation are

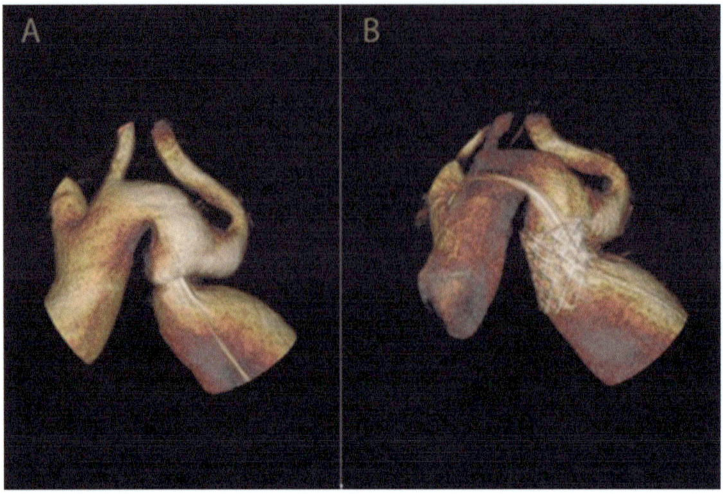

Fig. 13.5 (**a**) Rotational angiography with 3-D volume rendering demonstrating focal coarctation distal to an ectatic left subclavian artery. (**b**) Uncovered stent placement with resolution of the stenosis and minimal overlap with the ostium of the left subclavian artery

preferable. The balloon should be centered at the coarctation and should be inflated until the waist disappears or until maximum inflation pressure is achieved which is usually around 6 atm. The inflation time is approximately 10–15 s. The balloon should be kept away from the carotid and vertebral arteries. Once the balloon is rapidly deflated and removed, a catheter is then used to assess gradient across the coarctation and repeat angiography to ensure no dissection, aneurysm, or perforation/rupture has occurred.

Stent selection is based on the severity, length, and location of the narrowing. Large diameter uncovered hepatobiliary stents (Palmaz XL, Palmaz Genesis, ITI Mega and Max LD) are widely utilized and come in a variety of lengths and potential diameters (Fig. 13.5). Attempts should be made to avoid "jailing" the subclavian artery or the carotid artery, but there is little data to suggest that doing so is associated with significant obstruction to flow in these vessels. The diameter of the aorta at the diaphragm is typically used as the goal diameter to which the stent should be expanded; however, in order to minimize the risk of rupture or dissection, care should be taken to avoid increasing the coarctation diameter by more than 2.5-fold when using uncovered stents. A long large diameter sheath (10–14 Fr) is favored for stent deployment. A number of large diameter balloons are commercially available for stent deployment; however, the favored balloon is the NuMED balloon in balloon (BIB), which allows for expansion of a smaller inner balloon followed by a larger outer balloon. This technique allows for more precise stent positioning during deployment and minimizes the risk of stent deformation during expansion. Rapid ventricular pacing (at 160–200 bpm) may be used to produce transient decrease in systolic blood pressure (to <50 mmHg) to avoid stent movement or migration during inflation. Further dilation with larger balloons may be performed to achieve a satisfactory hemodynamic and anatomic result. The stent is often expanded 70–80 % of the diameter of the aorta at the level of the diaphragm to reduce the potential for complications including dissection and rupture. After balloon withdrawal, gradient measurements and repeat angiography should be performed to assess hemodynamic success and rule out any major vascular complications.

Despite the lack of proven efficacy in this setting, but based on known efficacy in coronary stenting, aspirin is often used for a minimum of 6 months post-stent placement. We recommend continuing long-term aspirin if a portion of the stent covers the arch vessels or if the stent is not well apposed to the proximal or distal aortic wall. Antibiotics are administered at the time of stent placement. Repeat imaging is indicated at approximately 3–6 weeks post procedure to exclude dissection, aneurysm formation, recoarctation, stent migration, or thrombosis and should be performed at regular intervals with echocardiography and Doppler [51]. We recommend performing a follow-up chest CT angiogram or MRI within 1–2 years of stent placement or sooner if there are concerning clinical examination, echocardiographic, or chest X-ray findings.

13.3 Outcomes of Intervention for Aortic Coarctation and Stent Choice

Outcomes of balloon angioplasty compared to surgery are available mostly in the pediatric population, where both intervention methods provided similar acute gradient reduction and decrease in systolic blood pressure, with lower procedure-related complications and shorter hospital stay in the angioplasty group but with higher recoarctation and aneurysm formation [42, 52, 53]. Factors predicting worse acute results included transverse arch hypoplasia, higher initial gradient, and older age [48–50, 53–63].

Long-term outcomes post-balloon angioplasty also highlight the increased risk of aneurysm formation and need for re-intervention post angioplasty compared to surgery. It is important to note however that surgical approach for patient with recoarctation is associated with an increased mortality as high as 7 % relative to native coarctation [41, 48–50, 55, 64–74].

The pathophysiology behind the higher rate of recoarctation and aneurysm formation post angioplasty is thought to be secondary to the stretch caused by the inflating balloon leading to wall damage and disruption of the aortic wall elastic properties. The intimal and medial tears are the recognized mechanism of angioplasty [75, 48]. However, the degree of stretch and aortic wall disruption, as well as the degree of underlying medial abnormality, thinning, and calcification, will increase the risk of adverse outcomes post angioplasty [4, 6, 76].

In order to address the significant rates of recoarctation and aneurysm formation with balloon angioplasty [66, 53], stenting has now become the mainstay of percutaneous intervention in aortic coarctation, with the exception of young infants and children where surgery and balloon angioplasty are still the preferred methods. Outcomes post stenting prove that it is a safe and effective approach to aortic coarctation and recoarctation with a significant reduction in gradient and systolic blood pressure, as well as a decreased risk of restenosis, dissection, and aneurysm formation. It is important to note, however, that in the adult population, the initial gradient may not reflect the severity of the obstruction due to the presence of collaterals; hence, the degree of gradient reduction post stenting is not a reliable measure of success. Also, studies have shown that some adult patients without residual stenosis will continue to be hypertensive, and that is thought to be due to underlying vascular disease and aortopathy [77–82].

There are three main types of stents:

1. Uncovered balloon expandable metallic stents
2. Covered balloon expandable stents (with a layer of PTFE)
3. Self-expanding covered stent grafts

Uncovered balloon expandable stents were developed for hepatobiliary interventions but are widely used for coarctation interventions. They are associated with improved procedural safety and efficacy when compared to balloon angioplasty alone; however, the incidence of aneurysm formation is persistent, and there is a low risk of stent fracture [83, 84]. Covered balloon expandable stents are now preferentially used in the treatment of aortic coarctation in much of the world but as of the time of the writing of this chapter are still not commercially available or approved as first-line therapy for aortic stenting in the United States (Figs. 13.6 and 13.7). They can be used to effectively treat dissections, aneurysms, or ruptures of

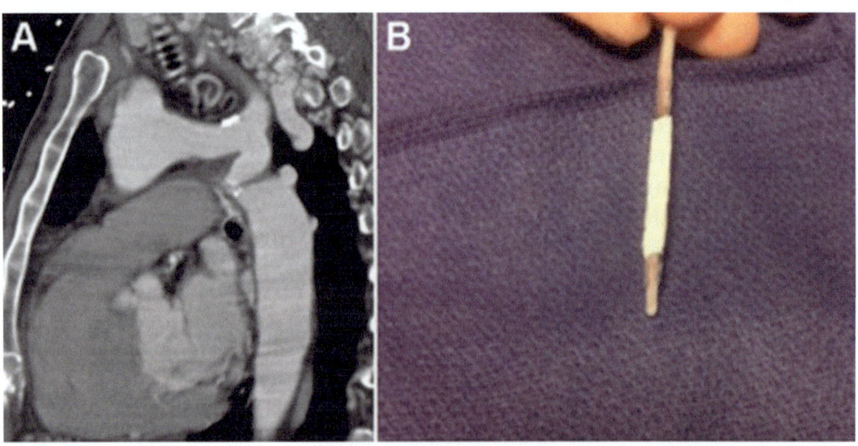

Fig. 13.6 (**a**) CT angiogram, sagittal view, demonstrating near interruption of the proximal descending thoracic aorta distal to the left subclavian artery in a 55-year-old man with coronary artery disease, multiple prior myocardial infarctions, and evidence of multiple arterial collaterals. (**b**) Balloon expandable covered stents are preferred to uncovered stents in order to minimize the risk of aortic rupture

the aorta caused during balloon angioplasty or uncovered stent deployment (Fig. 13.3). They are also strategic in cases with coarctation and a patent ductus arteriosus (PDA), where a covered stent would treat both, dilating the coarctation and occluding the PDA, as well as severe native coarctation or aortic interruption (Figs. 13.6 and 13.7) and older patients where there is a higher potential for dissection [85–91]. Careful positioning is critical to avoid occluding the spinal cord arterial branches, carotid arteries, and subclavian arteries (Fig. 13.3). The spinal cord branches originate at vertebra T9; this is oftentimes safely well below the level of the coarctation decreasing the risk of paraplegia, and pre-procedural imaging can help delineate the origin of the spinal cord vessels [92–94]. If occlusion of these branches does occur, perforation of the stent covering at the site of the branch can restore blood flow [24]. Other downsides to the use of covered stents include the need for larger sheaths, increasing the potential for femoral artery injury as well as the worse consequences of stent embolization with vessel occlusion such as with the renal and mesenteric vessels. Self-expanding stent grafts are widely used in aortic dissection and aneurysm formation in the adult population, and their use was extended in aortic coarctation, and some suggest that it is preferable in cases where there is an existing aneurysm and aortopathy, though it provides less radial strength compared to balloon expandable stents (Figs. 13.8 and 13.9) [92, 95, 96]. Multiple stent platforms can be utilized in sequence to achieve both coverage of aneurysms or dissections and adequate expansion of stenotic segments. For example, deployment of covered self-expanding stent grafts to cover an aneurysmal portion of the aorta followed by deployment of high radial force balloon mounted uncovered metallic stents can be used to provide greater radial force within the narrowed aorta (Figs. 13.8 and 13.9). The choice of stent ought to be individualized to the anatomy of each patient.

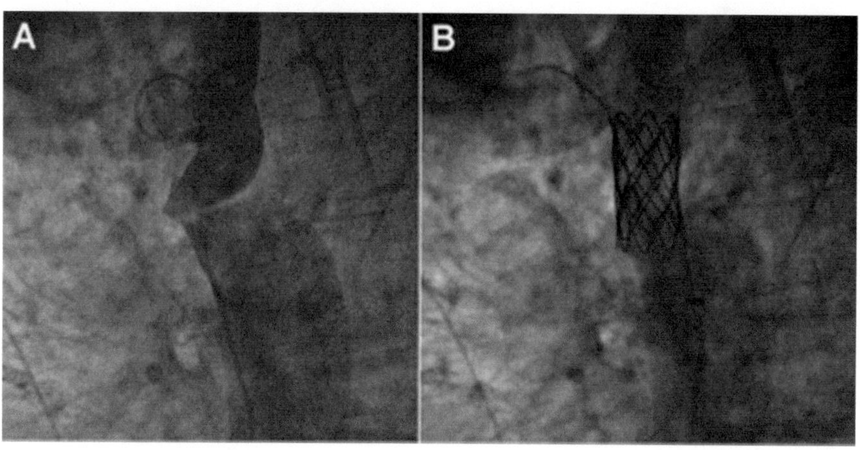

Fig. 13.7 The same patient from Fig. 13.5 with near interruption of the aorta. (**a**) Severe native coarctation noted on aortic angiography in a steep lateral anterior oblique view. (**b**) Resolution of the coarctation following deployment of a covered balloon expandable stent without evidence of aortic rupture or dissection

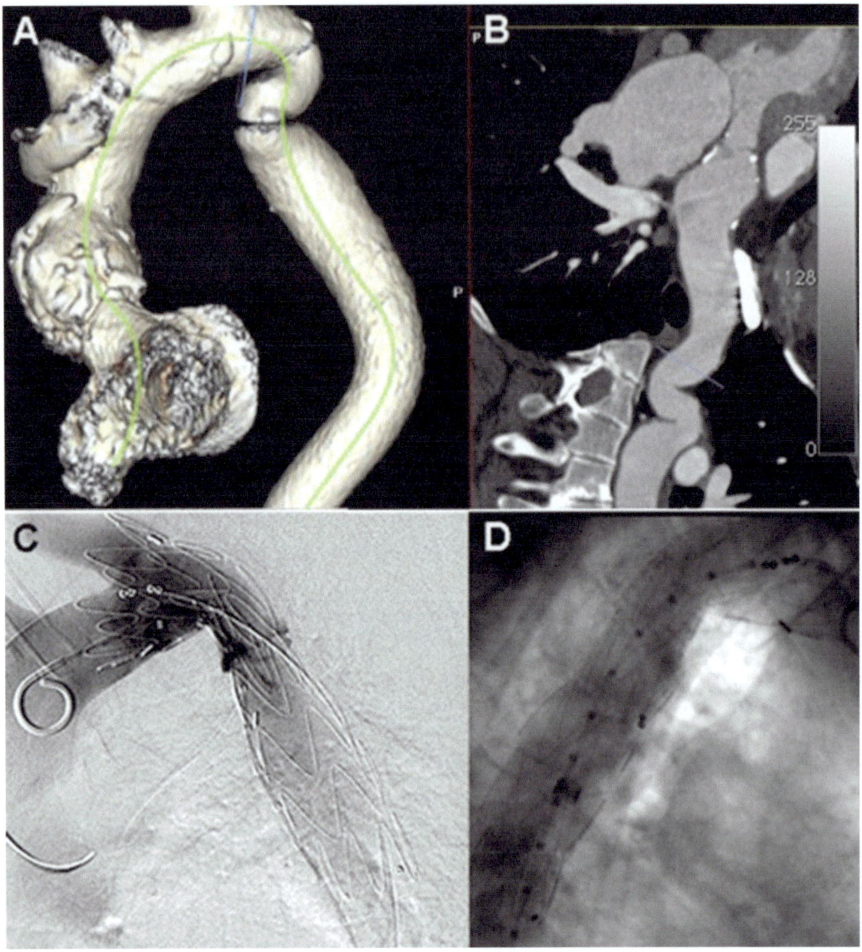

Fig. 13.8 (**a**) CT angiogram with 3-D volume rendering, left anterior oblique view, demonstrating a complex coarctation with severe tortuosity of the distal aortic arch and proximal descending thoracic aorta. (**b**) Multi-planar reconstruction of the aorta demonstrating the S-shaped tortuosity with multiple areas of stenosis. (**c**) Aortic angiogram with digital subtraction, left lateral view demonstrating a covered self-expanding stent graft within the distal arch and descending thoracic aorta with subsequent placement of a high radial force balloon expandable stent within the tortuous portion of the aorta. Note the resolution of aortic tortuosity and stenosis. (**d**) Aortic angiogram, right anterior oblique view, demonstrating resolution of stenosis and tortuosity

13.4 Complications

Complications of percutaneous interventions on aortic coarctation include dissection, rupture, aneurysm, pseudoaneurysm, and fistula formation at the arterial access site. It is important to remove the sheaths slowly to avoid avulsion of the

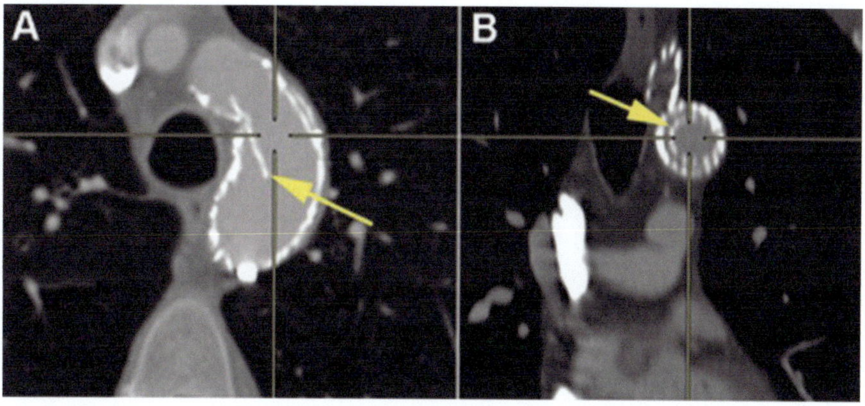

Fig. 13.9 (**a**) CT angiogram, axial view, demonstrating a self-expanding covered stent graft within the aortic arch and a high radial force uncovered balloon expandable stent (*yellow arrow*) within it at the site of the severest stenosis. This technique allows for aggressive dilation of severe and complex forms of coarctation using uncovered stainless steel stents within protective covered less rigid covered stent grafts. (**b**) Coronal view demonstrating the uncovered stent within the covered stent graft

femoral artery. Other complications include but are not limited to the following: stent migration, stent fracture, and thromboembolic complications. Paradoxical hypertension occurs more often in children, and less commonly compared to postsurgery [53, 48], and is managed medically. Endocarditis or aortitis is treated with intravenous antibiotics and usually does not require stent removal [82, 97–103]. Embolic stroke can also occur in up to 3.7 % of patients and can be minimized with antiplatelet therapy and meticulous care of wire, balloon, and stent positioning. Aneurysm formation may occur in up to 17 % of cases with uncovered stents; it is postulated that it's due to the medial injury during dilation; this incidence has decreased in occurrence with the use of covered stents. Pseudoaneurysm formation is associated with overdilation; this can be if stent dilation is limited to 70 % of the reference vessel diameter and less than 2.5 times the minimal luminal diameter at the site of coarctation. Fatal complications include aortic rupture; however, this complication can be managed with rapid placement of covered stents. Death from percutaneous intervention of aortic coarctation has been reported in 0–1.4 % of cases [26, 39, 51, 60, 87, 104–113]. An underappreciated adverse consequence of stenting is the insertion of a noncompliant, nonpulsatile stent in the aorta that can affect dynamic blood pressure control in the future [114–116].

13.5 Conclusion

Stenting is a significant advancement in the treatment of aortopathies, especially aortic coarctation. Stenting is the preferred method for management of aortic coarctation in adults and older children. The advent of covered stent platforms decreases the risk of serious complications such as rupture, pseudoaneurysm formation, and dissection.

References

1. Knight L, Edwards JE (1974) Right aortic arch: types and associated cardiac anomalies. Circulation 50(5):1047–1051. doi:10.1161/01.cir.50.5.1047
2. Damjanov I (2005) Robbins and cotran pathologic basis of disease, 7th edition. Shock 23 (5):482–483. doi:10.1097/00024382-200505000-00016
3. Kingwell B, Boutouyrie P (2007) Genetic influences on the arterial wall. Clin Exp Pharmacol Physiol 34(7):652–657. doi:10.1111/j.1440-1681.2007.04655.x
4. Isner JM, Donaldson RF, Fulton D, Bhan I, Payne DD, Cleveland RJ (1987) Cystic medial necrosis in coarctation of the aorta: a potential factor contributing to adverse consequences observed after percutaneous balloon angioplasty of coarctation sites. Circulation 75 (4):689–695. doi:10.1161/01.cir.75.4.689
5. Nicol ED, Gatzoulis M, Padley SPG, Rubens M (2007) Assessment of adult congenital heart disease with multi-detector computed tomography – beyond coronary lumenography. Clin Radiol 62(6):518–527. doi:10.1016/j.crad.2007.01.003
6. Niwa K, Perloff JK, Bhuta SM, Laks H, Drinkwater DC, Child JS, Miner PD (2001) Structural abnormalities of great arterial walls in congenital heart disease : light and electron microscopic analyses. Circulation 103(3):393–400. doi:10.1161/01.cir.103.3.393
7. Rudolph AM, Heymann MA, Spitznas U (1972) Hemodynamic considerations in the development of narrowing of the aorta. Am J Cardiol 30(5):514–525. doi:10.1016/0002-9149(72) 90042-2
8. Vogt M (2005) Impaired elastic properties of the ascending aorta in newborns before and early after successful coarctation repair: proof of a systemic vascular disease of the prestenotic arteries? Circulation 111(24):3269–3273. doi:10.1161/circulationaha.104.529792
9. Aboulhosn J, Child JS (2006) Left ventricular outflow obstruction: subaortic stenosis, bicuspid aortic valve, supravalvar aortic stenosis, and coarctation of the aorta. Circulation 114(22):2412–2422. doi:10.1161/circulationaha.105.592089
10. Fyler DC, Buckley LP, Hellenbrand WE, Cohn HE, Nadas AS (1978) 104 New England Regional Infant Cardiac Program (NERICP) effects on care delivery. Pediatr Res 12:381–381. doi:10.1203/00006450-197804001-00109
11. Gotzsche CO, Krag-Olsen B, Nielsen J, Sorensen KE, Kristensen BO (1994) Prevalence of cardiovascular malformations and association with karyotypes in Turner's syndrome. Arch Dis Child 71(5):433–436. doi:10.1136/adc.71.5.433
12. Matura LA, Ho VB, Rosing DR, Bondy CA (2007) Aortic dilatation and dissection in turner syndrome. Circulation 116(15):1663–1670. doi:10.1161/circulationaha.106.685487
13. McBride KL, Pignatelli R, Lewin M, Ho T, Fernbach S, Menesses A, Lam W, Leal SM, Kaplan N, Schliekelman P, Towbin JA, Belmont JW (2005) Inheritance analysis of congenital left ventricular outflow tract obstruction malformations: segregation, multiplex relative risk, and heritability. Am J Med Genet 134A(2):180–186. doi:10.1002/ajmg.a.30602

14. Nihoyannopoulos P, Karas S, Sapsford RN, Hallidie-Smith K, Foale R (1987) Accuracy of two-dimensional echocardiography in the diagnosis of aortic arch obstruction. J Am Coll Cardiol 10(5):1072–1077. doi:10.1016/s0735-1097(87)80348-0
15. Wessels MW, Berger RMF, Frohn-Mulder IME, Roos-Hesselink JW, Hoogeboom JJM, Mancini GS, Bartelings MM, Rd K, Wladimiroff JW, Niermeijer MF, Grossfeld P, Willems PJ (2005) Autosomal dominant inheritance of left ventricular outflow tract obstruction. Am J Med Genet 134A(2):171–179. doi:10.1002/ajmg.a.30601
16. Crafóörd C (1982) First resection of coarctation of aorta. Indian J Thorac Cardiovasc Surg 1 (1):54–55. doi:10.1007/bf02664147
17. Sos T, Sniderman K, Rettek-Sos B, Strupp A, Alonso D (1979) Percutaneous transluminal dilatation of coarctation of thoracic aorta post mortem. Lancet 314(8149):970–971. doi:10.1016/s0140-6736(79)92675-8
18. Singer MI, Rowen M, Dorsey TJ (1982) Transluminal aortic balloon angioplasty for coarctation of the aorta in the newborn. Am Heart J 103(1):131–132. doi:10.1016/0002-8703(82)90539-7
19. O'Laughlin MP, Perry SB, Lock JE, Mullins CE (1991) Use of endovascular stents in congenital heart disease. Circulation 83(6):1923–1939. doi:10.1161/01.cir.83.6.1923
20. Warnes CA, Williams RG, Bashore TM, Child JS, Connolly HM, Dearani JA, Del Nido P, Fasules JW, Graham TP Jr, Hijazi ZM, Hunt SA, King ME, Landzberg MJ, Miner PD, Radford MJ, Walsh EP, Webb GD (2008) ACC/AHA 2008 guidelines for the management of adults with congenital heart disease: executive summary: a report of the American College of Cardiology/American Heart Association Task Force on Practice Guidelines (writing committee to develop guidelines for the management of adults with congenital heart disease). Circulation 118(23):2395–2451. doi:10.1161/CIRCULATIONAHA.108.190811
21. Baumgartner H, Bonhoeffer P, De Groot NMS, de Haan F, Deanfield JE, Galie N, Gatzoulis MA, Gohlke-Baerwolf C, Kaemmerer H, Kilner P, Meijboom F, Mulder BJM, Oechslin E, Oliver JM, Serraf A, Szatmari A, Thaulow E, Vouhe PR, Walma E, Vahanian A, Auricchio A, Bax J, Ceconi C, Dean V, Filippatos G, Funck-Brentano C, Hobbs R, Kearney P, McDonagh T, Popescu BA, Reiner Z, Sechtem U, Sirnes PA, Tendera M, Vardas P, Widimsky P, McDonagh T, Swan L, Andreotti F, Beghetti M, Borggrefe M, Bozio A, Brecker S, Budts W, Hess J, Hirsch R, Jondeau G, Kokkonen J, Kozelj M, Kucukoglu S, Laan M, Lionis C, Metreveli I, Moons P, Pieper PG, Pilossoff V, Popelova J, Price S, Roos-Hesselink J, Uva MS, Tornos P, Trindade PT, Ukkonen H, Walker H, Webb GD, Westby J (2010) ESC guidelines for the management of grown-up congenital heart disease (new version 2010): The Task Force on the Management of Grown-up Congenital Heart Disease of the European Society of Cardiology (ESC). Eur Heart J 31(23):2915–2957. doi:10.1093/eurheartj/ehq249
22. Boshoff D, Budts W, Mertens L, Eyskens B, Delhaas T, Meyns B, Daenen W, Gewillig M (2006) Stenting of hypoplastic aortic segments with mild pressure gradients and arterial hypertension. Heart 92(11):1661–1666. doi:10.1136/hrt.2005.084822
23. Pushparajah K, Sadiq M, Brzezińska-Rajszys G, Thomson J, Rosenthal E, Qureshi SA (2013) Endovascular stenting in transverse aortic arch hypoplasia. Cathet Cardiovasc Intervent 82 (4):E491–E499. doi:10.1002/ccd.24735
24. Tsai SF, Hill SL, Cheatham JP (2009) Treatment of aortic arch aneurysm with a NuMED-covered stent and restoration of flow to excluded left subclavian artery: perforation and dilation of e-PTFE can be done! Cathet Cardiovasc Intervent 73:385–389. doi:10.1002/ccd.21825
25. Keen G (1987) Spinal cord damage and operations for coarctation of the aorta: aetiology, practice, and prospects. Thorax 42(1):11–18. doi:10.1136/thx.42.1.11
26. Holzer R, Qureshi S, Ghasemi A, Vincent J, Sievert H, Gruenstein D, Weber H, Alday L, Peirone A, Zellers T, Cheatham J, Slack M, Rome J (2010) Stenting of aortic coarctation: acute, intermediate, and long-term results of a prospective multi-institutional registry-

Congenital cardiovascular interventional study consortium (CCISC). Catheter Cardiovasc Interv 76(4):553–563. doi:10.1002/ccd.22587
27. Botta L, Russo V, Grigioni F, Arpesella G, Rocchi G, Di Bartolomeo R, Fattori R (2006) Unusual rapid evolution of Type B aortic dissection in a Marfan patient following heart transplantation: successful endovascular treatment. Eur J Vasc Endovasc Surg 32 (4):358–360. doi:10.1016/j.ejvs.2006.04.014
28. Fleck TM, Hutschala D, Tschernich H, Rieder E, Czerny M, Wolner E, Grabenwoger M (2003) Stent graft placement of the thoracoabdominal aorta in a patient with Marfan syndrome. J Thorac Cardiovasc Surg 125(6):1541–1543. doi:10.1016/s0022-5223(02)73606-4
29. Groenink M, Lohuis TAJ, Tijssen JGP, Naeff MSJ, Hennekam RCM, van der Wall EE, Mulder BJM (1999) Survival and complication free survival in Marfan's syndrome: implications of current guidelines. Heart 82(4):499–504. doi:10.1136/hrt.82.4.499
30. Roselli EE, Idrees JJ, Lowry AM, Masabni K, Soltesz EG, Johnston DR, Kalahasti V, Blackstone EH, Sabik JF, Lytle BW, Svensson LG (2016) Beyond the aortic root: staged open and endovascular repair of arch and descending aorta in patients with connective Tissue disorders. Ann Thorac Surg 101(3):906–912. doi:10.1016/j.athoracsur.2015.08.011
31. Ehrlich MP, Nienaber CA, Rousseau H, Beregi J-P, Piquet P, Schepens M, Bartoli J-M, Schillinger M, Fattori R (2008) Short-term conversion to open surgery after endovascular stent-grafting of the thoracic aorta: the talent thoracic registry. J Thorac Cardiovasc Surg 135 (6):1322–1326. doi:10.1016/j.jtcvs.2007.09.036
32. Eid-Lidt G, Gaspar J, Meléndez-Ramírez G, Cervantes SJ, González-Pacheco H, Dámas de Los Santos F, Meave-González A, Ramírez Marroquín S (2013) Endovascular treatment of type B dissection in patients with marfan syndrome: mid-term outcomes and aortic remodeling. Catheter Cardiovasc Interv 82(7):E898–E905. doi:10.1002/ccd.24725
33. Nordon IM, Hinchliffe RJ, Holt PJ, Morgan R, Jahangiri M, Loftus IM, Thompson MM (2009) Endovascular management of chronic aortic dissection in patients with Marfan syndrome. J Vasc Surg 50(5):987–991. doi:10.1016/j.jvs.2009.05.056
34. Waterman AL, Feezor RJ, Lee WA, Hess PJ, Beaver TM, Martin TD, Huber TS, Beck AW (2012) Endovascular treatment of acute and chronic aortic pathology in patients with Marfan syndrome. J Vasc Surg 55(5):1234–1241. doi:10.1016/j.jvs.2011.11.089
35. Svensson LG, Kouchoukos NT, Miller DC, Bavaria JE, Coselli JS, Curi MA, Eggebrecht H, Elefteriades JA, Erbel R, Gleason TG, Lytle BW, Mitchell RS, Nienaber CA, Roselli EE, Safi HJ, Shemin RJ, Sicard GA, Sundt TM, Szeto WY, Wheatley GH (2008) Expert consensus document on the treatment of descending thoracic aortic disease using endovascular stent-grafts has been supported by unrestricted educational grants from Cook, Inc and Medtronic, Inc. Ann Thorac Surg 85(1):S1–S41. doi:10.1016/j.athoracsur.2007.10.099
36. Grabenwoger M, Alfonso F, Bachet J, Bonser R, Czerny M, Eggebrecht H, Evangelista A, Fattori R, Jakob H, Lonn L, Nienaber CA, Rocchi G, Rousseau H, Thompson M, Weigang E, Erbel R (2012) Thoracic Endovascular Aortic Repair (TEVAR) for the treatment of aortic diseases: a position statement from the European Association for Cardio-Thoracic Surgery (EACTS) and the European Society of Cardiology (ESC), in collaboration with the European Association of Percutaneous Cardiovascular Interventions (EAPCI). Eur J Cardiothorac Surg 42(1):17–24. doi:10.1093/ejcts/ezs107
37. Sohn S, Rothman A, Shiota T, Luk G, Tong A, Swensson RE, Sahn DJ (1994) Acute and follow-up intravascular ultrasound findings after balloon dilation of coarctation of the aorta. Circulation 90(1):340–347. doi:10.1161/01.cir.90.1.340
38. De Lezo JS, Sancho M, Pan M, Romero M, Olivera C, Luque M (1989) Angiographic follow-up after balloon angioplasty for coarctation of the aorta. J Am Coll Cardiol 13(3):689–695. doi:10.1016/0735-1097(89)90612-8
39. Fletcher SE, Cheatham JP, Froeming S (1998) Aortic aneurysm following primary balloon angioplasty and secondary endovascular stent placement in the treatment of native coarctation of the aorta. Catheter Cardiovasc Diagn 44(1):40–44. doi:10.1002/(sici)1097-0304 (199805)44:1<40::aid-ccd10>3.3.co;2-y

40. Fletcher SE, Nihill MR, Grifka RG, O'Laughlin MP, Mullins CE (1995) Balloon angioplasty of native coarctation of the aorta: midterm follow-up and prognostic factors. J Am Coll Cardiol 25(3):730–734. doi:10.1016/0735-1097(94)00437-u
41. Rao PS, Galal O, Smith PA, Wilson AD (1996) Five- to nine-year follow-up results of balloon angioplasty of native aortic coarctation in infants and children. J Am Coll Cardiol 27 (2):462–470. doi:10.1016/0735-1097(95)00479-3
42. Shaddy RE, Boucek MM, Sturtevant JE, Ruttenberg HD, Jaffe RB, Tani LY, Judd VE, Veasy LG, McGough EC, Orsmond GS (1993) Comparison of angioplasty and surgery for unoperated coarctation of the aorta. Circulation 87(3):793–799. doi:10.1161/01.cir.87.3.793
43. Ohkubo M, Takahashi K, Kishiro M, Akimoto K, Yamashiro Y (2004) Histological findings after angioplasty using conventional balloon, radiofrequency thermal balloon, and stent for experimental aortic coarctation. Pediatr Int 46(1):39–47. doi:10.1111/j.1328-0867.2004.t01-1-.x
44. Trent MS, Parsonnet V, Shoenfeld R, Brener BJ, Eisenbud DE, Novick AS, Campbell AY, Ferrara-Ryan M, Villanueva A (1990) A balloon-expandable intravascular stent for obliterating experimental aortic dissection. J Vasc Surg 11(5):707–717. doi:10.1016/0741-5214(90) 90218-y
45. Bank ER, Aisen AM, Rocchini AP, Hernandez RJ (1987) Coarctation of the aorta in children undergoing angioplasty: pretreatment and posttreatment MR imaging. Radiology 162 (1):235–240. doi:10.1148/radiology.162.1.2947263
46. Oliver JM, Gallego P, Gonzalez A (2005) Risk factors for aortic complications in adults with coarctation of the aorta. ACC Curr J Rev 14(2):93–94. doi:10.1016/j.accreview.2004.12.157
47. Kaine SF, O'Brian Smith E, Mott AR, Mullins CE, Geva T (1996) Quantitative echocardiographic analysis of the aortic arch predicts outcome of balloon angioplasty of native coarctation of the aorta. Circulation 94(5):1056–1062. doi:10.1161/01.cir.94.5.1056
48. Ovaert C, McCrindle BW, Nykanen D, MacDonald C, Freedom RM, Benson LN (2000) Balloon angioplasty of native coarctation: clinical outcomes and predictors of success. J Am Coll Cardiol 35(4):988–996. doi:10.1016/s0735-1097(99)00646-4
49. Reich O, Tax P, Bartakova H, Tomek V, Gilik J, Lisy J, Radvansky J, Matejka T, Tlaskal T, Svobodova I, Chaloupecky V, Skovranek J (2008) Long-term (up to 20 years) results of percutaneous balloon angioplasty of recurrent aortic coarctation without use of stents. Eur Heart J 29(16):2042–2048. doi:10.1093/eurheartj/ehn251
50. Yetman AT, Nykanen D, McCrindle BW, Sunnegardh J, Adatia I, Freedom RM, Benson L (1997) Balloon angioplasty of recurrent coarctation: A 12-year review. J Am Coll Cardiol 30 (3):811–816. doi:10.1016/s0735-1097(97)00228-3
51. Forbes TJ, Moore P, Pedra CAC, Zahn EM, Nykanen D, Amin Z, Garekar S, Teitel D, Qureshi SA, Cheatham JP, Ebeid MR, Hijazi ZM, Sandhu S, Hagler DJ, Sievert H, Fagan TE, Ringwald J, Du W, Tang L, Wax DF, Rhodes J, Johnston TA, Jones TK, Turner DR, Pass R, Torres A, Hellenbrand WE (2007) Intermediate follow-up following intravascular stenting for treatment of coarctation of the aorta. Catheter Cardiovasc Interv 70(4):569–577. doi:10.1002/ccd.21191
52. Hernández-González M, Solorio S, Conde-Carmona I, Rangel-Abundis A, Ledesma M, Munayer J, David F, Ortegón J, Jiménez S, Sánchez-Soberanis AN, Meléndez C, Claire S, Gomez J, Teniente-Valente R, Alva C (2003) Intraluminal aortoplasty vs. surgical aortic resection in congenitalaortic coarctation. Arch Med Res 34(4):305–310. doi:10.1016/s0188-4409(03)00055-9
53. Rodés-Cabau J, Miró J, Dancea A, Ibrahim R, Piette E, Lapierre C, Jutras L, Perron J, Tchervenkow CI, Poirier N, Dahdah NS, Houde C (2007) Comparison of surgical and transcatheter treatment for native coarctation of the aorta in patients $\geq$1 year old. The Quebec Native Coarctation of the Aorta Study. Am Heart J 154(1):186–192. doi:10.1016/j.ahj.2007.03.046

54. Anjos R, Qureshi SA, Rosenthal E, Murdoch I, Hayes A, Parsons J, Baker EJ, Tynan M (1992) Determinants of hemodynamic results of balloon dilation of aortic recoarctation. Am J Cardiol 69(6):665–671. doi:10.1016/0002-9149(92)90161-q
55. Cooper RS, Ritter SB, Rothe WB, Chen CK, Griepp R, Golinko RJ (1987) Angioplasty for coarctation of the aorta: long-term results. Circulation 75(3):600–604. doi:10.1161/01.cir.75.3.600
56. del Cerro MJ, Fernández-Ruiz A, Benito F, Rubio D, Castro MC, Moreno F (2005) Balloon angioplasty for native coarctation in children: immediate and medium-term results. Revista Española de Cardiología (English Edition) 58(9):1054–1061. doi:10.1016/s1885-5857(06)60438-6
57. Früh S, Knirsch W, Dodge-Khatami A, Dave H, Prêtre R, Kretschmar O (2011) Comparison of surgical and interventional therapy of native and recurrent aortic coarctation regarding different age groups during childhood. Eur J Cardiothorac Surg 39(6):898–904. doi:10.1016/j.ejcts.2010.09.048
58. Hellenbrand WE, Allen HD, Golinko RJ, Hagler DJ, Lutin W, Kan J (1990) Balloon angioplasty for aortic recoarctation: results of valvuloplasty and angioplasty of congenital anomalies registry. Am J Cardiol 65(11):793–797. doi:10.1016/0002-9149(90)91390-r
59. Hijazi ZM, Fahey JT, Kleinman CS, Hellenbrand WE (1991) Balloon angioplasty for recurrent coarctation of aorta. Immediate and long-term results. Circulation 84(3):1150–1156. doi:10.1161/01.cir.84.3.1150
60. McCrindle BW, Jones TK, Morrow WR, Hagler DJ, Lloyd TR, Nouri S, Latson LA (1996) Acute results of balloon angioplasty of native coarctation versus recurrent aortic obstruction are equivalent. J Am Coll Cardiol 28(7):1810–1817. doi:10.1016/s0735-1097(96)00379-8
61. Morrow WR, Vick GW, Nihill MR, Rokey R, Johnston DL, Hedrick TD, Mullins CE (1988) Balloon dilation of unoperated coarctation of the aorta: Short- and intermediate-term results. J Am Coll Cardiol 11(1):133–138. doi:10.1016/0735-1097(88)90178-7
62. Siblini G, Rao PS, Nouri S, Ferdman B, Jureidini SB, Wilson AD (1998) Long-term follow-up results of balloon angioplasty of postoperative aortic recoarctation. Am J Cardiol 81(1):61–67. doi:10.1016/s0002-9149(97)00805-9
63. Tynan M (1980) Book reviews heart disease in infancy and childhood. By KeithJ. D., RoweR. D. and VladP., 3rd ed. 1978 (Macmillan, New York/Toronto/London), £36·00. ISBN 0–02–36220–2. Br J Radiol 53(630):579–579. doi:10.1259/0007-1285-53-630-579-b
64. Bouzguenda I, Marini D, Ou P, Boudjemline Y, Bonnet D, Agnoletti G (2009) Percutaneous treatment of neonatal aortic coarctation presenting with severe left ventricular dysfunction as a bridge to surgery. Cardiol Young 19(03):244. doi:10.1017/s1047951109003837
65. Burrows PE, Benson LN, Babyn P, MacDonald C (1994) Magnetic resonance imaging of the iliofemoral arteries after balloon dilation angioplasty of aortic arch obstructions in children. Circulation 90(2):915–920. doi:10.1161/01.cir.90.2.915
66. Cowley CG (2005) Long-term, randomized comparison of balloon angioplasty and surgery for native coarctation of the aorta in childhood. Circulation 111(25):3453–3456. doi:10.1161/circulationaha.104.510198
67. Fawzy ME, Fathala A, Osman A, Badr A, Mostafa MA, Mohamed G, Dunn B (2008) Twenty-two years of follow-up results of balloon angioplasty for discreet native coarctation of the aorta in adolescents and adults. Am Heart J 156(5):910–917. doi:10.1016/j.ahj.2008.06.037
68. Fiore AC, Fischer LK, Schwartz T, Jureidini S, Balfour I, Carpenter D, Demello D, Virgo KS, Pennington DG, Johnson RG (2005) Comparison of angioplasty and surgery for neonatal aortic coarctation. Ann Thorac Surg 80(5):1659–1665. doi:10.1016/j.athoracsur.2005.03.143
69. Ino T, Ohkubo M (1997) Dilation mechanism, causes of restenosis and stenting in balloon coarctation angioplasty. Acta Paediatr 86(4):367–371. doi:10.1111/j.1651-2227.1997.tb09024.x

70. Lee C-L, Lin J-F, Hsieh K-S, Lin C-C, Huang T-C (2007) Balloon angioplasty of native coarctation and comparison of patients younger and older than 3 months. Circ J 71 (11):1781–1784. doi:10.1253/circj.71.1781
71. Park Y, Lucas VW, Sklansky MS, Kashani IA, Rothman A (1997) Balloon angioplasty of native aortic coarctation in infants 3 months of age and younger. Am Heart J 134(5):917–923. doi:10.1016/s0002-8703(97)80015-4
72. Rao PS, Chopra PS, Koscik R, Smith PA, Wilson AD (1994) Surgical versus balloon therapy for aortic coarctation in infants $\leq$ 3 months old. J Am Coll Cardiol 23(6):1479–1483. doi:10.1016/0735-1097(94)90395-6
73. Walhout RJ, Suttorp MJ, Mackaij GJ, Ernst JMPG, Plokker HWM (2009) Long-term outcome after balloon angioplasty of coarctation of the aorta in adolescents and adults: Is aneurysm formation an issue? Catheter Cardiovasc Interv 73(4):549–556. doi:10.1002/ccd.21842
74. Wright GE, Nowak CA, Goldberg CS, Ohye RG, Bove EL, Rocchini AP (2005) Extended resection and end-to-end anastomosis for aortic coarctation in infants: results of a tailored surgical approach. Ann Thorac Surg 80(4):1453–1459. doi:10.1016/j.athoracsur.2005.04.002
75. Ino T, Ohkubo M, Akimoto K, Nishimoto K, Yabuta K, Kawasaki S, Watanabe M, Hosoda A (1996) Angiographic assessment of the stretch-recoil-gain relation after balloon coarctation angioplasty and its relation to late restenosis. Jpn Circ J 60(2):102–107. doi:10.1253/jcj.60.102
76. Oliver JM, Gallego P, Gonzalez A, Aroca A, Bret M, Mesa JM (2004) Risk factors for aortic complications in adults with coarctation of the aorta. J Am Coll Cardiol 44(8):1641–1647. doi:10.1016/j.jacc.2004.07.037
77. Bulbul ZR, Bruckheimer E, Love JC, Fahey JT, Hellenbrand WE (1996) Implantation of balloon-expandable stents for coarctation of the aorta: implantation data and short-term results. Catheter Cardiovasc Diagn 39(1):36–42. doi:10.1002/(sici)1097-0304(199609)39:1<36::aid-ccd7>3.3.co;2-z
78. Gardiner HM, Celermajer DS, Sorensen KE, Georgakopoulos D, Robinson J, Thomas O, Deanfield JE (1994) Arterial reactivity is significantly impaired in normotensive young adults after successful repair of aortic coarctation in childhood. Circulation 89(4):1745–1750. doi:10.1161/01.cir.89.4.1745
79. Guenthard J, Zumsteg U, Wyler F (1996) Arm-leg pressure gradients on late follow-up after coarctation repair: possible causes and implications. Eur Heart J 17(10):1572–1575. doi:10.1093/oxfordjournals.eurheartj.a014723
80. Gunthard J, Buser PT, Miettunen R, Hagmann A, Wyler F (1996) Effects of morphologic restenosis, defined by MRI after coarctation repair, on blood pressure and arm-leg and Doppler gradients. Angiology 47(11):1073–1080. doi:10.1177/000331979604701107
81. Kaemmerer H, Oelert F, Bahlmann J, Blücher S, Meyer G, Mügge A (1998) Arterial hypertension in adults after surgical treatment of aortic coarctation. Thorac Cardiovasc Surg 46(03):121–125. doi:10.1055/s-2007-1010207
82. Magee AG, Brzezinska-Rajszys G, Qureshi SA, Rosenthal E, Zubrzycka M, Ksiazyk J, Tynan M (1999) Stent implantation for aortic coarctation and recoarctation. Heart 82 (5):600–606. doi:10.1136/hrt.82.5.600
83. Carrozza M, Santoro G, Giovanna Russo M, Caianiello G, Calabrò R (2006) Stress stent fracture: Is stent angioplasty really a safe therapeutic option in native aortic coarctation? Int J Cardiol 113(1):127–128. doi:10.1016/j.ijcard.2005.08.041
84. Golden AB, Hellenbrand WE (2007) Coarctation of the aorta: stenting in children and adults. Catheter Cardiovasc Interv 69(2):289–299. doi:10.1002/ccd.21009
85. Gunn J, Cleveland T, Gaines P (1999) Covered stent to treat co-existent coarctation and aneurysm of the aorta in a young man. Heart 82(3):351–351. doi:10.1136/hrt.82.3.351
86. Sadiq M, Malick NH, Qureshi SA (2003) Simultaneous treatment of native coarctation of the aorta combined with patent ductus arteriosus using a covered stent. Catheter Cardiovasc Interv 59(3):387–390. doi:10.1002/ccd.10501

87. Tzifa A, Ewert P, Brzezinska-Rajszys G, Peters B, Zubrzycka M, Rosenthal E, Berger F, Qureshi SA (2006) Covered cheatham-platinum stents for aortic coarctation. J Am Coll Cardiol 47(7):1457–1463. doi:10.1016/j.jacc.2005.11.061
88. Forbes T, Matisoff D, Dysart J, Aggarwal S (2003) Treatment of coexistent coarctation and aneurysm of the aorta with covered stent in a pediatric patient. Pediatr Cardiol 24 (3):289–291. doi:10.1007/s00246-002-0262-9
89. Ewert P, Abdul-Khaliq H, Peters B, Nagdyman N, Schubert S, Lange PE (2004) Transcatheter therapy of long extreme subatretic aortic coarctations with covered stents. Catheter Cardiovasc Interv 63(2):236–239. doi:10.1002/ccd.20119
90. Pedra CAC, Fontes VF, Esteves CA, Arrieta SR, Braga SLN, Justino H, Kambara AM, Moreira SM, Sousa JER (2004) Use of covered stents in the management of coarctation of the aorta. Pediatr Cardiol 26(4):431–439. doi:10.1007/s00246-004-0814-2
91. Tan J-L, Mullen M (2005) Emergency stent graft deployment for acute aortic rupture following primary stenting for aortic coarctation. Catheter Cardiovasc Interv 65 (2):306–309. doi:10.1002/ccd.20370
92. Kato N, Dake MD, Miller DC, Semba CP, Mitchell RS, Razavi MK, Kee ST (1997) Traumatic thoracic aortic aneurysm: treatment with endovascular stent-grafts. Radiology 205(3):657–662. doi:10.1148/radiology.205.3.9393517
93. Mitchell RS, Dake MD, Semba CP, Fogarty TJ, Zarins CK, Liddell RP, Miller DC (1996) Endovascular stent–graft repair of thoracic aortic aneurysms. J Thorac Cardiovasc Surg 111 (5):1054–1062. doi:10.1016/s0022-5223(96)70382-3
94. Rousseau H, Soula P, Perreault P, Bui B, d'Othee BJ, Massabuau P, Meites G, Concina P, Mazerolles M, Joffre F, Otal P (1999) Delayed treatment of traumatic rupture of the thoracic aorta with endoluminal covered stent. Circulation 99(4):498–504. doi:10.1161/01.cir.99.4.498
95. Dake MD, Miller DC, Semba CP, Mitchell RS, Walker PJ, Liddell RP (1994) Transluminal placement of endovascular stent-grafts for the treatment of descending thoracic aortic aneurysms. N Engl J Med 331(26):1729–1734. doi:10.1056/nejm199412293312601
96. Kenny D, Margey R, Turner MS, Tometzki AJ, Walsh KP, Martin RP (2008) Self-expanding and balloon expandable covered stents in the treatment of aortic coarctation with or without aneurysm formation. Catheter Cardiovasc Interv 72(1):65–71. doi:10.1002/ccd.21559
97. Brzezinska-Rajszys G, Qureshi SA, Ksiazyk J, Zubrzycka M, Kosciesza A, Kubicka K, Tynan M (1999) Middle aortic syndrome treated by stent implantation. Heart 81 (2):166–170. doi:10.1136/hrt.81.2.166
98. Marshall AC, Perry SB, Keane JF, Lock JE (2000) Early results and medium-term follow-up of stent implantation for mild residual or recurrent aortic coarctation. Am Heart J 139 (6):1054–1060. doi:10.1067/mhj.2000.106616
99. Mohan UR, Danon S, Levi D, Connolly D, Moore JW (2009) Stent implantation for coarctation of the aorta in children <30 kg. J Am Coll Cardiol Intv 2(9):877–883. doi:10.1016/j.jcin.2009.07.002
100. Oechslin EN (2008) Does a stent cure hypertension? Heart 94(7):828–829. doi:10.1136/hrt.2007.130013
101. Pihkala J, Pedra CAC, Nykanen D, Benson LN (2000) Implantation of endovascular stents for hypoplasia of the transverse aortic arch. Cardiol Young 10(01). doi:10.1017/s1047951100006302
102. Suárez de Lezo J, Pan M, Romero M, Medina A, Segura J, Pavlovic D, Martinez C, Tejero I, Navero JP, Torres F, Lafuente M, Hernández E, Melián F, Concha M (1995) Balloon-expandable stent repair of severe coarctation of aorta. Am Heart J 129(5):1002–1008. doi:10.1016/0002-8703(95)90123-x
103. Thanopoulos BD (2000) Stent treatment for coarctation of the aorta: intermediate term follow up and technical considerations. Heart 84(1):65–70. doi:10.1136/heart.84.1.65

104. Benson LN, Freedom RM, Wilson GJ, Halliday WC (1986) Cerebral complications following balloon angioplasty of coarctation of the aorta. Cardiovasc Intervent Radiol 9(4):184–186. doi:10.1007/bf02577937
105. Butera G, Piazza L, Chessa M, Negura DG, Rosti L, Abella R, Delogu A, Condoluci C, Magherini A, Carminati M (2007) Covered stents in patients with complex aortic coarctations. Am Heart J 154(4):795–800. doi:10.1016/j.ahj.2007.06.018
106. Qureshi SA (2009) Use of covered stents to treat coarctation of the aorta. Korean Circ J 39 (7):261. doi:10.4070/kcj.2009.39.7.261
107. Forbes TJ, Garekar S, Amin Z, Zahn EM, Nykanen D, Moore P, Qureshi SA, Cheatham JP, Ebeid MR, Hijazi ZM, Sandhu S, Hagler DJ, Sievert H, Fagan TE, Ringewald J, Du W, Tang L, Wax DF, Rhodes J, Johnston TA, Jones TK, Turner DR, Pedra CAC, Hellenbrand WE (2007) Procedural results and acute complications in stenting native and recurrent coarctation of the aorta in patients over 4 years of age: a multi-institutional study. Catheter Cardiovasc Interv 70(2):276–285. doi:10.1002/ccd.21164
108. Godart F (2011) Intravascular stenting for the treatment of coarctation of the aorta in adolescent and adult patients. Arch Cardiovasc Dis 104(12):627–635. doi:10.1016/j.acvd.2011.08.005
109. Harrison DA (2001) Endovascular stents in the management of coarctation of the aorta in the adolescent and adult: one year follow up. Heart 85(5):561–566. doi:10.1136/heart.85.5.561
110. Mahadevan VS, Vondermuhll IF, Mullen MJ (2006) Endovascular aortic coarctation stenting in adolescents and adults: angiographic and hemodynamic outcomes. Catheter Cardiovasc Interv 67(2):268–275. doi:10.1002/ccd.20585
111. Qureshi AM, McElhinney DB, Lock JE, Landzberg MJ, Lang P, Marshall AC (2007) Acute and intermediate outcomes, and evaluation of injury to the aortic wall, as based on 15 years experience of implanting stents to treat aortic coarctation. Cardiol Young 17(03):307. doi:10.1017/s1047951107000339
112. Rao PS (1993) Aortic rupture after balloon angioplasty of aortic coarctation. Am Heart J 125 (4):1205–1206. doi:10.1016/0002-8703(93)90150-8
113. Balaji S, Oommen R, Rees PG (1991) Fatal aortic rupture during balloon dilatation of recoarctation. Heart 65(2):100–101. doi:10.1136/hrt.65.2.100
114. Chen SSM, Donald AE, Storry C, Halcox JP, Bonhoeffer P, Deanfield JE (2008) Impact of aortic stenting on peripheral vascular function and daytime systolic blood pressure in adult coarctation. Heart 94(7):919–924. doi:10.1136/hrt.2006.109389
115. Eicken A (2005) The fate of systemic blood pressure in patients after effectively stented coarctation. Eur Heart J 27(9):1100–1105. doi:10.1093/eurheartj/ehi748
116. Xu J, Shiota T, Omoto R, Zhou X, Kyo S, Ishii M, Rice MJ, Sahn DJ (1997) Intravascular ultrasound assessment of regional aortic wall stiffness, distensibility, and compliance in patients with coarctation of the aorta. Am Heart J 134(1):93–98. doi:10.1016/s0002-8703 (97)70111-x

Part III
Various Disorders That Represent Aortopathy

Chapter 14
The Marfan Syndrome

Romy Franken and Barbara J.M. Mulder

Abstract Marfan syndrome is an autosomal dominant disorder of connective tissue in which abnormalities in the cardiovascular, skeletal, and ocular systems may be present to a highly variable degree. Marfan syndrome is caused by mutations in the *FBN1* gene, which affect the structural integrity of the extracellular matrix and weaken the connective tissues. Prevalence has been estimated at 2–3 per 10,000 individuals and about 25 % of patients represent new mutations. Prognosis is mainly determined by progressive dilation of the aorta, which may lead to aortic dissection and death at a young age. Therefore, early identification of patients with Marfan syndrome is of considerable importance, and regular imaging of the aortic root and all other parts of the aorta is crucial in the follow-up. To prevent premature death, prophylactic aortic root surgery is performed in a person with normal body surface area when reaching a certain threshold (45–50 mm), and β-blockers are prescribed to reduce the aortic wall stress, reduce aortic dilation rate, and subsequently delay the time to prophylactic surgery. Currently, losartan treatment is evaluated as a novel pharmacological treatment strategy to prevent aortic dilation and aortic complications. Patients should be advised to avoid situations that increase blood pressure and heart rate dramatically.

Keywords Aortic dilation • Connective tissue • Dissection • Surgery • Treatment

---

R. Franken
Department of Cardiology, Academic Medical Center Amsterdam, Meibergdreef 9 room B2-240, 1105 AZ Amsterdam, The Netherlands

B.J.M. Mulder (✉)
Department of Cardiology, Academic Medical Center Amsterdam, Meibergdreef 9 room B2-240, 1105 AZ Amsterdam, The Netherlands

Interuniversity Cardiology Institute of the Netherlands, Utrecht, The Netherlands
e-mail: b.j.mulder@amc.uva.nl

K. Niwa, H. Kaemmerer (eds.), *Aortopathy*, DOI 10.1007/978-4-431-56071-5_14

14.1 Natural History and Clinical Presentation

14.1.1 Diagnosis

Marfan syndrome is an autosomal dominant disorder of connective tissue in which abnormalities in the cardiovascular, skeletal, and ocular systems may be present to a highly variable degree. Prevalence has been estimated at 2–3 per 10,000 individuals and about 25 % of patients represent new mutations. Prognosis is mainly determined by progressive dilation of the aorta, which may lead to aortic dissection and premature death [1]. Therefore, early identification and establishment of the diagnosis in patients with Marfan syndrome and subsequently performing prophylactic surgery to prevent aortic dissection and rupture are of considerable importance. Elucidation of the molecular mechanisms behind Marfan syndrome will allow improvement in diagnostic testing, but so far genetic testing mainly plays a supporting role alongside the clinical diagnostic guidelines, following the revised Ghent criteria (Table 14.1) [2].

The diagnosis requires the coexistence of aortic root aneurysm or aortic dissection together with either a pathogenic *FBN1* mutation, ectopia lentis, or a positive family history. The remaining cardinal manifestations of Marfan syndrome are incorporated in a systemic score, where a systemic score >7 also contributes to the diagnosis (Table 14.2) [2].

Marfan syndrome considerably overlaps with other heritable connective tissue disorders, such as Loeys-Dietz syndrome, familial ectopia lentis, and Ehlers-Danlos syndrome. The variability in clinical expression and presence of *FBN1* mutations in the different fibrillinopathies require a multidisciplinary approach in a Marfan screening center for complete evaluation and counseling.

Table 14.1 The revised Ghent criteria for diagnosis of Marfan syndrome

Family history	Aortic dilation ($Z \geq 2$) or dissection	Ectopia lentis	Systemic score (≥7 of 20)	Pathogenic *FBN1* mutation
	X	X		
	X		X	
	X			X
		X		Xao
X	X			
X		X		
X			X	

Each line represents a possible combination leading to Marfan syndrome
Xao: *FBN1* mutation associated with aortic pathology

Table 14.2 Scoring of the systemic features

Feature	Score
Wrist and thumb sign	3 (wrist or thumb: 1)
Pectus carinatum deformity	2 (pectus excavatum or chest asymmetry: 1)
Hindfoot deformity	2 (plain pes planus: 1)
Pneumothorax	2
Dural ectasia	2
Protrusio acetabuli	2
Reduced upper segment/lower segment ratio *and* increased arm/height *without* severe scoliosis	1
Scoliosis or thoracolumbar kyphosis	1
Reduced elbow extension	1
Facial features (3/5): dolichocephaly, enophthalmus, downslanting palpebral fissures, malar hypoplasia, retrognathia	1
Skin striae	1
Myopia >3 diopters	1
Mitral valve prolapse (all types)	1

14.1.2 Clinical Cardiovascular Findings

Mean survival of untreated patients was about 40 years in historic series. Prognosis and premature death of Marfan patients is mainly determined by aortic dissection. The risk of type A dissection clearly increases with larger aortic root diameter at the level of the sinuses of Valsalva, which is found in up to 80 % of the Marfan patients. However, aortic dissection may occasionally occur in patients with no or only mild aortic dilation [3]. Not only the aortic root but also other parts of the aorta may be dilated [4]. Additional predictors for aortic dissection are aortic elasticity and aortic tortuosity [5–8]. Decreased aortic elasticity determined by noninvasive measurement of local distensibility and flow wave velocity with magnetic resonance imaging (MRI) has been an individual predictor. In addition, increased elongation of the aorta, leading to a curved and tortuous aorta, has been found to correlate with increasing aortic diameter and independently predicts aortic dissections in Marfan patients as well [9].

The definition of aortic dilation in the diagnostic criteria for adults relies on a Z-score above 2, which may be calculated with different Z-score equations [10]. Different methods are used for aortic dilation in different publications. Currently, the Z-score normalized for height is recommended [11].

A dilated aorta is often asymptomatic. The presence of significant aortic, tricuspid, or mitral regurgitation may lead to symptoms of ventricular volume overload. Some patients with Marfan syndrome have a slightly impaired left and right ventricular ejection fraction without significant valvular regurgitation, which may be due to a fibrillin defect in the myocardium [12], especially patients with a non-missense fibrillin-1 mutation had left ventricular dilation [13]. However, the left ventricular dimensions and systolic function were found to be normal in most Marfan patients, and none fulfilled the criteria for dilated cardiomyopathy [14].

The combination of increased height and a structural abnormality of the blood vessels may cause impaired orthostatic tolerance, leading to fatigue and orthostatic hypotension [15]. To counteract orthostatic drops in blood pressure, patients can be educated in physical maneuvers, such as leg crossing and muscle tensing.

14.1.3 Late Outcome

Life expectancy of Marfan patients has improved substantially up to a median survival of 60–70 years, due to the advances in medical and surgical therapy [16]. In about 15 % of the patients, the first aortic event occurs in the distal aorta [17, 18]. However, the aortic root is mostly the first site to be affected. The 18-year survival rate after aortic root replacement has been reported to be 76 % [19]. After aortic root replacement, patients deserve intensive surveillance because of an increased risk of developing aneurysms and dissections distal to the site of the graft [3, 17, 20, 21]. The increased risk of postsurgical complications may be a more advanced disease in patients undergoing aortic surgery, hemodynamic factors and altered wall mechanics due to the impact of intervention at the level of the root, or tissue damage because of clamping of the aorta during the operation.

In a small series of 40 patients with Marfan syndrome, MRI showed coronary ostial aneurysms in 27 (43 %) patients after 3 months to 19 years after elective aortic root surgery [22]. Coronary ostial aneurysms are usually not progressive and may be developed due to perioperative stretch of the weakened wall of the coronary ostium. However, follow-up studies are needed to confirm that these aneurysms are not clinically relevant.

14.2 Genetics

Marfan syndrome is caused by mutations in the *FBN1* gene on chromosome 15q21 encoding fibrillin-1, a large glycoprotein in the extracellular matrix [1]. *FBN1* mutations induce abnormal or deficient fibrillin-1 protein synthesis, which affects the structural integrity of the extracellular matrix and weakens the supporting tissues. Fibrillin-1 normally binds to a large latent complex, which comprises the inactive form of transforming growth factor-β (TGF-β) [23]. *FBN1* mutations or the damaged extracellular matrix seems to lead to an increased plasma TGF-β level [24], which is associated with aortic root dilation in a mouse model of Marfan syndrome [25], as well as with aortic dilation rate in Marfan patients [26].

In approximately 90 % of the Marfan patients, an *FBN1* mutation is identified, and almost all of the currently 3000 registered *FBN1* mutations are unique to an affected individual or family. Genotype-phenotype correlations have been complicated by this large number of unique mutations and clinical heterogeneity among family members. One interesting classification is based on the effect of the *FBN1* mutation on the fibrillin-1 protein, referred to as dominant negative or haploinsufficient mutations [27]. Dominant negative mutations, such as cysteine substitutions, lead to a disturbed protein folding and generally a higher prevalence of ectopia lentis. On the other hand, haploinsufficient mutations, such as premature termination codon mutations, lead to a lower production of normal fibrillin-1 protein and generally more often to skeletal features and cardiovascular involvement, such as aortic dissection [28, 29].

14.3 Treatment

14.3.1 Surgical Treatment

The threshold diameter for aortic surgery is 50 mm for any level of the aorta, or 45 mm for the aortic root in combination with either a family history of dissection, progressive dilation of more than 2 mm/year by repetitive measurement using the same imaging technique, severe aortic or mitral valve regurgitation, or if pregnancy is desired. Lower thresholds for intervention may be considered according to the lower body surface area (BSA) in patients of small stature or according to patient's preference [30]. On average, women have a smaller aorta (by 5 mm), which is only partly explained by a smaller BSA [31]. An indexed aortic diameter (adjusted for BSA) could be useful for operative decision-making [32]; surgery then would be indicated at an aortic diameter of 4.5 cm in patients with a BSA of 1.65 m^2, 5.0 cm at a BSA of 1.8 m^2, and 5.5 cm at a BSA of 2 m^2.

Over the past 30 years, the composite replacement of the aortic valve and ascending aorta ("Bentall procedure") has been a low-risk and very durable operation for aortic root aneurysm in Marfan patients. In a series of 675 Marfan patients undergoing aortic root surgery, the operative mortality rate was 1.5 % for elective operations and 11.7 % for emergency operations [33]. However, in patients with initially normal aortic valves, valve-sparing operations with root replacement by a Dacron prosthesis and reimplantation of the coronary arteries into the prosthesis (the David procedure) have now become the preferred choice of surgery. Either type of aortic root replacement appears to be safe, reproducible, and associated with excellent 5–10-year results. Freedom from reoperation of the aortic valve after the David procedure was 94.8 %, with a slow progressive deterioration of aortic valve function after long-term follow-up [19]. A homograft or bioprosthetic valve may also be considered to avoid anticoagulant therapy.

Information concerning the outcomes of endovascular stenting in Marfan patients is scarce. In Marfan patients with aortic dissection, the use of endovascular stenting should only be considered in life-threatening emergencies as a bridge to definite therapy, since these aortas demand close clinical and imaging surveillance to detect progressive dilation, resulting in high endoleak rates, a 12 % mortality rate, and a 14–18 % need of a new surgical procedure [34–36].

Personalized external aortic root support (PEARS) is a novel surgical approach, stabilizing the aortic root and decreasing the risk of aortic dissection in patients with Marfan syndrome. Although prospective follow-up data is currently lacking, in the first 30 selected patients operated with PEARS, the perioperative burden was less without any aortic or valvular event after 1.4–8.8 years of follow-up [37].

14.3.2 Medical Treatment

In patients with Marfan syndrome, and especially in patients with aortic dissection, rigorous antihypertensive medical treatment is important, aiming at a systolic blood pressure less than 120 mm Hg. The most commonly prescribed drugs are β-adrenergic blockers, which reduce the aortic dilation rate in patients with Marfan syndrome, due to its effects in reducing the blood pressure and the force on the left ventricular ejection [38, 39]. Losartan, an angiotensin II receptor 1 blocker, might be an alternative or complementary therapy to β-blockers, since losartan reduces arterial pressure and potentially interferes with the pathophysiology of Marfan syndrome by TGF-β antagonism. After evidence for effectiveness of losartan in a mouse model of Marfan syndrome [40], a small pilot study in children and adults demonstrated a beneficial effect of losartan combined with β-blockers ($n = 15$) on aortic dilation rate compared with β-blockers alone ($n = 13$) after 35 months of echocardiographic follow-up [41]. Subsequently, eight randomized clinical trials were initiated to test losartan effectiveness; so far, four studies have been published [42]. The COMPARE trial demonstrated a beneficial effect of losartan on top of β-blockers on aortic root dilation rate in a larger cohort ($n = 145$) as measured by MRI and additionally demonstrated the beneficial effect of losartan on the distal part of the aorta after aortic root surgery [43]. The Marfan Sartan trial evaluated the benefit of adding losartan to a high dose of β-blockers. Remarkably, in this cohort of 292 children and adults, aortic dilation rate was similar for the losartan- and placebo-treated group after 3.5 years of echocardiographic follow-up [44]. The Pediatric Heart Network study demonstrated that both losartan and atenolol were equally effective in reducing aortic dilatation rate in a large, blinded trial including 608 children during 3 years by echocardiography [45]. The last published trial so far demonstrated in 140 Marfan patients aged 5–60 years that losartan was not inferior in respect to atenolol and tended to be more favorable in the losartan monotherapy group when corrected for BSA or Z-score measured by MRI over 3 years of follow-up [46]. The discrepancies in outcome between the studies may be explained by the different study designs [42]. Until the results of the ongoing three trials and meta-analysis are known, we can conclude that losartan does not seem to be more effective in reducing the aortic dilation rate than a high dosage of β-blockers, but that losartan can safely be administered as an alternative or as an additive to β-blocker therapy, especially in patients with intolerance or side effects of β-blockers [42].

14.4 Outpatient Assessment

14.4.1 Follow-Up

Optimal long-term outcome demands lifelong follow-up with imaging of the aortic root by means of echocardiography and the entire aorta by means of MRI at regular intervals. This is particularly true if a dissection has occurred and its stability is being monitored. Patients with mitral valve prolapse and moderate or severe mitral regurgitation should also be followed with yearly echocardiography. Antihypertensive medical treatment, aiming at a systolic blood pressure less than 120 mm Hg, is important in all patients with Marfan syndrome. After aortic dissection, systolic blood pressure should not exceed 110 mm Hg. Lifelong and regular follow-up of these patients requires involvement of trained specialists with ample expertise in a tertiary referral center.

Regular imaging of the aortic root and all other parts of the aorta is crucial in the follow-up of patients with Marfan syndrome (Table 14.3).

Echocardiography in the parasternal long-axis view is mostly used for measurement of the aortic root (Fig. 14.1). By means of Doppler echocardiography, the presence and hemodynamic consequences of aortic regurgitation, mitral valve

Table 14.3 Different imaging modalities

	Transthoracic echocardiography	Transesophageal echocardiography	Magnetic resonance imaging or computed tomography
Aortic root dilation	x		x
Presence and severity of aortic regurgitation	x	x	
Presence and severity of mitral regurgitation	x	x	
Reparability of mitral and aortic valves		x	
Dilation of the pulmonary trunk	x		x
Evidence of endocarditis	x	x	x
Presence of ascending aortic dissection	x	x	x
Intraoperative evaluation of aortic and mitral valve surgery		x	
Dimensions of major branches and arteries			x
Presence of lumbosacral dural ectasia			x
Aortic elasticity and tortuosity			x

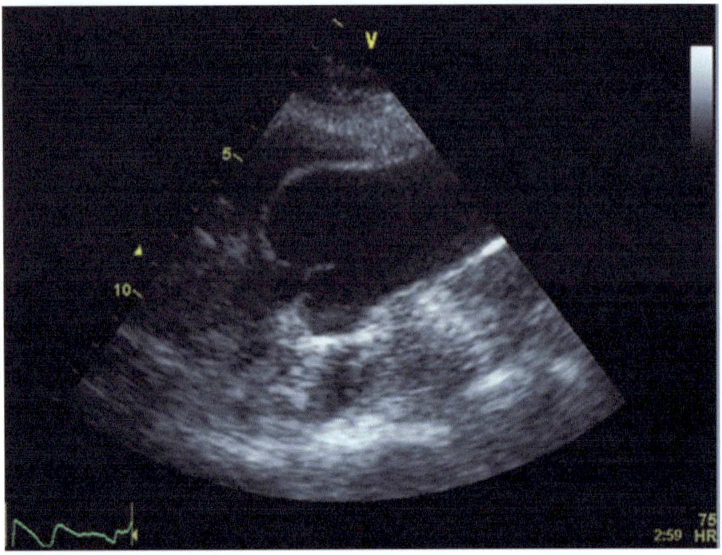

Fig. 14.1 Long-axis echocardiography showing a dilated aortic root in a patient with Marfan syndrome (From Mulder [4])

prolapse, mitral regurgitation, and occasionally tricuspid valve prolapse can be assessed. MRI is particularly useful for imaging of the entire aorta, for patients with deformation of the chest wall and asymmetrical aortic roots (Fig. 14.2) [47]. Imaging of the entire aorta should be performed in every patient. When parts of the aorta are dilated, regular follow-up should be performed at least once every year. Even when the aorta shows no abnormalities, imaging should be repeated within 5 years. Computed tomography (CT) may be used when MRI cannot be performed because of contraindications or unavailability. With MRI, aortic elasticity can be measured and is often reduced. Aortic elasticity of the thoracic descending aorta appeared to be an independent predictor for progressive descending aortic dilation [14]. Holter monitoring should be performed in symptomatic patients, because ventricular arrhythmias, conduction disturbances, and sudden cardiac death may occasionally occur.

14.4.2 Lifestyle Advices

Patients should be advised to avoid both physical and emotional situations that increase blood pressure and heart rate dramatically. Furthermore, patients should be advised to avoid exertion at maximal capacity, competitive sports, contact sports, and isometric sports.

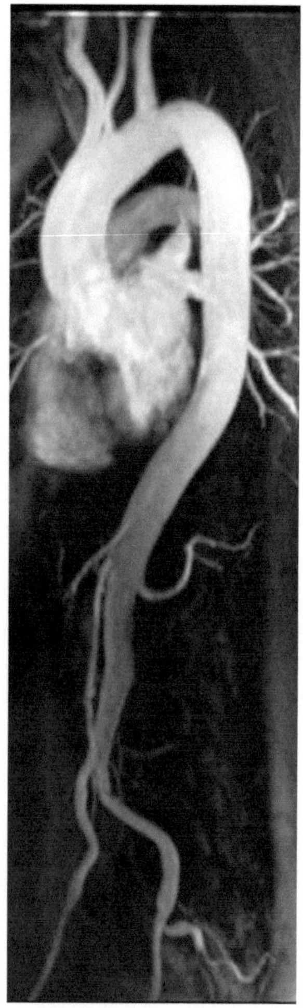

Fig. 14.2 MR image of a dilated aortic root and aorta in a patient with Marfan syndrome (From Franken et al. [1])

14.4.3 Endocarditis Prophylaxis

According to contemporary IE prevention guidelines, endocarditis prophylaxis is only recommended in patients with a prosthetic valve, in patients with previous endocarditis, and in patients with complete repair using prosthetic material (surgical or percutaneous) for up to 6 months after the procedure (until endothelialization) and ongoing only when a residual defect persists at the site of prosthetic material [48].

14.4.4 Pregnancy

For women with Marfan syndrome, pregnancy presents a twofold problem: a 50 % chance that the child will be affected and an increased risk of aortic dissection during or (especially) shortly after pregnancy. Women with an aortic diameter above 45 mm are strongly discouraged from becoming pregnant before surgical repair. An aortic diameter below 40 mm rarely presents a problem, although a completely safe diameter does not exist. With an aorta between 40 and 45 mm, recent aortic growth and a family history of aortic events are important for advising pregnancy with or without preconception aortic repair [49]. A recent study on 55 pregnancies in 35 women with Marfan syndrome showed an increased aortic dilation rate of 0.3 mm/month. This increased aortic dilation rate decreased after delivery, but remained higher than the pre-pregnancy dilation rate [50]. Two other smaller studies have reported no difference between the baseline and the pregnancy aortic dilation rate [51, 52]. Pregnancy, however, did influence long-term growth rate in Marfan women with an aortic root diameter above 40 mm (0.36 mm/year vs. 0.14 mm/year in the childless Marfan women) [51]. In addition to cardiovascular complications, pregnancy in women with Marfan syndrome is associated with a high rate of premature deliveries, preterm premature rupture of membranes, and increased mortality in the offspring [51]. Especially the use of β-blockers is associated with intrauterine growth retardation [53].

References

1. Franken R, den Hartog AW, Singh M et al (2012) Marfan syndrome: progress report. Prog Pediatr Cardiol 34:9–14
2. Loeys BL, Dietz HC, Braverman AC et al (2010) The revised Ghent nosology for the Marfan syndrome. J Med Genet 47:476–485
3. den Hartog AW, Franken R, Zwinderman AH et al (2015) The risk for type B aortic dissection in Marfan syndrome. J Am Coll Cardiol 65:246–254
4. Mulder BJM (2008) The distal aorta in the Marfan syndrome. Neth Heart J 16:382–386
5. Adams JN, Brooks M, Redpath TW et al (1995) Aortic distensibility and stiffness index measured by magnetic resonance imaging in patients with Marfan's syndrome. Br Heart J 73:265–269
6. Groenink M, De Roos A, Mulder BJ et al (2001) Biophysical properties of the normal-sized aorta in patients with Marfan syndrome: evaluation with MR flow mapping. Radiology 219:535–540
7. Hirata K, Triposkiadis F, Sparks E et al (1991) The Marfan syndrome: abnormal aortic elastic properties. J Am Coll Cardiol 18:57
8. Nollen GJ, Groenink M, Tijssen JGP et al (2004) Aortic stiffness and diameter predict progressive aortic dilation in patients with Marfan syndrome. Eur Heart J 25:1146–1152
9. Franken R, El Morabit A, de Waard V et al (2015) Increased aortic tortuosity indicates a more severe aortic phenotype in adults with Marfan syndrome. Int J Cardiol 194:7–12
10. van Kimmenade RRJ, Kempers M, de Boer MJ et al (2013) A clinical appraisal of different Z-score equations for aortic root assessment in the diagnostic evaluation of Marfan syndrome. Genet Med 15:528–532

11. Devereux RB, de Simone G, Arnett DK et al (2012) Normal limits in relation to age, body size and gender of two-dimensional echocardiographic aortic root dimensions in persons =15 years of age. Am J Cardiol 110:1189–1194
12. de Witte P, Aalberts JJ, Radonic T et al (2011) Intrinsic biventricular dysfunction in Marfan syndrome. Heart 97:2063–2068
13. Aalbert JJ, van Tintelen JP, Meijboom LJ et al (2014) Relation between genotype and left-ventricular dilatation in patients with Marfan syndrome. Gene 534:40–43
14. Meijboom LJ, Timmermans J, Van Tintelen JP et al (2005) Evaluation of left ventricular dimensions and function in Marfan's syndrome without significant valvular regurgitation. Am J Cardiol 95:795–797
15. Van Dijk N, Boer MC, Mulder BJM et al (2008) Is fatigue in Marfan syndrome related to orthostatic intolerance? Clin Auton Res 18:187–193
16. Silverman DI, Gray JG, Roman MJ et al (1995) Family history of severe cardiovascular disease in Marfan syndrome is associated with increased aortic diameter and decreased survival. J Am Coll Cardiol 26:1062–1067
17. Engelfriet PM, Boersma E, Tijssen JGP et al (2006) Beyond the root: dilation of the distal aorta in the Marfan's syndrome. Heart 92:1238–1243
18. Finkbohner R, Johnston D, Crawford ES et al (1995) Marfan syndrome: long-term survival and complications after aortic aneurysm repair. Circulation 91:728–733
19. David TE, Feindel CM, David CM, Manlhiot C (2014) A quarter of a century of experience with aortic valve-sparing operations. J Thorac Cardiovasc Surg 148:872–879
20. Engelfriet P, Boersma E, Oechslin E et al (2005) The spectrum of adult congenital heart disease in Europe: morbidity and mortality in a 5 year follow-up period. The Euro Heart Survey on adult congenital heart disease. Eur Heart J 26:2325–2333
21. Kawamoto S, Bluemke DA, Traill TA, Zerhouni EA (1997) Thoracoabdominal aorta in Marfan syndrome: MR imaging findings of progression of vasculopathy after surgical repair. Radiology 203:727–732
22. Meijboom LJ, Nollen GJ, Merchant N et al (2002) Frequency of coronary ostial aneurysms after aortic root surgery in patients with the Marfan syndrome. Am J Cardiol 89:1135–1138
23. Ramirez F, Dietz HC (2007) Marfan syndrome: from molecular pathogenesis to clinical treatment. Curr Opin Genet Dev 17:252–258
24. Franken R, Radonic T, den Hartog AW et al (2015) The revised role of TGF-β in aortic aneurysms in Marfan syndrome. Neth Heart J 23:116–121
25. Neptune ER, Frischmeyer PA, Arking DE et al (2003) Dysregulation of TGF-beta activation contributes to pathogenesis in Marfan syndrome. Nat Genet 33:407–411
26. Franken R, den Hartog AW, de Waard V et al (2013) Circulating transforming growth factor-β as a prognostic biomarker in Marfan syndrome. Int J Cardiol 168:2441–2446
27. Franken R, den Hartog AW, Radonic T et al (2015) Beneficial outcome of losartan therapy depends on type of FBN1 mutation in Marfan syndrome. Circ Cardiovasc Genet 8:383–388
28. Franken R, Heesterbeek TJ, de Waard V et al (2014) Diagnosis and genetics of Marfan syndrome. Expert Opin Orphan Drugs 2:1–14
29. Franken R, Groenink M, de Waard V et al (2016) Genotype impacts survival in Marfan syndrome. Eur Heart J
30. Erbel R, Aboyans V, Boileau C et al (2014) 2014 ESC guidelines on the diagnosis and treatment of aortic diseases. Eur Heart J 34:2873–2926
31. Meijboom LJ, Timmermans J, Zwinderman AH et al (2005) Aortic root growth in men and women with the Marfan's syndrome. Am J Cardiol 96:1441–1444
32. Davies RR, Gallo A, Coady MA et al (2006) Novel measurement of relative aortic size predicts rupture of thoracic aortic aneurysms. Ann Thorac Surg 81:169–177
33. Gott VL, Greene PS, Alejo DE et al (1990) Replacement of the aortic root in patients with Marfan's syndrome. N Engl J Med 340:1307–1313
34. Nordon IM, Hinchliffe RJ, Holt PJ et al (2009) Endovascular management of chronic aortic dissection in patients with Marfan syndrome. J Vasc Surg 5:987–991

35. Pacini D, Parolari A, Berretta P et al (2013) Endovascular treatment for type B dissection in Marfan syndrome: is it worthwhile? Ann Thorac Surg 2:737–749
36. Preventza O, Mohammed S, Cheong BY et al (2014) Endovascular therapy in patients with genetically triggered thoracic aortic disease: applications and short- and mid-term outcomes. Eur J Cardiothorac Surg 2:248–253
37. Treasure T, Takkenberg JJ, Golesworthy T et al (2014) Personalised external aortic root support (PEARS) in Marfan syndrome: analysis of 1–9 year outcomes by intention-to-treat in a cohort of the first 30 consecutive patients to receive a novel tissue and valve-conserving procedure, compared with the published results of aortic root replacement. Heart 100:969–975
38. Shores J, Berger KR, Murphy EA, Pyeritz RE (1994) Progression of aortic dilation and the benefit of long-term beta-adrenergic blockade in Marfan's syndrome. N Engl J Med 330:1335–1341
39. Engelfriet P, Mulder BJM (2007) Is there benefit of beta-blocking agents in the treatment of patients with the Marfan syndrome? Int J Cardiol 114:300–302
40. Habashi JP, Judge DP, Holm TM et al (2006) Losartan, an AT1 antagonist, prevents aortic aneurysm in a mouse model of Marfan syndrome. Science 312:117–121
41. Chiu HH, Wu MH, Wang JK et al (2013) Losartan added to β-blockade therapy for aortic root dilation in Marfan syndrome: a randomized, open-label pilot study. Mayo Clin Proc 88:271–276
42. Franken R, Mulder BJ (2015) Aortic disease: Losartan versus atenolol in the Marfan aorta-how to treat? Nat Rev Cardiol 12:447–448
43. Groenink M, den Hartog AW, Franken R et al (2013) Losartan reduces aortic dilatation rate in adults with Marfan syndrome: a randomized, open-label study. Eur Heart J 34:3491–3500
44. Milleron O, Arnoult F, Ropers J et al (2015) Marfan Sartan: a randomized, double-blind, placebo-controlled trial. Eur Heart J 36:2160–2166
45. Lacro RV, Dietz HC, Sleeper LA et al (2014) Atenolol versus losartan in children and young adults with Marfan's syndrome. N Engl J Med 27:2061–2071
46. Forteza A, Evangelista A, Sánchez V et al (2015) Efficacy of losartan vs. atenolol for the prevention of aortic dilation in Marfan syndrome: a randomized clinical trial. Eur Heart J. doi:10.1093/eurheartj/ehv575
47. Meijboom LJ, Groenink M, Van der Wall EE et al (2000) Aortic root asymmetry in Marfan patients; evaluation by magnetic resonance imaging and comparison with standard echocardiography. Int J Card Imaging 16:161–168
48. Nishimura RA, Carabello BA, Faxon DP (2008) American College of Cardiology/American Heart Association Task Force, 2008 ACC/AHA 2008 guideline update on valvular heart disease: focused update on infective endocarditis: a report of the American College of Cardiology/American Heart Association Task Force on Practice Guidelines: endorsed by the Society of Cardiovascular Anesthesiologists, Society for Cardiovascular Angiography and Interventions, and Society of Thoracic Surgeons. Circulation 118:887–896
49. Meijboom LJ, Vos FE, Timmermans J et al (2005) Pregnancy and aortic root growth in the Marfan syndrome: a prospective study. Eur Heart J 26:914–920
50. Donnelly RT, Pinto NM, Kocolas I, Yetman AT (2012) The immediate and long-term impact of pregnancy on aortic growth rate and mortality in woman with Marfan syndrome. J Am Coll Cardiol 60:224–229
51. Meijboom LJ, Drenthen W, Pieper PG et al (2006) Obstetric complications in Marfan syndrome. Int J Cardiol 110:53–59
52. Rossiter JP, Repke JT, Morales AJ, Murphy EA (1995) A prospective longitudinal evaluation of pregnancy in the Marfan syndrome. Am J Obstet Gynecol 173:1599–1606
53. Ersbøll A, Hedegaard M, Søndergaard L et al (2014) Treatment with oral beta-blockers during pregnancy complicated by maternal heart disease increases the risk of fetal growth restriction. BJOG An Int J Obstet Gynaecol 121:618–625

Chapter 15
Bicuspid Aortic Valve

Yskert von Kodolitsch and Harald Kaemmerer

Abstract Bicuspid aortic valve (BAV) has a prevalence of 0.5–1.39% in the general population. The prevalence of BAV in aortic dissection is 3.5–11.8%. Unfortunately, the incidence of aortic dissection in BAV remains unknown. The etiology of BAV is polygenetic, where environmental factors and unknown genetic factors seem to interact to cause BAV. In some instances, chromosomal aberrations or defined gene defects cause BAV.

Congenital BAV must be distinguished from acquired BAV. Congenital aortic valve malformations differ by number of cusps, ranging from one to five. BAV cusps can be subclassified according to patterns of calcification, severity of calcification, presence of a raphe, and fusion of cusps. We tend to perceive BAV as an isolated congenital heart defect. However, we identified 20 well-defined syndromic, complex, or isolated congenital heart defects that are associated with BAV disease, some of which are apparently quite frequent.

BAV aortopathy can be classified according to presence and type of aortic valve dysfunction, shape of the proximal aorta, aortic arch involvement, and coexistence with coarctation of the aorta.

Factors that may increase the risk for aneurysmal formation, aortic rupture, or dissection in BAV comprise aortic valve characteristics, comorbidities of BAV, and behavioral factors. Candidates for biomarkers of BAV aortopathy comprise a family history with early dissection or death, increased aortic growth rates, proximal aortic shape, aortic stiffness and aortic elasticity markers, aortic wall shear stress, endothelial dysfunction, and serological biomarkers.

Keywords Bicuspid aortic valve • Aortic dilatation • Aortic regurgitation • Aortic stenosis • Aortopathy • Genetics

---

Y. von Kodolitsch, M.D., M.B.A.
Department of Cardiology/Angiology, Centre of Cardiology and Cardiovascular Surgery, University Hospital Hamburg – Eppendorf, Hamburg, Germany

H. Kaemmerer, M.D. (✉)
Klinik für Kinderkardiologie und angeborene Herzfehler, Deutsches Herzzentrum München, Technische Universität München, Lazarettstr. 36, D-80636 München, Germany
e-mail: Kaemmerer@dhm.mhn.de

K. Niwa, H. Kaemmerer (eds.), *Aortopathy*, DOI 10.1007/978-4-431-56071-5_15

List of Abbreviations

AOA	Aortic arch
ASC	Ascending aorta
AVA	Aortic valve annulus (anatomical ventriculo-arterial junction)
AVR	Aortic valve replacement
BAV	Bicuspid aortic valve
BAV-COA	Coexistence of bicuspid aortic valve and coarctation of the aorta
BAV-I	BAV with predominant insufficiency
BAV-LN	BAV with fusion of the left and noncoronary cusp
BAV-MO	BAV morphotype
BAV-RI	BAV with balanced stenosis and insufficiency
BAV-RL	BAV with fusion of the right and left coronary cusp
BAV-RN	BAV with fusion of the right and noncoronary cusp
BAV-S	BAV with predominant stenosis
CHD	Congenital heart defect
COA	Coarctation of the aorta
DESC	Descending thoracic aorta
HTN	Arterial hypertension
SOV	Sinus of valsalva
STJ	Sinotubular junction
TAV	Tricuspid aortic valve

15.1 Introduction

Bicuspid aortic valve (BAV) may simply be viewed as "an aortic valve that has two cusps instead of three," and BAV aortopathy may simply be considered as "post-stenotic dilatation of the ascending aorta."

More than 500 years ago, Leonardo da Vinci explained and depicted BAV for the first time. Paget recalled in 1844 the tendency of the BAV to develop disease, Peacock mentioned the tendency of these valves to develop obstructions or regurgitation early, Osler described the predilection of these valves to infective endocarditis, and Victor Babes (1891), in Germany, and 3 decades later Maude Abbott, in North America (1927), commented on an association between congenital BAV and aortic aneurysm, dissection, and rupture, and since Abbott described aortopathy in BAV [1]. Since then, the literature on BAV disease has grown into complex field on detailed and conflicting knowledge.

15.2 Frequency of BAV and BAV Aortopathy

Besides mitral valve prolapse, BAV is the most frequent congenital heart defect in the general population. Autopsy studies and echocardiographic screening studies yield strikingly similar results on the frequency of BAV in the general population. The prevalence ranges from 0.5 to 1.39% at autopsy and between 0.5 and 0.9% on echocardiographic screening. Autopsy studies and a clinical register of aortic dissection assess the prevalence of BAV in individuals with aortic dissection. Both types of studies report BAV in 7.5–11.2% and 3.5–11.8% of aortic dissections. Nistri et al. found aortic dilatation, which they defined with diameters >2 standard deviation above normal, in 68.9% of young Italian conscripts with BAV at echocardiographic screening [2]. The widely cited 2% prevalence of BAV appears to stem from a single autopsy study published in 1923 [3]. Cohort studies that register aortic events in BAV report on 0.5–0.8% incidence of aortic dissection with various difference of intervals of follow-up, treatment standards, reasons for inclusion, and ages at inclusion into the cohort. Hence, the accurate prevalence and natural history of BAV aortopathy are difficult to interpret in these studies (Table 15.1).

15.3 Classification of BAV: Etiology

BAV is a congenital heart anomaly, and to the best of our knowledge, the literature reports exclusively genetic causes of BAV. However, other causes of BAV such as intrauterine infection or intoxication appear to be a possible cause. Moreover, the

Table 15.1 Frequency of BAV and BAV aortopathy

Type of study	Frequency of BAV in the general population	Frequency of aortopathy in BAV
Autopsy	0.5–1.39% (meta-analysis of necropsy studies) [4]	7.5–11.2% of fatal aortic dissections have BAV [5–7]
	Roberts mentioned in one study where BAV was diagnosed in 18/800 autopsies (2) [3]	
Population screening with transthoracic echocardiography	0.5–0.9% (screening of neonates, primary school students, military) [2, 4, 8–10]	68.9% of BAV exhibits dilatation of proximal aorta [2]
Registry of aortic dissection		3.5–11.8% of aortic dissections have BAV [11, 12]
Cohort studies [13–17]		0.5–0.8% incidence of aortic dissection during follow-up in BAV [13, 15, 18]. The frequency of aortic dissection was 0.1% per patient-year of follow-up [15] and 3.1 cases per 10,000 patient-years, respectively [18]

BAV phenotype is highly variable, and epigenetic modifiers and environmental factors are likely to play an important role in BAV disease event when a distinct causative genetic defect can be identified [19].

We classify the genetic causes of BAV according to frequency and mechanisms (Table 15.2). First, male predominance and familial occurrence of BAV are found in BAV, which argue for a genetic mechanism in a majority of individuals with BAV. Second, only a small fraction of individuals with BAV have chromosomal disorders. However, some chromosomal disorders, such as Turner syndrome, have BAV in up to 30%. Third, BAV may be a monogenetic disease, where autosomal dominant traits are most frequent, but where other traits, such as autosomal recessive or X-linked traits, may occur. Monogenetic BAV can occur sporadically [20].

NOTCH1, *TGFBR1*, and *FBN1* are examples for genes, where series of patients suggest a causative relationship between gene defect and BAV phenotype. Conversely, *ACTA2* and *SMAD6* are examples for genes, where studies of individual patients or studies of relatives suggest such a causative relationship. In most of these genes, the pathogenic mechanism is unclear, and the association of mutation with phenotype is not firmly established. The *NOTCH1*, however, is a good example for a gene, where the association with BAV is well established, whereas the *FBN1* gene or the *DMD* gene is an example, where this relationship has been questioned. In all putatively causative genes however, the BAV phenotype and the associated cardiovascular and systemic phenotype are variable.

The etiology of BAV is polygenetic, where environmental factors and unknown genetic factors seem to interact. In some instances, chromosomal aberrations or defined gene defects cause BAV.

15.4 Classification of BAV: Valve Anatomy

An aortic valve may be considered "bicuspid" when we identify two cusps instead of three. However, numerous classification systems are available to further differentiate or classify BAV on the basis of anatomical criteria (Table 15.3).

First, anatomical classifications distinguish BAV from other anatomical variants of the aortic valve. These classifications include differentiation of congenital from acquired BAV and differentiation of BAV from unicuspid (UAV), quadricuspid (QAV), or pentacuspid (PAV) aortic valves according to the number of aortic valve cusps.

Second, anatomical classifications subclassify congenital BAV according to anatomical features of the aortic valve. Such classifications distinguish BAV according to patterns of valve calcification and the grade of valve calcification. However, most anatomical classifications focus on characterizing BAV according to which cusps are fused to one cusp and whether a raphe is present or absent. Unfortunately, there are many variants of such anatomical classifications, where some use the same expression to characterize different types of valves. We believe

Table 15.2 Classification of BAV according to etiology

Etiology (syndrome)	Percent of BAV per etiology (number of individuals with BAV per number of individuals with etiology)
Familial occurrence of BAV	
Familial BAV	10.1% (21/207) of siblings of 181 children have BAV [21]
	4.6% (16/348) [22], 8% (4/52) [23], and 9.1% (17/186) [24] of first-degree relatives have BAV
Chromosomal disorders	
Monosomy X (Turner) [25, 26]	11.5% (28/244) [27], 12.5% (74/594) [28], 12.8% (15/117) [29], 14% (25/179) [30], 17.5% (7/40) [31], 29.6% (74/250) [32], and 22.6% (47/208) [33]
22q11.2 deletion (DiGeorge, velocardiofacial, VCF)	3.2% (3/93) [33] and 16.7% (1/6) [34]
7q11.23 deletion (Williams) [35, 36]	3% (1/32) [36]
1q21.1 microdeletion [20]	4.8% (1/21) individuals with 1q21.1 microdeletion [37]
17q21.31 deletion (Koolen-De Vries)	18.2% (2/11) [38]
9q subtelomeric deletion (Kleefstra)	6.7% (1/15) [39]
Trisomy 21 (Down) [35]	4% (2/55), but unclear whether BAV or pulmonary bicuspid valve [40]
Monogenetic disorders: gene symbol (syndrome)	
1. Disorders with evidence from case series	
NOTCH1 (aortic valve disease 1, AOVD1)	4.2% (2/48) with sporadic BAV [41]
	10.4% (4/48) with BAV and aortic aneurysm [42]
	18.2% (2/11) of BAV had NOTCH1 mutation [43]
KMT2D, KDM6A (Kabuki) [44]	20% (4/20) [44]
	15.4% (2/13) [45]
GATA5 (non-syndromal BAV) [46]	4% (4/100) with non-synonymous GATA5 variants in 100 BAV cases [46]
FLN1 (periventricular nodular heterotopia)	9% (1/11) [47]
PTPN11, SOS1, KRAS, RAF1 (Noonan) [48]	0.8% (1/118) [49]
CREBBP (Rubinstein-Taybi)	2% (3/138) [50]
TGFBR1, TGFBR2 (Loeys-Dietz) [51, 52]	50% (2/4) families with TGFBR1 mutation [52]
	One report of an individual with BAV with a TGFBR2 mutation [51]
FBN1	4.7% (12/257) individuals with clinical diagnosis of Marfan syndrome (an FBN1 mutation is some); a BAV was present [53]
KCNJ2 (Anderson; long QT syndrome 7)	7.1% (3/42) of one kindred with autosomal dominant segregation of ventricular arrhythmias [54]
2. Disorders with evidence from case reports	
ACTA2 (familial thoracic aortic aneurysm) [55]	BAV in four families with ACTA2 mutation [55, 56]

(continued)

Table 15.2 (continued)

Etiology (syndrome)	Percent of BAV per etiology (number of individuals with BAV per number of individuals with etiology)
FLNB (Larsen)	One report of an individual with BAV with Larsen syndrome [57]
SMAD6 (aortic valve disease 2, AOVD2)	One report of an individual with BAV, aortic valve stenosis, and coarctation with calcification of the aorta [58]
GATA6	One report of carrier of the mutation with BAV in a family with GATA6 mutation [59]
Autosomal dominant heart-hand syndrome	One report of an individual with BAV, patent ductus arteriosus, and hand anomalies [60]
DMD (Becker's muscular dystrophy) [61]	One report of an individual with BAV with Becker's muscular dystrophy [61]

that a uniform classification system should be used. Buchner et al. distinguished BAV with raphe, where they classify BAV-RL, BAV-RN, and BAV-LN, depending on which aortic cusps, the right (R), left (L), or noncoronary (N), are fused, from BAV without raphe, where BAV-LA designated BAV with lateral orientation of the free edge of cusps and BAV-AP with anterior-posterior orientation. This classification covers all other classification systems and it is simple.

Third, we tabulate classification systems that combine the above described anatomical classification of BAV with other features of BAV disease, such as valvular function or aortic shape. However, such classifications may yield >20 subtypes, which are complicated to use without offering the reward of improving clinical management. Moreover, these combi-classifications are only in use to describe all possible combination of BAV anatomy with additional BAV disease features rather than that they establish new disease entities (such as a typical aortopathy in LR-BAV), and hence they do not provide additional insight into BAV disease.

Congenital BAV must be distinguished from acquired BAV. Congenital aortic valve malformations differ by number of cusps, ranging from one to five. BAV cusps can be subclassified according to patterns of calcification, severity of calcification, presence of a raphe, and fusion of cusps. Combi-classifications, where anatomical subtypes of BAV are combined with additional features of BAV disease, may be too complex for routine clinical use.

15.5 Classification of BAV: Associated Congenital Heart Defect (CHD)

We classify BAV into four categories according to the presence of associated congenital heart defects (CHDs):

Table 15.3 Classification systems of BAV valve anatomy

Classification	Frequency
Classifying BAV as congenital versus acquired	
Angelini distinguished congenital from acquired BAV by anatomic characteristics as follows	
1. Congenital BAV has two cusps, two sinuses, and two interleaflet triangles	Congenital BAV: 10.9%
2. Acquired BAV has two cusps, three sinuses, and three interleaflet triangles [62]	Acquired BAV: 89.1% [62]
Classifying congenital aortic valve malformation by number of cusps	
Unicuspid aortic valve (UAV). Mookadam classified UAV according to anatomy as follows [63, 64]	0.02% of patients referred to echocardiography [65]
1. Uni-commissural type with slit-shaped UAV	Male/female ratio: 4:1 [63]
2. A-commissural type with pinhole-shaped UAV	Uni-commissural type seems more frequent than the a-commissural type [63]
	In 96 patients with aortic valve replacement, 100% and 0% of UAV, 77% and 12% of BAV, and 64% and 36% of TAV had aortic stenosis and pure valve regurgitation, respectively [66]
Quadricuspid aortic valve (QAV) [67]. Hurwitz and Roberts classified UAV according to seven anatomical types A–G [68], where A is QAV with four equal cusps; B, three equal and one smaller cusp; C, two equal larger and two equal smaller; and G, four unequal cusps	0.008–0.033% of autopsies and 0.043% of echocardiographies [67]
	Male/female ratio: 1.6:1.
	Type A: 12%
	Type B: 60%
	Type C: 15% [68]
Pentacuspid aortic valve (PAV) [69]	Six patients with PAV reported in the literature [70]
Classifying BAV by cusp calcification	
Thubrikar et al. classified aortic cusps by pattern of calcific deposits [66]:	Occurrence of calcification patterns per cusp in BAV
1. Any calcification deposits without pattern	11.4% without pattern
2. Coaptation pattern with deposits along the line of cusp coaptation	88.6% with pattern
3. Radial pattern with deposits as spokes spread inward from the cusp attachment to the center of the cusp	Raphe was always calcified
Beppu et al. assessed the sclerotic index in BAV on TTE by dividing each aortic cusp into three segments along the coaptation line (six segments in all), where they also scored the raphe, if present. They scored each segment and raphe as 4 with calcium >3 mm, 2 with presence of calcium, 1 with echo density less than calcium, and 0 with no increased echo density [71]. Warren et al. suggested an alternative grading of cusp calcification [72]	Sclerotic index ranged from 0 to 13 with good linear correlation with the patient's age [71]

(continued)

Table 15.3 (continued)

Classification	Frequency
Classifying BAV by cusp morphology	
Brandenburg et al. classify BAV according to cusp fusion and raphe [73]:	
Type 1 with fusion of right and left cusp (R-L),	Type 1 (R-L): 70–79.6%
Type 2 with fusion of right and noncoronary cusp (R-N)	Type 2 (R-N): 1 24.4%
Type 3 with fusion of left and noncoronary cusp (L-N)	Type 3 (L-N): 0.5% [74]
Beppu et al. assessed the eccentricity index of BAV as the ratio of the widths of each cusp measured as distance from edge of cusp to aortic wall. They classified BAV according to this index [71]:	
Eccentric valve: index ≥1.2	Eccentric aortic valve: 57.3%
Symmetric valve: index <1.2	Symmetric aortic valve: 42.7%
Sadee et al. classify three BAV groups [75]:	
Group 1: purely bicuspid BAV	Group 1: 23%
Group 2: BAV with a conjoined cusps containing a raphe	Group 2: 34%
Group 3: BAV with a conjoined cusps and central indentation of free cusp edge [75]	Group 3: 43% [75]
Tokunaga classify four types of BAV [76]:	
Type 1: two cusps are situated right and left; a coronary artery arises from each related sinus of Valsalva	Type 1 (44.7%)
Type 2: type 1 plus raphe in the right cusp	Type 2 (22.4%)
Type 3: one cusp is located anteriorly, the other is posteriorly, and both coronary arteries arise from anterior cusp	Type 3 (3.5%)
Type 4: type 3 + raphe in the anterior cusp	Type IV (29.4%)
Buchner classified five types of BAV according to presence and location of raphe [77]:	
BAV with raphe	
BAV-RL, fusion of the right and left coronary cusps	BAV-RL: 72.4%
BAV-RN, fusion of the right and noncoronary cusps	BAV-RN: 13.3%
BAV-LN, fusion of the left and noncoronary cups	BAV-LN: 0%
BAV without raphe	
BAV-LA, lateral orientation of the free edge of cusps	BAV-LA: 10.5%
BAV-AP, anterior-posterior orientation	BAV-AP: 3.8%

(continued)

Table 15.3 (continued)

Classification	Frequency
Sonoda et al. classified the BAV based on the cusp location in the short axis view of the valve on the transesophageal echocardiogram [78]	
A-P-BAV: BAV with leaflets arranged anteroposteriorly and commissures to the right and to the left	A-P-BAV: 66.7%
R-L-BAV: BAV with leaflets orientated laterally and commissures positioned anteriorly and posteriorly	R-L-BAV: 33.3%
Classifying BAV by cusp morphology plus other features (combi-classifications of BAV)	
Sievers classification combines three "blocks"—type, spatial position of the free edge of cusps, and valvular function:	
Type 0, no raphe; spatial subtype, orientation of the free edge of the cusps anteroposterior (ap) or lateral (lat)	Type 0, lat, I: 2%; type 0, lat, S: 2%; type 0, ap, I: 0.3%; type 0, ap, S: 2%; type 0, ap, B: 0.3%
Type 1, one raphe; spatial subtypes, L-R, R-N, N-L (see Brandenburg classification)	Type 1, L-R, I: 26%, type 1, L-R, S: 39%, type 1, L-R, B: 5%; type 1, R-N, I: 7%; type 1, R-N, S: 5%; type 1, R-N, B: 2%; type 1, R-N, No: 0.3%; type 1, N-L, I: 1%; type 1, N-L, S: 1%; type 1, N-L, B: 1%
Type 2, two raphes; spatial subtypes, L-R/R-N	Type 2, L-R/R-N, I: 2%; type 2, L-R/R-N, S: 2%; type 2, L-R/R-N, B: 1%
Subclassification according to functional status of the valve: predominant insufficiency (I), predominant stenosis (S), balanced insufficiency and stenosis (B), or no insufficiency and stenosis (No) [79]	
Schaefer et al. combine cusp morphology and aortic shape to classify BAV [80]:	
BAV classification:	
Type 1, fusion of right and left coronary cusp	BAV 1N: 60%
Type 2, right and noncoronary fusion	BAV 1A: 50%
Type 3, left and noncoronary fusion	BAV 1E: 5%
Aortic shape classification:	
Type N, normal shape	BAV 2N: 32%
Type E, sinus effacement	BAV 2A: 54%
Type A, with ascending dilatation	BAV 2E: 14%

1. Smaller series report on the presence of BAV in syndromic or complex CHD, such as Ebstein's anomaly, Shone's complex, hypoplastic left heart syndrome, double-outlet right ventricle, tetralogy of Fallot, or complete transposition of the great arteries.

Table 15.4 Classification of BAV according to associated congenital heart defect (CHD)

Associated CHD	Frequency of BAV
1. BAV in syndromic or complex CHD (≥ 2 additional cardiovascular malformations)	
Ebstein's anomaly [81]	0.8% (2/250) [81], 7.6% (8/106) [82], and 4.8% (5/104) of Ebstein patients [83]
Shone's complex [84, 85]	84.2% (16/19) [86] and 88.9% (24/27) in patients with operation for Shone's complex [87]
Hypoplastic left heart syndrome (HLHS) [81, 88–91]	11.2% (64/570) of HLHS or interrupted aortic arch (IAA) [81]
	12.1% (4/33) of relatives of a subset of infants with isolated HLHS [88]
Double-outlet right ventricle (DORV) [81]	0.7% (5/773) of DORV [81]
Tetralogy of Fallot (TOF) [81]	0.6 (7/1213) of TOF [81]
	1.7% (1/59) of TOF [92]
Complete transposition of the great arteries (TGA) [92]	0.1% (1/1567) of TGA [81]
	1.0% (1/103) of TGA [92]
BAV in combination with the other CHDs	
2. Association with evidence from larger series	
Coarctation of the aorta (COA) [92] [81, 93]	55.0% (459/835) of isolated COA [81]
	17.6% (111/629) of complex COA [81]
	31.4% (49/156) of BAV has a history of prior COA repair [94]
	25–85% of BAV has COA [95]
	59.6% (268/449) of COA has BAV [96]
Patent ductus arteriosus (PDA) [97, 98]	20.9% (53/253) of PDA [99]
	8.3% (1/12) of PDA [92]
Ventricular septal defect (VSD) [97] [92, 98]	20.5% (17/83) of isolated VSD [92]
	51.1% (24/47) of VSD and aortic arch obstruction [92]
Atrial septal defect (ASD) [100]	1% of 294 adults with ASD [101]
Complete atrioventricular septal defect (CAVC) [81]	1.0% (11/1074) of CAVC [81]
Total anomalous pulmonary venous return (TAPVR) [81]	0.8% (2/247) of TAPVR [81]
Partial anomalous pulmonary venous return (PAPVR)	0.9% (2/233) of PAPVR [81]
3. Rare association of BAV with CHD	
Coronary arterial anomaly [102]	Casuistic reports on BAV with anomalous origin of the:
	Right coronary artery between the left and right coronary sinus of Valsalva [22], from the left sinus of Valsalva [103–105], from the ascending aorta high above the left posterior sinus of Valsalva[106], from the left ventricle [107], or from the pulmonary artery (ARCAPA) [108]
	Left coronary artery arising from the right sinus of Valsalva [109, 110]
	Single coronary artery [111–114]
	26% of 59 BAVs have left coronary artery dominance and 44% of left coronary ostia origin at or above aortic sinotubular junction [102]

(continued)

Table 15.4 (continued)

Associated CHD	Frequency of BAV
Bicuspid pulmonary valve (BPV) [115]	0.75% (24/3216) of cases with congenital heart disease had bilaterally BPV [116]
	Main pulmonary artery (MPA) diameters are larger in 194 individuals with BAV but without BPV than in 178 controls [117]
Mitral valve anomalies	3.1% (8/257) of black patients with MVP have BAV [118]
	4.7% (9/192) of adults with BAV have a myxomatous mitral valve [80]
	Elongation of the AML in BAV [119]
	8.9% (16/180) of patients with combined aortic and mitral valve replacement had BAV [120]
Mitral valve atresia	11.5% (3/26) of mitral atresia [92]
4. Rare associations of BAV and CHD (casuistic reports)	
Myocardial abnormalities	Left ventricular noncompaction [121], outflow tract diverticula adjacent to the commissures of a BAV [122], septal diverticulum [123], subannular aneurysm [124], hypertrophic cardiomyopathy [125]
Familial aorto-cervicocephalic arterial dissections [126]	Three families with BAV and cervicocephalic arterial dissections [126]
Intracranial aneurysms (IA) [127]	10% (6/61) of IA [127]
	1.8% (1/56) with subarachnoid hemorrhage related to IA [128]
	0.6% (2/317) of IA [129]
Miscellaneous vascular anomalies	Circumaortic innominate vein [130], isolated spontaneous dissection of the celiac trunk [131], aortic diverticulum [132], lusory artery [133], aberrant right subclavian artery aneurysm [134], persistent left and absent right superior vena cava [135]

2. BAV frequently associates with one typical additional CHD, where coarctation of the aorta (COA), patent ductus arteriosus (PDA), ventricular septal defect (VSD), and atrial septal defect (ASD) are the most common associates of BAV.
3. Coronary arterial anomaly, bicuspid pulmonary valve (BPV), and mitral valve anomalies are rare in BAV, but their association with BAV is well established.
4. There are only sparse or conflicting data on the potential association of BAV with CHD or vascular malformation such as myocardial abnormalities, familial aorto-cervicocephalic arterial dissections, intracranial aneurysms, and various arterial or venous vascular anomalies (Table 15.4).

We tend to perceive BAV as an isolated CHD. However, we identified 20 well-defined syndromic, complex, or isolated congenital heart defects that are associated with BAV disease; some of them are apparently quite frequent.

15.6 Classification of BAV: Aortopathy

BAV may be associated with aortic dilatation or aneurysm of the proximal aorta, the aortic arch, the descending aorta, or the abdominal aorta. Some studies classified BAV into four groups by type of aortopathy. BAV aortopathy was classified:

1. Type and presence of aortic valve dysfunction
2. Geometrical configuration of the proximal part of the aorta
3. Involvement of the aortic arch
4. According to presence of coarctation of the aorta (COA)

None of these classifications have been applied prospectively in large cohorts of unselected individuals with BAV, and hence their overlap and comprehensiveness cannot be estimated properly. However, all classifications provide useful means to describe subtypes of BAV aortopathy for future assessment of prognosis (Table 15.5).

15.7 Classification of BAV Aortopathy: Risk Factors

Patients with BAV may exhibit additional factors that may increase diameter of the aorta and increase the risk of aortic aneurysm formation, aortic dissection, and rupture. We distinguish risk that may arise from three types of risk factors:

1. From aortic valve characteristics, such as BAV morphotype, BAV stenosis, and BAV regurgitation
2. From comorbidities of BAV, such as arterial hypertension (HTN), atherosclerosis, and coarctation of the aorta (BAV-COA), or from sleep apnea, comprising obstructive (OSA) and central sleep apnea (CSA)
3. From behavioral factors including pregnancy, sports, high-performance aviation with G-force exposure, and drug abuse comprising cocaine, methamphetamine, and sildenafil

The evidence for increased risk for aortic complications is not equally strong for all factors in BAV (Table 15.6).

15.8 Classification of BAV Aortopathy: Candidate Biomarkers

Biomarkers should provide information of the development and evolution of BAV aortopathy. Aortic diameters clearly provide the single most important information on presence and risk of BAV aortopathy. Therefore, guidelines base their recommendations of timing for elective surgery of the aortic root predominantly on

Table 15.5 Classifications of BAV according to aortopathy

Classification	Frequencies
1. According to BAV dysfunction	
Aydin et al. classified ascending aortic aneurysm (AAA) in relation to bicuspid aortic valve (BAV) dysfunction similar to Hahn et al. as follows [136, 137]:	
ACA with BAV severe stenosis	ACA with BAV stenosis: 50%
ACA with BAV severe regurgitation	ACA with BAV regurgitation: 26.9%
ACA without BAV dysfunction	ACA without BAV dysfunction: 23.1% [136]
2. According to shape of the proximal aorta	
Bauer et al. classified the configuration of proximal aortopathy according to diameter enlargement at level 1 (aortic annulus), level 2 (aortic sinus), level 3 (sinotubular junction), and level 4 (ascending aorta) as follows [138]:	
Normal: levels 1–4 normal	
Marfanoid: 1–3 enlarged, 4 normal	
Symmetric dilatation: 1–2 normal, 3–4 enlarged	
Asymmetric dilatation: 1–3 normal, 4 enlarged	
3. According to involvement of the aortic arch	
Fazel et al. classified the extent of BAV aortopathy based on cluster analysis as follows [139]:	
Cluster I, aortic root alone	Cluster I: 13%
Cluster II, tubular ascending aorta alone	Cluster II: 14%
Cluster III, tubular portion and transverse arch	Cluster III: 28%
Cluster IV, aortic root and tubular portion with tapering across the transverse arch	Cluster IV: 45%
4. According to coexistence with coarctation of the aorta (Co-COA)	
BAV aortopathy according to location and presence of COA (irrespective of previous COA repair) [140–142]:	
Type A: aneurysm of ascending aorta without COA	
Type A-COA: aneurysm of ascending aorta with COA	
Type B-COA: aneurysm of thoracic aorta in other locations than the ascending aorta	
Type C-COA: aneurysmal formation at the site of COA or previous COA repair	

diameters [176–178]. Nonetheless, aortic size has to be judged differently depending on sex, body size, body surface, and the individual tissue stability of the aortic wall [179]. Additional biomarkers may be helpful to further stratify the risk of acute aortic events in BAV aortopathy.

Candidates for biomarkers of BAV aortopathy comprise a family history with dissection or death at younger age, increased aortic growth rates, proximal aortic shape, biomarkers of aortic stiffness and aortic elasticity markers, biomarkers of

Table 15.6 Risk factors and predictors of BAV aortopathy

1. Aortic valve characteristics
Bicuspid aortic valve morphotype (BAV-MO)
BAV-RL was associated with enlarged SOV diameters [143–145], rapid growth of SOV diameters [94], and lower age at aortic operation [145]
BAV-RN was associated with enlarged diameters of ASC [143] and with rapid growth of ASC diameters [146]
Progression of cusp sclerosis was faster in BAV-RL than BAV-RN, and it was faster in eccentric cusps than symmetric cusps
Aortic valve pressure gradient increased approximately 18 mmHg by each decade, but in eccentric BAV and BAV-RL, aortic valve pressure gradient increased 27 mmHg per decade [71]
Bicuspid aortic valve stenosis (BAV-S)
BAV-S was a protective factor for SOV dilatation [147, 148]
BAV-S severity related to enlarged diameters of ASC [143, 149]
BAV-S gradient predicted growth of ASC diameters in children [146]
BAV-S had a higher risk of rupture, dissection, or death before operative repair than did those with normally functioning valves [16]
Bicuspid aortic valve regurgitation (BAV-I)
Absence of BAV-I or mild BAV-I/BAV-S lead to aortic surgery in only 5 $\pm$ 2%, without any aortic dissection during 20 years of follow-up [13]
BAV-I severity related to enlarged SOV diameters [149]
Moderate or severe BAV-I was not associated with rapid aortic dilatation in one study [94], but it was an independent determinant of SOV diameter in another study [143]
BAV-I was associated with extension of dilatation from ASC past the innominate artery into AOA and DESC [150]
BAV-I at AVR was associated with a tenfold higher risk of post-AVR aortic dissection compared with BAV-S [151]
2. Comorbidities
Arterial hypertension (HTN)
In the general population, 4–17% with HTN had dilatation of SOV [152]
In BAV, SOV diameter was significantly larger than individuals in the general population with HTN [143]
HTN (>140/90 mmHg) was associated univariately with rapid aortic dilatation [94]
Atherosclerosis
In the general population, distal aortic dilatation showed only weak association with risk factors for atherosclerosis and aortic atherosclerotic plaques [153]
BAV with coarctation of the aorta (BAV-COA)
BAV-COA after repair or with mild pressure gradients was the only predictor of ASC aneurysm [154]
Aortic dissection or rupture occurred exclusively in BAV-COA [154]
BAV-COA were younger at AVR and ASC surgery than isolated BAV [155]
In children with BAV-COA, SOV, and ASC, diameters were larger than isolated BAV [156]
Maximal velocity, secondary flow, pressure loss, time-averaged wall shear stress, and oscillatory shear index downstream of the COA in those with BAV-COA were higher [157] than isolated BAV
One study found that prior COA repair was protective against rapid aortic dilatation in BAV-COA [94]

(continued)

Table 15.6 (continued)

Sleep apnea
Obstructive (OSA) and central sleep apnea (CSA) are frequent in patients with aortic dissection and Marfan syndrome
Aortic diameters and stiffness are increased in sleep apnea [158–163]
Therefore, OSA and CSA are likely to increase the risk for aortic aneurysm and dissection in BAV
3. Behavioral factors
Pregnancy
One review of the literature identified that BAV was observed in 10% (4/40) of women with prepartum type A aortic dissection [164] and in 4.9% (6/122) of parturients with aortic dissection [165]
In a cohort of 88 women with BAV, there was no aortic dissection in 216 pregnancies and 186 deliveries [14]
Sports
2.5% (4/158) of trained athletes with sudden death had BAV with valve stenosis but no aortic dissection or rupture [166]
88 consecutive athletes with BAV had a significantly higher increase of aortic diameters than in 56 athletes with a normal tricuspid valve during 5 years of follow-up, but diameters remained within normal ranges [167]
High-performance aviation with G-force exposure
Exposure to G-force and anti-G maneuvers did not worsen cardiac and valve function in eight aviators with BAV [168]
Drug abuse
Cocaine
37% (14/38) of hospitalized patients with aortic dissection used cocaine in the minutes or hours preceding their presentation [169]
IRAD identified cocaine use in 0.5% (5/921) of individuals with aortic dissection (one type A, four type B) [170]
A literature analysis identified 15 patients with type A aortic dissection and 6 with type B dissection associated with a recent cocaine use [171] 69.2% (9/10) of aortic dissections in cocaine users had type B dissection, but none of them had BAV [172]
Methamphetamine
In 5.5% (6/109) of individuals with aortic dissection and 20% (6/30) of patients under the age of 50 with aortic dissection, acute aortic dissection was secondary to hypertensive crises from methamphetamine use [173]
In a population-based case-control study of 30,922,098 hospital discharges of persons, aged 18–49 years, significant association of amphetamine abuse/dependence and thoracic and thoracoabdominal aortic dissections was identified in 3116 individuals [174]
Sildenafil
There are casuistic reports on post-sildenafil aortic dissections, in one individual with BAV and post-sildenafil type A dissection [175]

Table 15.7 Candidate biomarkers of BAV aortopathy

1. Family history with dissection or death in the young
The ESC guideline considers a family history of dissection as a risk factor in BAV that justifies earlier surgical intervention for aortopathy [177]
Aortopathy was prevalent in relatives of BAV patients [180, 181]
32% of 48 first-degree relatives of individuals with BAV who had morphologically normal TAV exhibited functionally abnormal and dilated aortic roots [180]
First-degree relatives had a higher prevalence of thoracic aortic aneurysms and sudden death with a relative risks of thoracic aortic aneurysm development of 10.9 in brothers and 1.8 in fathers and sisters of index patients with BAV [182]
2. Increased aortic growth rates
Cohort studies of adults with BAV estimate mean annual rates of progression of diameters (mm/year) as 0.18 at AVA, 0.17 at SOV, 0.18 at STJ, and 0.37 at ASC [94] and as 0.5 at SOV, 0.5 at STJ, and 0.9 at proximal ASC [183] and as 0.2 at ASC [184]
Cohort studies with comparison of adults with BAV versus adults with TAV estimate mean annual rates of progression of diameters (mm/year) at ASC as 0.77 vs. 0.16 [185], 0.86 vs. 0.82 (n.s.) at SOV, 1.06 vs. 0.63 (n.s.) at STJ, and 0.81 vs. 0.75 at proximal ASC (n.s.) [17]. One study estimated annual aortic growth rates as 0.19 cm/year vs. 0.13 cm/year [16]
A cohort study of children aged <19 years (mean 8.5 ± 5.3) with isolated BAV and normal z-scores on initial examination estimated the rate of ASC diameter growth as 0.18 ± 0.30 z-score per year [146]. In a cohort study of 28 children with functionally normal BAVs and of 25 controls (mean age 9.0 ± 4.8 vs. 8.7 ± 6.1 years), aortic growth rates were 1.2 ± 0.08 vs. 0.6 ± 0.08 mm/year ($P < 0.0001$) [186]
3. Proximal aortic shape
Proximal aortic shape with extension of dilatation from SOV beyond STJ into ASC indicated increased risk for rupture and dissection in Marfan syndrome [187]
BAV-S with asymmetrical tubular dilatation was called "BAD-MATE syndrome," which may have a prognostic meaning [188]
An ellipsoidal or spherical shape of the proximal aorta may be the origin of a transverse tearing of the aortic intima as initiating event for acute dissection [189]
BAV-RL was associated with normal aortic shape but larger diameters of SOV (type N) and BAV-RN with larger distal ASC and AOA dimensions (type A) [80]
4. Aortic stiffness/aortic elasticity
Nine studies with comparison of adults with BAV and healthy adults with TAV who were matched for age and gender all identified increased aortic stiffness parameters in the following BAV groups (mean age in years ± standard deviation):
10 BAV individuals (47 ± 4) [190]
16 men (median age 31 years) with nonstenotic BAV and proximal ascending aortic diameters ≥40 mm [191]
20 individuals (27 ± 11 years) with nonstenotic BAVs with larger SOV diameters [192]
29 individuals with BAV-RL (mean age 41.5 years) and larger SOV diameters [144]
40 BAV individuals (44 ± 16 years) with larger SOV diameters [193]
49 males with BAV (19.4 ± 1.4 years) and larger SOV diameters [194]
50 individuals with BAVs (52 ± 14 years) without significant valve dysfunction but larger ascending aortic diameters [195]
50 individuals with BAV (median age 30; 16–56 years) with aortic diameter ≤4 cm [196]
127 BAV outpatients (23 ± 10 years) with no or mild valvular impairment but larger aortic diameters [197]

(continued)

Table 15.7 (continued)

Two studies with comparison of children with BAV and healthy children with TAV who were matched for age and gender both identified increased aortic stiffness parameters in BAV:
48 pediatric individuals (mean age 11.9 ± 4.8 years) with an isolated BAV and larger aortic root diameters [198]
53 consecutive pediatric individuals with BAV (mean age 16 ± 4 years) with mild aortic valve disease maximum rates [199]
Three studies showed that increased stiffness parameters were statistically independent of aortic dilatation [198–200]
In one study BAV-RL showed significantly stiffer and less distensible elasticity parameters than BAV-RN [198]
5. Aortic wall shear stress (AWASS) [201]
Four-dimensional flow MR imaging revealed nested helical flow at peak systole in ASC in 15 of 20 individuals with BAV but not in 25 patients with a TAV and not in 8 healthy volunteers. Helical flow was eccentric in all cases, it was present irrespective of aortic dilatation and BAV-S, and it was right-handed in 11 BAV-RL and left-handed in 4 BAV-RN [202]
Systolic flow displacement calculated from conventional 2D PC-MRI in the ASC related to future aortic growth in 17 adults with BAV-RL [203]
19 patients with BAV and eccentric systolic blood flow in ASC had significantly and asymmetrically elevated wall shear stress as compared to both 7 patients with BAV and normal flow and to 20 patients with TAV and no valvular disease [204]
Among 13 patients with BAV, 10 with abnormal flow patterns demonstrated significantly higher growth rates than those without, and 7 BAV with markedly eccentric flow exhibited more rapid growth than those without [205]
Patients with BAV had increased 99th percentile wall stress in ASC [206]
6. Endothelial dysfunction
16 men with nonstenotic BAV but dilated aortas had decreased brachial flow-mediated vasodilation to hyperemia as marker of endothelial dysfunction than both 16 men with BAV and nondilated aorta and 16 normal controls [191]
Flow-mediated dilatation (FMD) as marker of endothelial dysfunction was decreased in 43 individuals with BAV, but its decreases were unrelated to aortopathy [207]
7. Serological biomarkers reported in BAV (alphabetical order)
ACE insertion/deletion polymorphism [208]
ADMA (asymmetric dimethylarginine) [207]
α1AT (soluble alpha-1 antitrypsin) [209]
MicroRNA: miR-1 [210], miR-21 [210], miR-29b [211]
MMP-2, MMP-8, and MMP-9 [191, 209, 210, 212–214]
MPO (myeloperoxidase) [207]
OPG (osteoprotegerin) [215]
sRAGE (soluble receptor for advanced glycation end product) [216]
RANKL [215]
TGFb1 (transforming growth factor-beta1) [217]
TIMP [210, 214]
Transcript biomarkers FHL1, collagens α1(XI), α2(V), α1(III), and α1(I) [218]

aortic wall shear stress (AWASS), biomarkers of endothelial dysfunction, and serological biomarkers (Table 15.7).

No single candidate biomarker of BAV aortopathy has currently accumulated evidence enough for introduction into clinical routine. However, many of the candidate biomarkers exhibit promising data. Some of these markers are likely to improve future management of BAV disease.

References

1. Braverman AC, Guven H, Beardslee MA, Makan M, Kates AM et al (2005) The bicuspid aortic valve. Curr Probl Cardiol 30:470–522
2. Nistri S, Basso C, Marzari C, Mormino P, Thiene G (2005) Frequency of bicuspid aortic valve in young male conscripts by echocardiogram. Am J Cardiol 96:718–721
3. Roberts WC (1970) The congenitally bicuspid aortic valve. A study of 85 autopsy cases. Am J Cardiol 26:72–83
4. Basso C, Boschello M, Perrone C, Mecenero A, Cera A et al (2004) An echocardiographic survey of primary school children for bicuspid aortic valve. Am J Cardiol 93:661–663
5. Edwards WD, Leaf DS, Edwards JE (1978) Dissecting aortic aneurysm associated with congenital bicuspid valve. Circulation 57:1022
6. Larson EW, Edwards WD (1984) Risk factors for aortic dissection: a necropsy study of 161 cases. Am J Cardiol 53:849–855
7. Roberts CS, Roberts WC (1991) Dissection of the aorta associated with congenital malformation of the aortic valve. J Am Coll Cardiol 17:712–716
8. Gray GW, Salisbury DA, Gulino AM (1995) Echocardiographic and color flow Doppler findings in military pilot applicants. Aviat Space Environ Med 66:32–34
9. Tutar E, Ekici F, Atalay S, Nacar N (2005) The prevalence of bicuspid aortic valve in newborns by echocardiographic screening. Am Heart J 150:513–515
10. Strader JR, Harrell TW, Adair A, Kruyer WB (2008) Efficacy of echocardiographic screening of pilot applicants. Aviat Space Environ Med 79:514–517
11. Januzzi JL, Isselbacher EM, Fattori R, Cooper JV, Smith DE et al (2004) Characterizing the young patient with aortic dissection: results from the International Registry of Aortic Dissection (IRAD). J Am Coll Cardiol 43:665–669
12. Di Eusanio M, Trimarchi S, Patel HJ, Hutchison S, Suzuki T et al (2013) Clinical presentation, management, and short-term outcome of patients with type A acute dissection complicated by mesenteric malperfusion: observations from the International Registry of Acute Aortic Dissection. J Thorac Cardiovasc Surg 145:385–390.e1
13. Michelena HI, Desjardins VA, Avierinos JF, Russo A, Nkomo VT et al (2008) Natural history of asymptomatic patients with normally functioning or minimally dysfunctional bicuspid aortic valve in the community. Circulation 117:2776–2784
14. McKellar SH, MacDonald RJ, Michelena HI, Connolly HM, Sundt TM 3rd (2011) Frequency of cardiovascular events in women with a congenitally bicuspid aortic valve in a single community and effect of pregnancy on events. Am J Cardiol 107:96–99
15. Tzemos N, Therrien J, Yip J, Thanassoulis G, Tremblay S et al (2008) Outcomes in adults with bicuspid aortic valves. JAMA 300:1317–1325
16. Davies RR, Kaple RK, Mandapati D, Gallo A, Botta DM Jr et al (2007) Natural history of ascending aortic aneurysms in the setting of an unreplaced bicuspid aortic valve. Ann Thorac Surg 83:1338–1344

17. La Canna G, Ficarra E, Tsagalau E, Nardi M, Morandini A et al (2006) Progression rate of ascending aortic dilation in patients with normally functioning bicuspid and tricuspid aortic valves. Am J Cardiol 98:249–253
18. Michelena HI, Khanna AD, Mahoney D, Margaryan E, Topilsky Y et al (2011) Incidence of aortic complications in patients with bicuspid aortic valves. JAMA 306:1104–1112
19. Prakash SK, Bossé Y, Muehlschlegel JD, Michelena HI, Limongelli G et al (2014) A roadmap to investigate the genetic basis of bicuspid aortic valve and its complications insights from the International BAVCon (Bicuspid Aortic Valve Consortium). J Am Coll Cardiol 64:832–839
20. Moran R, Robin NH (2013) Chapter 46: Congenital heart defects. In: Rimoin D, Korf RP (eds) Emery and Rimoin's principles and practice of medical genetics, 6th edn. Academic, Oxford, pp 1–51
21. Hales AR, Mahle WT (2014) Echocardiography screening of siblings of children with bicuspid aortic valve. Pediatrics 133:e1212–e1217
22. Robledo-Carmona J, Rodríguez-Bailón I, Carrasco-Chinchilla F, Fernández B, Jiménez-Navarro M et al (2013) Hereditary patterns of bicuspid aortic valve in a hundred families. Int J Cardiol 168:3443–3449
23. Panayotova R, Macnab A, Waterworth PD (2013) A pilot project of familial screening in patients with bicuspid aortic valve disease. J Heart Valve Dis 22:150–155
24. Huntington K, Hunter AG, Chan KL (1997) A prospective study to assess the frequency of familial clustering of congenital bicuspid aortic valve. J Am Coll Cardiol 30:1809–1812
25. Carlson M, Silberbach M (2007) Dissection of the aorta in Turner syndrome: two cases and review of 85 cases in the literature. J Med Genet 44:745–749
26. Sybert VP, McCauley E (2004) Turner's syndrome. N Engl J Med 351:1227–1238
27. Sybert VP (1998) Cardiovascular malformations and complications in Turner syndrome. Pediatrics 101:E11
28. Mazzanti L, Cacciari E (1998) Congenital heart disease in patients with Turner's syndrome. Italian Study Group for Turner Syndrome (ISGTS). J Pediatr 133:688–692
29. Volkl TM, Degenhardt K, Koch A, Simm D, Dorr HG et al (2005) Cardiovascular anomalies in children and young adults with Ullrich-Turner syndrome the Erlangen experience. Clin Cardiol 28:88–92
30. Gotzsche CO, Krag-Olsen B, Nielsen J, Sorensen KE, Kristensen BO (1994) Prevalence of cardiovascular malformations and association with karyotypes in Turner's syndrome. Arch Dis Child 71:433–436
31. Dawson-Falk KL, Wright AM, Bakker B, Pitlick PT, Wilson DM et al (1992) Cardiovascular evaluation in Turner syndrome: utility of MR imaging. Australas Radiol 36:204–209
32. Sachdev V, Matura LA, Sidenko S, Ho VB, Arai AE et al (2008) Aortic valve disease in Turner syndrome. J Am Coll Cardiol 51:1904–1909
33. Olivieri LJ, Baba RY, Arai AE, Bandettini WP, Rosing DR et al (2013) Spectrum of aortic valve abnormalities associated with aortic dilation across age groups in Turner syndrome. Circ Cardiovasc Imaging 6:1018–1023
34. Ben-Shachar S, Ou Z, Shaw CA, Belmont JW, Patel MS et al (2008) 22q11.2 distal deletion: a recurrent genomic disorder distinct from DiGeorge syndrome and velocardiofacial syndrome. Am J Hum Genet 82:214–221
35. Lopez-Rangel E, Maurice M, McGillivray B, Friedman JM (1992) Williams syndrome in adults. Am J Med Genet 44:720–729
36. De Rubens FJ, Rodriguez LM, Hach JL, Del Castillo RV, Martinez HO (2008) Cardiovascular spectrum in Williams-Beuren syndrome: the Mexican experience in 40 patients. Tex Heart Inst J 35:279–285
37. Brunetti-Pierri N, Berg JS, Scaglia F, Belmont J, Bacino CA et al (2008) Recurrent reciprocal 1q21.1 deletions and duplications associated with microcephaly or macrocephaly and developmental and behavioral abnormalities. Nat Genet 40:1466–1471

38. Tan TY, Aftimos S, Worgan L, Susman R, Wilson M et al (2009) Phenotypic expansion and further characterisation of the 17q21.31 microdeletion syndrome. J Med Genet 46:480–489
39. Kleefstra T, van Zelst-Stams WA, Nillesen WM, Cormier-Daire V, Houge G et al (2009) Further clinical and molecular delineation of the 9q subtelomeric deletion syndrome supports a major contribution of EHMT1 haploinsufficiency to the core phenotype. J Med Genet 46:598–606
40. Tandon R, Edwards JE (1973) Cardiac malformations associated with Down's syndrome. Circulation 47:1349–1355
41. Mohamed SA, Aherrahrou Z, Liptau H, Erasmi AW, Hagemann C et al (2006) Novel missense mutations (p.T596 M and p.P1797H) in NOTCH1 in patients with bicuspid aortic valve. Biochem Biophys Res Commun 345:1460–1465
42. McKellar SH, Tester DJ, Yagubyan M, Majumdar R, Ackerman MJ et al (2007) Novel NOTCH1 mutations in patients with bicuspid aortic valve disease and thoracic aortic aneurysms. J Thorac Cardiovasc Surg 134:290–296
43. Foffa I, Ait Ali L, Panesi P, Mariani M, Festa P et al (2013) Sequencing of NOTCH1, GATA5, TGFBR1 and TGFBR2 genes in familial cases of bicuspid aortic valve. BMC Med Genet 14:44
44. Hughes HE, Davies SJ (1994) Coarctation of the aorta in Kabuki syndrome. Arch Dis Child 70:512–514
45. Yoon JK, Ahn KJ, Kwon BS, Kim GB, Bae EJ et al (2015) The strong association of left-side heart anomalies with Kabuki syndrome. Korean J Pediatr 58:256–262
46. Padang R, Bagnall RD, Richmond DR, Bannon PG, Semsarian C (2012) Rare non-synonymous variations in the transcriptional activation domains of GATA5 in bicuspid aortic valve disease. J Mol Cell Cardiol 53:277–281
47. Fox JW, Lamperti ED, Eksioglu YZ, Hong SE, Feng Y et al (1998) Mutations in filamin 1 prevent migration of cerebral cortical neurons in human periventricular heterotopia. Neuron 21:1315–1325
48. Romano AA, Allanson JE, Dahlgren J, Gelb BD, Hall B et al (2010) Noonan syndrome: clinical features, diagnosis, and management guidelines. Pediatrics 126:746–759
49. Burch M, Sharland M, Shinebourne E, Smith G, Patton M et al (1993) Cardiologic abnormalities in Noonan syndrome: phenotypic diagnosis and echocardiographic assessment of 118 patients. J Am Coll Cardiol 22:1189–1192
50. Stevens CA, Bhakta MG (1995) Cardiac abnormalities in the Rubinstein-Taybi syndrome. Am J Med Genet 59:346–348
51. Girdauskas E, Schulz S, Borger MA, Mierzwa M, Kuntze T (2011) Transforming growth factor-beta receptor type II mutation in a patient with bicuspid aortic valve disease and intraoperative aortic dissection. Ann Thorac Surg 91:e70–e71
52. Loeys BL, Chen J, Neptune ER, Judge DP, Podowski M et al (2005) A syndrome of altered cardiovascular, craniofacial, neurocognitive and skeletal development caused by mutations in TGFBR1 or TGFBR2. Nat Genet 37:275–281
53. Nistri S, Porciani MC, Attanasio M, Abbate R, Gensini GF et al (2012) Association of Marfan syndrome and bicuspid aortic valve: frequency and outcome. Int J Cardiol 155:324–325
54. Andelfinger G, Tapper AR, Welch RC, Vanoye CG, George AL Jr et al (2002) KCNJ2 mutation results in Andersen syndrome with sex-specific cardiac and skeletal muscle phenotypes. Am J Hum Genet 71:663–668
55. Guo DC, Pannu H, Tran-Fadulu V, Papke CL, Yu RK et al (2007) Mutations in smooth muscle alpha-actin (ACTA2) lead to thoracic aortic aneurysms and dissections. Nat Genet 39:1488–1493
56. Guo DC, Papke CL, Tran-Fadulu V, Regalado ES, Avidan N et al (2009) Mutations in smooth muscle alpha-actin (ACTA2) cause coronary artery disease, stroke, and Moyamoya disease, along with thoracic aortic disease. Am J Hum Genet 84:617–627
57. Liang CD, Hang CL (2001) Elongation of the aorta and multiple cardiovascular abnormalities associated with larsen syndrome. Pediatr Cardiol 22:245–246

58. Tan HL, Glen E, Töpf A, Hall D, O'Sullivan JJ et al (2012) Nonsynonymous variants in the SMAD6 gene predispose to congenital cardiovascular malformation. Hum Mutat 33:720–727
59. Lin X, Huo Z, Liu X, Zhang Y, Li L et al (2010) A novel GATA6 mutation in patients with tetralogy of Fallot or atrial septal defect. J Hum Genet 55:662–667
60. Gelb BD, Zhang J, Sommer RJ, Wasserman JM, Reitman MJ et al (1999) Familial patent ductus arteriosus and bicuspid aortic valve with hand anomalies: a novel heart-hand syndrome. Am J Med Genet 87:175–179
61. Feeley C, Rasbridge S (2006) Cardiomyopathy with a unique finding of bicuspid aortic valve in Becker's muscular dystrophy. Cardiovasc Pathol Off J Soc Cardiovasc Pathol 15:347–351
62. Angelini A, Ho SY, Anderson RH, Devine WA, Zuberbuhler JR et al (1989) The morphology of the normal aortic valve as compared with the aortic valve having two leaflets. J Thorac Cardiovasc Surg 98:362–367
63. Mookadam F, Thota VR, Garcia-Lopez AM, Emani UR, Alharthi MS et al (2010) Unicuspid aortic valve in adults: a systematic review. J Heart Valve Dis 19:79–85
64. Mookadam F, Thota VR, Lopez AM, Emani UR, Tajik AJ (2010) Unicuspid aortic valve in children: a systematic review spanning four decades. J Heart Valve Dis 19:678–683
65. Novaro GM, Mishra M, Griffin BP (2003) Incidence and echocardiographic features of congenital unicuspid aortic valve in an adult population. J Heart Valve Dis 12:674–678
66. Thubrikar MJ, Aouad J, Nolan SP (1986) Patterns of calcific deposits in operatively excised stenotic or purely regurgitant aortic valves and their relation to mechanical stress. Am J Cardiol 58:304–308
67. Khan SK, Tamin SS, Araoz PA (2011) Quadricuspid aortic valve by cardiac magnetic resonance imaging: a case report and review of the literature. J Comput Assist Tomogr 35:637–641
68. Hurwitz LE, Roberts WC (1973) Quadricuspid semilunar valve. Am J Cardiol 31:623–626
69. Cemri M, Cengel A, Timurkaynak T (2000) Pentacuspid aortic valve diagnosed by transoesophageal echocardiography. Heart 84:e9
70. Kuroki H, Hirooka K, Ohnuki M (2012) Pentacuspid aortic valve causing severe aortic regurgitation. J Thorac Cardiovasc Surg 143:e11–e12
71. Beppu S, Suzuki S, Matsuda H, Ohmori F, Nagata S et al (1993) Rapidity of progression of aortic stenosis in patients with congenital bicuspid aortic valves. Am J Cardiol 71:322–327
72. Warren BA, Yong JL (1997) Calcification of the aortic valve: its progression and grading. Pathology 29:360–368
73. Brandenburg RO Jr, Tajik AJ, Edwards WD, Reeder GS, Shub C et al (1983) Accuracy of 2-dimensional echocardiographic diagnosis of congenitally bicuspid aortic valve: echocardiographic-anatomic correlation in 115 patients. Am J Cardiol 51:1469–1473
74. Yuan SM (2011) The anatomopathology of bicuspid aortic valve. Folia Morphol (Warsz) 70:217–227
75. Sadee AS, Becker AE, Verheul HA, Bouma B, Hoedemaker G (1992) Aortic valve regurgitation and the congenitally bicuspid aortic valve: a clinico-pathological correlation. Br Heart J 67:439–441
76. Tokunaga H, Koyanagi H, Hashimoto A, Nakano K, Hirayama T et al (1992) [Classification of congenitally bicuspid aortic valve and its angiographic and surgical significance]. [Zasshi] [Journal] Nihon Kyobu Geka Gakkai 40:467–71; discussion 71–72
77. Buchner S, Hulsmann M, Poschenrieder F, Hamer OW, Fellner C et al (2010) Variable phenotypes of bicuspid aortic valve disease: classification by cardiovascular magnetic resonance. Heart 96:1233–1240
78. Sonoda M, Takenaka K, Uno K, Ebihara A, Nagai R (2008) A larger aortic annulus causes aortic regurgitation and a smaller aortic annulus causes aortic stenosis in bicuspid aortic valve. Echocardiography 25:242–248
79. Sievers HH, Schmidtke C (2007) A classification system for the bicuspid aortic valve from 304 surgical specimens. J Thorac Cardiovasc Surg 133:1226–1233

80. Schaefer BM, Lewin MB, Stout KK, Gill E, Prueitt A et al (2008) The bicuspid aortic valve: an integrated phenotypic classification of leaflet morphology and aortic root shape. Heart 94:1634–1638
81. Fernandes SM, Sanders SP, Khairy P, Jenkins KJ, Gauvreau K et al (2004) Morphology of bicuspid aortic valve in children and adolescents. J Am Coll Cardiol 44:1648–1651
82. Attenhofer Jost CH, Connolly HM, O'Leary PW, Warnes CA, Tajik AJ et al (2005) Left heart lesions in patients with Ebstein anomaly. Mayo Clin Proc 80:361–368
83. Barbara DW, Edwards WD, Connolly HM, Dearani JA (2008) Surgical pathology of 104 tricuspid valves (2000–2005) with classic right-sided Ebstein's malformation. Cardiovasc Pathol Off J Soc Cardiovasc Pathol 17:166–171
84. Bolling SF, Iannettoni MD, Dick M 2nd, Rosenthal A, Bove EL (1990) Shone's anomaly: operative results and late outcome. Ann Thorac Surg 49:887–893
85. Popescu BA, Jurcut R, Serban M, Parascan L, Ginghina C (2008) Shone's syndrome diagnosed with echocardiography and confirmed at pathology. Eur J Echocardiogr 9:865–867
86. Brauner RA, Laks H, Drinkwater DC Jr, Scholl F, McCaffery S (1997) Multiple left heart obstructions (Shone's anomaly) with mitral valve involvement: long-term surgical outcome. Ann Thorac Surg 64:721–729
87. Brown JW, Ruzmetov M, Vijay P, Hoyer MH, Girod D et al (2005) Operative results and outcomes in children with Shone's anomaly. Ann Thorac Surg 79:1358–1365
88. Brenner JI, Berg KA, Schneider DS, Clark EB, Boughman JA (1989) Cardiac malformations in relatives of infants with hypoplastic left-heart syndrome. Am J Dis Child 143:1492–1494
89. Hinton RB Jr, Martin LJ, Tabangin ME, Mazwi ML, Cripe LH et al (2007) Hypoplastic left heart syndrome is heritable. J Am Coll Cardiol 50:1590–1595
90. Hinton RB, Martin LJ, Rame-Gowda S, Tabangin ME, Cripe LH et al (2009) Hypoplastic left heart syndrome links to chromosomes 10q and 6q and is genetically related to bicuspid aortic valve. J Am Coll Cardiol 53:1065–1071
91. Roberts WC, Morrow AG, Braunwald E (1962) Complete interruption of the aortic arch. Circulation 26:39–59
92. Duran AC, Frescura C, Sans-Coma V, Angelini A, Basso C et al (1995) Bicuspid aortic valves in hearts with other congenital heart disease. J Heart Valve Dis 4:581–590
93. Perloff JK (2010) The variant associations of aortic isthmic coarctation. Am J Cardiol 106:1038–1041
94. Thanassoulis G, Yip JW, Filion K, Jamorski M, Webb G et al (2008) Retrospective study to identify predictors of the presence and rapid progression of aortic dilatation in patients with bicuspid aortic valves. Nat Clin Pract Cardiovasc Med 5:821–828
95. Folger GM Jr, Stein PD (1984) Bicuspid aortic valve morphology when associated with coarctation of the aorta. Catheter Cardiovasc Diagn 10:17–25
96. Teo LL, Cannell T, Babu-Narayan SV, Hughes M, Mohiaddin RH (2011) Prevalence of associated cardiovascular abnormalities in 500 patients with aortic coarctation referred for cardiovascular magnetic resonance imaging to a tertiary center. Pediatr Cardiol 32:1120–1127
97. Deshpande J, Kinare SG (1991) The bicuspid aortic valve – an autopsy study. Indian J Pathol Microbiol 34:112–118
98. Suzuki T, Nagai R, Kurihara H, Kurihara Y, Yamazaki T et al (1994) Stenotic bicuspid aortic valve associated with a ventricular septal defect in an adult presenting with congestive heart failure: a rare observation. Eur Heart J 15:402–403
99. Hutchins GM (1971) Coarctation of the aorta explained as a branch-point of the ductus arteriosus. Am J Pathol 63:203–209
100. Siu SC, Silversides CK (2010) Bicuspid aortic valve disease. J Am Coll Cardiol 55:2789–2800
101. Eichhorn P, Vogt P, Ritter M, Widmer V, Jenni R (1995) Abnormalities of the atrial septum in adults: kind, prevalence and clinical relevance. Schweiz Med Wochenschr 125:1336–1341

102. Lerer PK, Edwards WD (1981) Coronary arterial anatomy in bicuspid aortic valve. Necropsy study of 100 hearts. Br Heart J 45:142–147
103. Cho S, Jeon KN, Bae K (2015) Anomalous origin and aneurysm of the right coronary artery associated with congenital bicuspid aortic valve: MDCT findings. SpringerPlus 4:426
104. Ayusawa M, Sato Y, Kanamaru H, Kunimasa T, Sumitomo N et al (2010) MDCT of the anomalous origin of the right coronary artery from the left sinus of Valsalva associated with bicuspid aortic valve. Int J Cardiol 143:e45–e47
105. Aoyagi S, Suzuki S, Kosuga K, Ohishi K (1991) Anomalous origin of the right coronary artery associated with congenital bicuspid aortic valve. Kurume Med J 38:199–202
106. Palomo AR, Schrager BR, Chahine RA (1985) Anomalous origin of the right coronary artery from the ascending aorta high above the left posterior sinus of Valsalva of a bicuspid aortic valve. Am Heart J 109:902–904
107. Kang N, Tan SY, Ding ZP, Chua YL (2013) Abnormal origin of right coronary artery from left ventricle with bicuspid aortic stenosis. Ann Thorac Surg 96:e43–e45
108. Bossert T, Walther T, Doll N, Gummert JF, Kostelka M et al (2005) Anomalous origin of the right coronary artery from the pulmonary artery combined with aortic valve stenosis. Ann Thorac Surg 79:347–348
109. Tejada JG, Albarran A, Hernandez F, Jimenez S, Tascon JC (2001) Anomalous coronary artery origin associated with bicuspid aortic valve in a patient with rheumatic mitral stenosis: a case report. Angiology 52:649–652
110. Schang SJ, Pepine CJ, Bemiller CR (1975) Anomalous coronary artery origin and bicuspid aortic valve. Vasc Surg 9:67–72
111. Ishida N, Shimabukuro K, Matsuno Y, Ogura H, Takemura H (2014) Single coronary artery with bicuspid aortic valve stenosis and aneurysm of the ascending aorta: report of a case. Surg Today 44:550–552
112. Stajic Z, Mijailovic Z (2013) Single coronary artery associated with severe bicuspid aortic valve stenosis. J Saudi Heart Assoc 25:277–278
113. Rashid A, Saucedo JF, Hennebry TA (2005) Association of single coronary artery and congenital bicuspid aortic valve with review of literature. J Interv Cardiol 18:389–391
114. Morimoto K, Taniguchi I, Miyasaka S, Marumoto A (2005) Bicuspid aortic valve stenosis with single coronary artery. Ann Thorac Cardiovasc Surg 11:267–269
115. Kemaloglu Oz T, Karadeniz FO, Gundlapalli H, Erer B, Sharma RK et al (2014) Coexisting bicuspid aortic and pulmonary valves with normally related great vessels diagnosed by live/real time three-dimensional transesophageal echocardiography. Echocardiography 31:218–221
116. Ghez OY, Chetaille PM, Campbell BJ, Van Praagh R, Metras D (2002) Tetralogy of Fallot with aortic valvular stenosis: surgical correction in one case. Ann Thorac Surg 73:967–969
117. Kutty S, Kaul S, Danford CJ, Danford DA (2010) Main pulmonary artery dilation in association with congenital bicuspid aortic valve in the absence of pulmonary valve abnormality. Heart 96:1756–1761
118. Chisholm JC (1981) Mitral valve prolapse syndrome associated with congenital bicuspid aortic valve. J Natl Med Assoc 73:921–923
119. Charitos EI, Hanke T, Karluss A, Hilker L, Stierle U et al (2013) New insights into bicuspid aortic valve disease: the elongated anterior mitral leaflet. Eur J Cardiothorac Surg 43:367–370
120. Roberts WC, Janning KG, Vowels TJ, Ko JM, Hamman BL et al (2012) Presence of a congenitally bicuspid aortic valve among patients having combined mitral and aortic valve replacement. Am J Cardiol 109:263–271
121. Wrigley BJ, Rosin M, Banerjee P (2009) Replacement of a congenital bicuspid aortic valve in a patient with left ventricular noncompaction. Tex Heart Inst J 36:241–243
122. Krishnan U, Kilner PJ, Money-Kyrle A, Ramrakha P (2006) Two diverticula of the left ventricular outflow tract adjacent to the commissures of a bicuspid aortic valve. Congenit Heart Dis 1:332–334

123. Yildirir A, Batur MK, Kabakci G (2001) Left ventricular septal aneurysm in association with bicuspid aortic valve – a case report. Angiology 52:73–76
124. Vanelli P, Carro C, Scrofani R, Turiel M, Antona C et al (2002) Subannular left ventricular aneurysm in a patient with bicuspid aortic valve stenosis. Italian Heart J Off J Ital Fed Cardiol 3:608–610
125. Feizi O, Farrer Brown G, Emanuel R (1978) Familial study of hypertrophic cardiomyopathy and congenital aortic valve disease. Am J Cardiol 41:956–964
126. Schievink WI, Mokri B (1995) Familial aorto-cervicocephalic arterial dissections and congenitally bicuspid aortic valve. Stroke 26:1935–1940
127. Schievink WI, Raissi SS, Maya MM, Velebir A (2010) Screening for intracranial aneurysms in patients with bicuspid aortic valve. Neurology 74:1430–1433
128. Shaulov A, Leibowitz D, Rott D (2012) Prevalence of bicuspid aortic valve in patients presenting with subarachnoid hemorrhage related to an intracerebral aneurysm. Int J Cardiol 157:142–143
129. Goyal MS, Gottumukkala R, Bhalla S, Kates A, Zipfel GJ et al (2015) Bicuspid aortic valves and thoracic aortic aneurysms in patients with intracranial aneurysms. Neurology 84:46–49
130. Gupta P, Theut SB, Joshi A, Aggarwal S (2011) Circumaortic innominate vein in a patient with bicuspid aortic valve and coarctation. Ann Thorac Surg 92:e37
131. Zeina AR, Nachtigal A, Troitsa A, Admon G, Avshovich N (2010) Isolated spontaneous dissection of the celiac trunk in a patient with bicuspid aortic valve. Vasc Health Risk Manag 6:383–386
132. Westaby S, Bradlow WM, Newton JD, Mahesh B, Jin XY et al (2011) Rupture of an aneurysmal aortic diverticulum associated with coarctation and bicuspid aortic valve. Circulation 123:102–103
133. Di Martino L, Correale M, Cocco D, Di Biase M, Brunetti ND (2013) Bicuspid aortic valve and lusory artery: an unusual association. Intern Emerg Med 8:539–540
134. Kono T, Kitahara H, Watanabe T, Takano T, Sakaguchi M et al (2004) Successful repair of aberrant right subclavian artery aneurysm combined with bicuspid aortic valve through a median sternotomy. Ann Thorac Surg 77:2196–2197
135. Mandila C, Papanikolaou J, Saranteas T, Dounis G, Kostopanagiotou G et al (2009) Bicuspid aortic valve associated with persistent left and absent right superior vena cava. J Cardiothorac Vasc Anesth 23:579–580
136. Aydin A, Desai N, Bernhardt AM, Treede H, Detter C et al (2013) Ascending aortic aneurysm and aortic valve dysfunction in bicuspid aortic valve disease. Int J Cardiol 164:301–305
137. Hahn RT, Roman MJ, Mogtader AH, Devereux RB (1992) Association of aortic dilation with regurgitant, stenotic and functionally normal bicuspid aortic valves. J Am Coll Cardiol 19:283–288
138. Bauer M, Gliech V, Siniawski H, Hetzer R (2006) Configuration of the ascending aorta in patients with bicuspid and tricuspid aortic valve disease undergoing aortic valve replacement with or without reduction aortoplasty. J Heart Valve Dis 15:594–600
139. Fazel SS, Mallidi HR, Lee RS, Sheehan MP, Liang D et al (2008) The aortopathy of bicuspid aortic valve disease has distinctive patterns and usually involves the transverse aortic arch. J Thorac Cardiovasc Surg 135:901–907, 907.e1–907.e2
140. Preventza O, Livesay JJ, Cooley DA, Krajcer Z, Cheong BY et al (2013) Coarctation-associated aneurysms: a localized disease or diffuse aortopathy. Ann Thorac Surg 95:1961–1967; discussion 7
141. von Kodolitsch Y, Aydin AM, Bernhardt AM, Habermann C, Treede H et al (2010) Aortic aneurysms after correction of aortic coarctation: a systematic review. VASA 39:3–16
142. von Kodolitsch Y, Aydin AM, Koschyk DH et al (2002) Predictors of aneurysm formation after surgical correction of aortic coarctation. J Am Coll Cardiol 39:617–624
143. Della Corte A, Bancone C, Dialetto G, Covino FE, Manduca S et al (2014) Towards an individualized approach to bicuspid aortopathy: different valve types have unique determinants of aortic dilatation. Eur J Cardiothorac Surg 45:e118–e124

144. Schaefer BM, Lewin MB, Stout KK, Byers PH, Otto CM (2007) Usefulness of bicuspid aortic valve phenotype to predict elastic properties of the ascending aorta. Am J Cardiol 99:686–690
145. Russo CF, Cannata A, Lanfranconi M, Vitali E, Garatti A et al (2008) Is aortic wall degeneration related to bicuspid aortic valve anatomy in patients with valvular disease? J Thorac Cardiovasc Surg 136:937–942
146. Holmes KW, Lehmann CU, Dalal D, Nasir K, Dietz HC et al (2007) Progressive dilation of the ascending aorta in children with isolated bicuspid aortic valve. Am J Cardiol 99:978–983
147. Della Corte A, Bancone C, Quarto C, Dialetto G, Covino FE et al (2007) Predictors of ascending aortic dilatation with bicuspid aortic valve: a wide spectrum of disease expression. Eur J Cardiothorac Surg 31:397–404; discussion –5
148. Kang JW, Song HG, Yang DH, Baek S, Kim DH et al (2013) Association between bicuspid aortic valve phenotype and patterns of valvular dysfunction and bicuspid aortopathy: comprehensive evaluation using MDCT and echocardiography. JACC Cardiovasc Imaging 6:150–161
149. Kim YG, Sun BJ, Park GM, Han S, Kim DH et al (2012) Aortopathy and bicuspid aortic valve: haemodynamic burden is main contributor to aortic dilatation. Heart 98:1822–1827
150. Westhoff-Bleck M, Meyer GP, Lotz J, Tutarel O, Weiss T et al (2005) Dilatation of the entire thoracic aorta in patients with bicuspid aortic valve: a magnetic resonance angiography study. VASA 34:181–185
151. Girdauskas E, Rouman M, Disha K, Espinoza A, Misfeld M et al (2015) Aortic dissection after previous aortic valve replacement for bicuspid aortic valve disease. J Am Coll Cardiol 66:1409–1411
152. Milan A, Avenatti E, Tosello F, Iannaccone A, Leone D et al (2013) Aortic root dilatation in essential hypertension: prevalence according to new reference values. J Hypertens 31:1189–1195
153. Agmon Y, Khandheria BK, Meissner I, Schwartz GL, Sicks JD et al (2003) Is aortic dilatation an atherosclerosis-related process? Clinical, laboratory, and transesophageal echocardiographic correlates of thoracic aortic dimensions in the population with implications for thoracic aortic aneurysm formation. J Am Coll Cardiol 42:1076–1083
154. Oliver JM, Alonso-Gonzalez R, Gonzalez AE, Gallego P, Sanchez-Recalde A et al (2009) Risk of aortic root or ascending aorta complications in patients with bicuspid aortic valve with and without coarctation of the aorta. Am J Cardiol 104:1001–1006
155. Bauer M, Bauer U, Siniawski H, Hetzer R (2007) Differences in clinical manifestations in patients with bicuspid and tricuspid aortic valves undergoing surgery of the aortic valve and/or ascending aorta. Thorac Cardiovasc Surg 55:485–490
156. Quenot JP, Boichot C, Petit A, Falcon-Eicher S, d'Athis P et al (2005) Usefulness of MRI in the follow-up of patients with repaired aortic coarctation and bicuspid aortic valve. Int J Cardiol 103:312–316
157. Keshavarz-Motamed Z, Garcia J, Kadem L (2013) Fluid dynamics of coarctation of the aorta and effect of bicuspid aortic valve. PLoS One 8:e72394
158. Kohler M, Pitcher A, Blair E, Risby P, Senn O et al (2013) The impact of obstructive sleep apnea on aortic disease in Marfan's syndrome. Respiration 86:39–44
159. Hata M, Yoshitake I, Wakui S, Unosawa S, Takahashi K et al (2012) Sleep disorders and aortic dissection in a working population. Surg Today 42:403–405
160. Rybczynski M, Koschyk D, Karmeier A, Gessler N, Sheikhzadeh S et al (2010) Frequency of sleep apnea in adults with the Marfan syndrome. Am J Cardiol 105:1836–1841
161. Keles T, Durmaz T, Bayram NA, Ciftci B, Yeter E et al (2009) Effect of continuous positive airway pressure therapy on aortic stiffness in patients with obstructive sleep apnea syndrome. Echocardiography 26:1217–1224
162. Serizawa N, Yumino D, Takagi A, Gomita K, Kajimoto K et al (2008) Obstructive sleep apnea is associated with greater thoracic aortic size. J Am Coll Cardiol 52:885–886
163. Sampol G, Romero O, Salas A, Tovar JL, Lloberes P et al (2003) Obstructive sleep apnea and thoracic aorta dissection. Am J Respir Crit Care Med 168:1528–1531

164. Immer FF, Bansi AG, Immer-Bansi AS, McDougall J, Zehr KJ et al (2003) Aortic dissection in pregnancy: analysis of risk factors and outcome. Ann Thorac Surg 76:309–314
165. Yuan SM (2013) Aortic dissection during pregnancy: a difficult clinical scenario. Clin Cardiol 36:576–584
166. Maron BJ, Shirani J, Poliac LC, Mathenge R, Roberts WC, Mueller FO (1996) Sudden death in young competitive athletics. Clinical, and pathologic profiles. JAMA 276:199–204
167. Galanti G, Stefani L, Toncelli L, Vono MC, Mercuri R et al (2010) Effects of sports activity in athletes with bicuspid aortic valve and mild aortic regurgitation. Br J Sports Med 44:275–279
168. Carter D, Pokroy R, Azaria B, Matetzky S, Prokopetz A et al (2007) Effect of G-force on bicuspid aortic valve in aviators. Cardiology 108:124–127
169. Hsue PY, Salinas CL, Bolger AF, Benowitz NL, Waters DD (2002) Acute aortic dissection related to crack cocaine. Circulation 105:1592–1595
170. Eagle KA, Isselbacher EM, DeSanctis RW (2002) Cocaine-related aortic dissection in perspective. Circulation 105:1529–1530
171. Palmiere C, Burkhardt S, Staub C, Hallenbarter M, Paolo Pizzolato G et al (2004) Thoracic aortic dissection associated with cocaine abuse. Forensic Sci Int 141:137–142
172. Singh S, Trivedi A, Adhikari T, Molnar J, Arora R et al (2007) Cocaine-related acute aortic dissection: patient demographics and clinical outcomes. Can J Cardiol 23:1131–1134
173. Wako E, LeDoux D, Mitsumori L, Aldea GS (2007) The emerging epidemic of methamphetamine-induced aortic dissections. J Card Surg 22:390–393
174. Westover AN, Nakonezny PA (2010) Aortic dissection in young adults who abuse amphetamines. Am Heart J 160:315–321
175. Tiryakioglu SK, Tiryakioglu O, Turan T, Kumbay E (2009) Aortic dissection due to sildenafil abuse. Interact Cardiovasc Thorac Surg 9:141–143
176. Boodhwani M, Andelfinger G, Leipsic J, Lindsay T, McMurtry MS et al (2014) Canadian Cardiovascular Society position statement on the management of thoracic aortic disease. Can J Cardiol 30:577–589
177. Erbel R, Aboyans V, Boileau C, Bossone E, Di Bartolomeo R et al (2014) ESC Guidelines on the diagnosis and treatment of aortic diseases: document covering acute and chronic aortic diseases of the thoracic and abdominal aorta of the adult. The Task Force for the Diagnosis and Treatment of Aortic Diseases of the European Society of Cardiology (ESC). Eur Heart J 2014
178. Hiratzka LF, Bakris GL, Beckman JA, Bersin RM, Carr VF et al (2010) ACCF/AHA/AATS/ACR/ASA/SCA/SCAI/SIR/STS/SVM guidelines for the diagnosis and management of patients with thoracic aortic disease: a report of the American College of Cardiology Foundation/American Heart Association Task Force on Practice Guidelines, American Association for Thoracic Surgery, American College of Radiology, American Stroke Association, Society of Cardiovascular Anesthesiologists, Society for Cardiovascular Angiography and Interventions, Society of Interventional Radiology, Society of Thoracic Surgeons, and Society for Vascular Medicine. Circulation 121:e266–e369
179. von Kodolitsch Y, Robinson P, Berger J (2014) When should surgery be performed in Marfan syndrome and other connective tissue disorders to protect against type a dissection? In: Bonser RS, Pagano D, Haverich A, Mascaro J (eds) Controversies in aortic dissection and aneurysmal disease. Springer, London, pp 17–47
180. Biner S, Rafique AM, Ray I, Cuk O, Siegel RJ et al (2009) Aortopathy is prevalent in relatives of bicuspid aortic valve patients. J Am Coll Cardiol 53:2288–2295
181. Martin LJ, Hinton RB, Zhang X, Cripe LH, Benson DW (2011) Aorta measurements are heritable and influenced by bicuspid aortic valve. Front Genet 2:61
182. Biddinger A, Rocklin M, Coselli J, Milewicz DM (1997) Familial thoracic aortic dilatations and dissections: a case control study. J Vasc Surg 25:506–511
183. Ferencik M, Pape LA (2003) Changes in size of ascending aorta and aortic valve function with time in patients with congenitally bicuspid aortic valves. Am J Cardiol 92:43–46

184. Novaro GM, Griffin BP (2004) Congenital bicuspid aortic valve and rate of ascending aortic dilatation. Am J Cardiol 93:525–526
185. Etz CD, Zoli S, Brenner R, Roder F, Bischoff M et al (2010) When to operate on the bicuspid valve patient with a modestly dilated ascending aorta. Ann Thorac Surg 90:1884–1890; discussion 91–92.
186. Beroukhim RS, Kruzick TL, Taylor AL, Gao D, Yetman AT (2006) Progression of aortic dilation in children with a functionally normal bicuspid aortic valve. Am J Cardiol 98:828–830
187. Roman MJ, Rosen SE, Kramer-Fox R, Devereux RB (1993) Prognostic significance of the pattern of aortic root dilation in the Marfan syndrome. J Am Coll Cardiol 22:1470–1476
188. Cotrufo M, Della Corte A (2009) The association of bicuspid aortic valve disease with asymmetric dilatation of the tubular ascending aorta: identification of a definite syndrome. J Cardiovasc Med (Hagerstown) 10:291–297
189. Robicsek F, Thubrikar MJ (1994) Hemodynamic considerations regarding the mechanism and prevention of aortic dissection. Ann Thorac Surg 58:1247–1253
190. Warner PJ, Al-Quthami A, Brooks EL, Kelley-Hedgepeth A, Patvardhan E et al (2013) Augmentation index and aortic stiffness in bicuspid aortic valve patients with non-dilated proximal aortas. BMC Cardiovasc Disord 13:19
191. Tzemos N, Lyseggen E, Silversides C, Jamorski M, Tong JH et al (2010) Endothelial function, carotid-femoral stiffness, and plasma matrix metalloproteinase-2 in men with bicuspid aortic valve and dilated aorta. J Am Coll Cardiol 55:660–668
192. Grotenhuis HB, Ottenkamp J, Westenberg JJ, Bax JJ, Kroft LJ et al (2007) Reduced aortic elasticity and dilatation are associated with aortic regurgitation and left ventricular hypertrophy in nonstenotic bicuspid aortic valve patients. J Am Coll Cardiol 49:1660–1665
193. Aydin A, Mortensen K, Rybczynski M, Sheikhzadeh S, Willmann S et al (2011) Central pulse pressure and augmentation index in asymptomatic bicuspid aortic valve disease. Int J Cardiol 147:466–468
194. Nistri S, Sorbo MD, Basso C, Thiene G (2002) Bicuspid aortic valve: abnormal aortic elastic properties. J Heart Valve Dis 11:369–373; discussion 73–74
195. Shim CY, Cho IJ, Yang WI, Kang MK, Park S et al (2011) Central aortic stiffness and its association with ascending aorta dilation in subjects with a bicuspid aortic valve. J Am Soc Echocardiogr 24:847–852
196. Jackson V, Petrini J, Caidahl K, Eriksson MJ, Liska J et al (2011) Bicuspid aortic valve leaflet morphology in relation to aortic root morphology: a study of 300 patients undergoing open-heart surgery. Eur J Cardiothorac Surg 40:e118–e124
197. Nistri S, Grande-Allen J, Noale M, Basso C, Siviero P et al (2008) Aortic elasticity and size in bicuspid aortic valve syndrome. Eur Heart J 29:472–479
198. Pees C, Michel-Behnke I (2012) Morphology of the bicuspid aortic valve and elasticity of the adjacent aorta in children. Am J Cardiol 110:1354–1360
199. Donato Aquaro G, Ait-Ali L, Basso ML, Lombardi M, Pingitore A et al (2011) Elastic properties of aortic wall in patients with bicuspid aortic valve by magnetic resonance imaging. Am J Cardiol 108:81–87
200. Oulego-Erroz I, Alonso-Quintela P, Mora-Matilla M, Gautreaux Minaya S, de Armentia SLL (2012) Ascending aorta elasticity in children with isolated bicuspid aortic valve. Int J Cardiol 168(2):1143–1146
201. Hope MD, Hope TA (2013) Functional and molecular imaging techniques in aortic aneurysm disease. Curr Opin Cardiol 28:609–618
202. Hope MD, Hope TA, Meadows AK, Ordovas KG, Urbania TH et al (2010) Bicuspid aortic valve: four-dimensional MR evaluation of ascending aortic systolic flow patterns. Radiology 255:53–61
203. Burris NS, Sigovan M, Knauer HA, Tseng EE, Saloner D et al (2014) Systolic flow displacement correlates with future ascending aortic growth in patients with bicuspid aortic valves undergoing magnetic resonance surveillance. Investig Radiol 49:635–639

204. Hope MD, Hope TA, Crook SE, Ordovas KG, Urbania TH et al (2011) 4D flow CMR in assessment of valve-related ascending aortic disease. JACC Cardiovasc Imaging 4:781–787
205. Hope MD, Wrenn J, Sigovan M, Foster E, Tseng EE et al (2012) Imaging biomarkers of aortic disease: increased growth rates with eccentric systolic flow. J Am Coll Cardiol 60:356–357
206. Nathan DP, Xu C, Plappert T, Desjardins B, Gorman JH 3rd et al (2011) Increased ascending aortic wall stress in patients with bicuspid aortic valves. Ann Thorac Surg 92:1384–1389
207. Ali OA, Chapman M, Nguyen TH, Chirkov YY, Heresztyn T et al (2014) Interactions between inflammatory activation and endothelial dysfunction selectively modulate valve disease progression in patients with bicuspid aortic valve. Heart 100:800–805
208. Foffa I, Murzi M, Mariani M, Mazzone AM, Glauber M et al (2012) Angiotensin-converting enzyme insertion/deletion polymorphism is a risk factor for thoracic aortic aneurysm in patients with bicuspid or tricuspid aortic valves. J Thorac Cardiovasc Surg 144:390–395
209. Kilickesmez KO, Abaci O, Kocas C, Yildiz A, Kaya A et al (2012) Dilatation of the ascending aorta and serum alpha 1-antitrypsin level in patients with bicuspid aortic valve. Heart Vessel 27:391–397
210. Ikonomidis JS, Ivey CR, Wheeler JB, Akerman AW, Rice A et al (2013) Plasma biomarkers for distinguishing etiologic subtypes of thoracic aortic aneurysm disease. J Thorac Cardiovasc Surg 145:1326–1333
211. Boon RA, Seeger T, Heydt S, Fischer A, Hergenreider E et al (2011) MicroRNA-29 in aortic dilation: implications for aneurysm formation. Circ Res 109:1115–1119
212. Schmoker JD, McPartland KJ, Fellinger EK, Boyum J, Trombley L et al (2007) Matrix metalloproteinase and tissue inhibitor expression in atherosclerotic and nonatherosclerotic thoracic aortic aneurysms. J Thorac Cardiovasc Surg 133:155–161
213. Boyum J, Fellinger EK, Schmoker JD, Trombley L, McPartland K et al (2004) Matrix metalloproteinase activity in thoracic aortic aneurysms associated with bicuspid and tricuspid aortic valves. J Thorac Cardiovasc Surg 127:686–691
214. Wang Y, Wu B, Dong L, Wang C, Wang X et al (2014) Circulating matrix metalloproteinase patterns in association with aortic dilatation in bicuspid aortic valve patients with isolated severe aortic stenosis. Heart Vessels 31:189–197
215. Irtiuga OB, Zhiduleva EV, Dubrovskaia OB, Moiseeva OM (2014) Concentration of osteoprotegerin and RANKL in blood serum of patients with aortic stenosis. Kardiologiia 54:44–48
216. Branchetti E, Bavaria JE, Grau JB, Shaw RE, Poggio P et al (2014) Circulating soluble receptor for advanced glycation end product identifies patients with bicuspid aortic valve and associated aortopathies. Arterioscler Thromb Vasc Biol 34:2349–2357
217. Hillebrand M, Millot N, Sheikhzadeh S, Rybczynski M, Gerth S et al (2014) Total serum transforming growth factor-beta1 is elevated in the entire spectrum of genetic aortic syndromes. Clin Cardiol 37:672–679
218. Black KM, Masuzawa A, Hagberg RC, Khabbaz KR, Trovato ME et al (2013) Preliminary biomarkers for identification of human ascending thoracic aortic aneurysm. J Am Heart Assoc 2:e000138

Chapter 16
Aortic Coarctation

Allard T. van den Hoven and Jolien W. Roos-Hesselink

Abstract In this chapter the anatomy, epidemiology, pathogenesis, clinical aspects, and genetic associations of aortic coarctation will be discussed. Depending on the balance between the degree of flow disturbance and the compensatory mechanisms available to overcome it, the clinical presentation may vary from the critically ill neonate in heart failure to the asymptomatic child or adult with hypertension. Untreated coarctation carries a poor prognosis with average survival age of 35 years in historic cohorts.

Imaging is essential to diagnose coarctation of the aorta in time and to follow up the patient after treatment. We discuss the indication for treatment and the various treatment options and the advantages and disadvantages of percutaneous and surgical intervention. Lifelong surveillance is warranted, also after successful operative or interventional treatment, since patients remain at risk, particularly for hypertension, recoarctation, and aneurysm formation.

In the last section, we describe the myriad of syndromes that include aortic coarctation in their cardiovascular phenotype. It is important to see aortic coarctation as part of a more generalized aortopathy instead of a stand-alone defect.

Keywords Aortic coarctation • Aortic aneurysm

16.1 Background/Introduction

Aortic coarctation, a congenital stenosis usually located in juxta-ductal position [1–3], has been recognized since its first description in 1760 by Morgagni during his autopsy of a monk [4]. It was more formally recognized as a clinical entity after its description in 1928 [5]; the first surgical correction was performed in 1945 [6]. Nowadays it is generally accepted to be part of a general aortopathy, linked with other left-sided heart defects such as a bicuspid aortic valve (BAV) [7]. The coarctation can vary in severity from quite discrete to a severe long hypoplastic

A.T. van den Hoven • J.W. Roos-Hesselink (✉)
Department of Cardiology, Erasmus University Medical Center, Room Ba-583a, P.O. Box 2040, 3000 Rotterdam, CA, The Netherlands
e-mail: j.roos@erasmusmc.nl

K. Niwa, H. Kaemmerer (eds.), *Aortopathy*, DOI 10.1007/978-4-431-56071-5_16

aortic segment. The incidence of CoA is approximately 4 per 10,000 live births and constitutes 5–8 % of all congenital heart disease (CHD) [8]. Nowadays, aortic coarctation is preferably repaired surgically at an early age, but catheter intervention has become a valid alternative, especially in outgrown children and adults. Lifelong surveillance is warranted, also after successful repair, since patients remain at risk, particularly for hypertension, recoarctation, and aneurysm formation [9–11]. According to historic studies, when left untreated, most patients die before the age of 50 mainly due to coronary artery disease, stroke, or intracranial hemorrhage. Nowadays, 72 % of patients are alive 30 years after operation [10]. Even in patients with satisfactory repair, major complications do occur.

16.2 Anatomy, Epidemiology, and Pathogenesis

16.2.1 Anatomy

Aortic coarctation is defined as a narrowing of the aortic isthmus, often juxta-ductal in position. Three main types can be distinguished depending on the anatomical position of the infolding of the aortic wall relative to the ductus arteriosus (DA): pre-ductal, post-ductal, or at the site of the ductus [Fig. 16.1]. In 90 % of cases, the infolding is directly opposite to the DA. The pre-ductal or infant type is a cyanotic and duct-dependent lesion. After birth the closure of the DA will result in hypoperfusion of the lower extremities. Also, coarctation has been described in anecdotal cases to present in the abdominal aorta, which is however more likely to be inflammatory or autoimmune in origin. Aortic coarctation can even be traumatic when aortic dissection compromises the true lumen of the aorta.

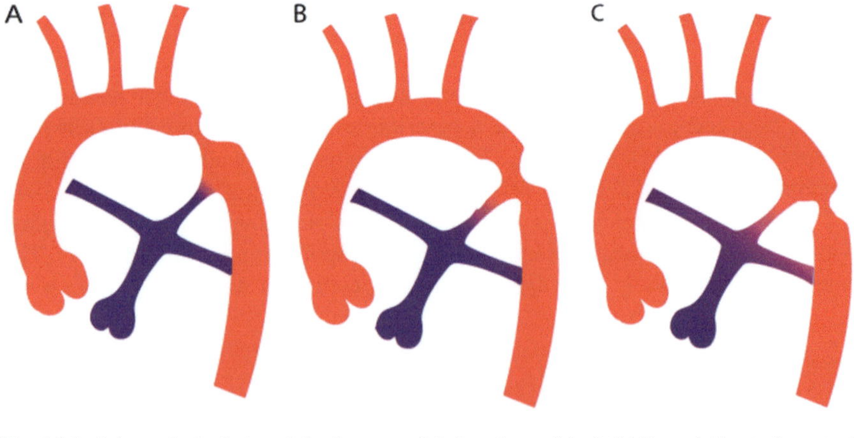

Fig. 16.1 Schematic depiction of the three possible locations of the infolding relative to the patent ductus arteriosus (PDA). (**a**) Pre-ductal coarctation. (**b**) Para-ductal coarctation. (**c**) Post-ductal coarctation

16.2.2 Epidemiology

Aortic coarctation is a relatively frequent congenital heart defect (CHD) and is found in approximately 3–4 per 10,000 live births and constitutes 5 % of all CHD [8]. It occurs more often in males than in females in a ratio between 1.27 and 1.74 and 1 [12, 13]. In most patients it is diagnosed shortly after birth, depending on the subtype and clinical symptoms.

16.2.3 Etiology

There are three possible theories explaining the development of coarctation. There is the ductal tissue theory, which suggests that ductal muscular tissue extends into the wall of the thoracic aorta, causing the aorta to constrict postnatally simultaneous with the ductus arteriosus. Several studies have confirmed the presence of ductal tissue in the aortic wall [14, 15].

Another theory is the developmental theory, which suggests coarctation formation starts with a fault in early fetal development. A part of the fetal circulation involutes to form the separate dorsal aorta and right subclavian artery. A small segment of the fetal dorsal aorta will erroneously involute and will subsequently move cranially with the left subclavian artery [16]. This would then form the coarctation.

The third theory is based on hemodynamical changes. During fetal development the aortic isthmus is a naturally occurring narrow segment because it doesn't have to conduct a large flow of blood. This segment will then later be widened to facilitate the increased blood flow. If the increase in blood flow remains absent, this narrow area will persist and a coarctation will be formed. This could also partly explain the association with BAV, as a diminished forward flow and increased post-ductal flow can predispose to development of CoA as well.

The etiology of CoA remains enigmatic, but it is generally assumed that coarctation is in fact part of a general aortopathy, linked with bicuspid aortic valve, aortic dissection, and even intracranial aneurysms [7]. More research is clearly needed to discern cause and effect.

16.2.4 Histology

Comparatively little attention has been directed to the prevalence, range, or degree of histological changes in the aortic wall (arterial media) of patients with CoA.

Small studies have compared pre- and post-stenotic tissue to assess the histological abnormalities and tried to account for the influence of blood pressure. There is evidence to support an inherent vessel wall weakness that occurs separately from hemodynamical changes [17]. The underlying cause of these histological abnormalities is most probably so-called cystic media necrosis [18]. More research has been conducted on the aortic vessel wall in BAV, which often coincides with CoA as discussed below. In BAV too aortic wall changes seem to take place at least partly independent from hemodynamics [19]. BAV patients have structural changes of the aortic media such as thinner elastic lamellae and greater distance between the lamellae [20]. Apoptosis of smooth muscle cells might contribute to weakness of the wall which might explain the high cardiovascular morbidity in BAV patients [21]. As BAV and CoA are two related abnormalities with both origins in the neural crest cells, they seem to be part of a broader aortopathy.

16.3 Clinical Picture

16.3.1 Pathophysiology

The main pathophysiological mechanism by which aortic coarctation causes morbidity and mortality is the afterload increase of the left ventricle (LV). This occurs when the arterial duct closes postnatally and starts a causal chain in which increased left ventricular pressures lead to compensatory hypertrophy and eventually (diastolic) dysfunction. When the coarctation is severe enough, this can be an acute process, leading to hypoperfusion distal to the coarctation, presenting in neonates with signs of shock, but also to a "backward failure," where the rapid increase in LV systolic afterload, increased wall stress, and compensatory left ventricular hypertrophy may cause increased pulmonary venous pressures with pulmonary congestion, followed by elevated pulmonary arterial pressures, right ventricular pressure overload, and subsequently heart failure. The foramen ovale might be opened by the sudden increase in pressure causing left to right shunting of blood.

In less pronounced cases, this process will be less rapid, and collaterals can develop, bypassing the coarcted segment and delaying the onset of clinical signs.

In addition to ductal tissue in the aortic wall, other histological wall changes are present in CoA patients. Wall stiffness is increased and distensibility is decreased [22]. There is more collagen but less smooth muscle tissue in the prestenotic aortic wall when compared to post-stenotic aortic wall. Cystic medial necrosis, the depletion or disarray of elastic tissue, is also seen.

The effects of coarctation are not yet fully explained, as patients with a relieved coarctation often still suffer from hypertension, requiring pharmacological treatment. No clear association could be established between the remaining gradient over the CoA and the occurrence of hypertension. Therefore, the involvement of the renin-angiotensin-aldosterone system is supposed, although also other mechanisms, such as baroreceptor resetting, may be involved.

16.3.2 Complications

The natural history has been described in coarctation patients before correction became imperative. These patients often suffer from left heart failure, intracranial hemorrhage, infective endocarditis, aortic dissection and rupture, and coronary artery and cerebrovascular disease [2, 10]. Nowadays, after intervention the most common complications are hypertension, recurrent coarctation, aortic aneurysm or rupture, early coronary artery disease, and cardiomyopathy. When the coarctation is relieved at a very early age, the risk of recoarctation increases, while repair at older age is associated with hypertension. Risk for complications increases with age, and BAV is an independent additional risk factor for complications as is age [23]. BAV itself is associated with ascending aortic dilatation and higher risk of aortic dissection and rupture, which possibly explains the increased risk when present in addition to CoA. Intracranial berry aneurysms are reported in patients with coarctation. It is however unclear if there is a common pathophysiological ground to this association and whether it is due to secondary modifiable risk factors, such as blood pressure.

16.3.3 Diagnosis

The clinical presentation of CoA varies greatly with age. When CoA becomes evident shortly after birth, it presents as a severe cyanotic heart defect, with poor feeding, tachypnea, lethargy, symptoms of congestive heart failure, or shock. The onset of symptoms will coincide with closure of the ductus arteriosus. When CoA presents later, during childhood or even in adulthood, the clinical symptoms will mainly be due to high blood pressure in the upper extremities and may include nosebleeds, intracranial hemorrhage, dizziness, tinnitus, and shortness of breath. Also symptoms from low blood pressure in the lower extremities may become evident including abdominal angina, claudication, leg cramps, exertional leg fatigue, and cold feet [24]. A blood pressure gradient can often be seen as a high upper body systolic hypertension, in combination with a relative lower body hypotension. However, when large collaterals exist, this may be absent.

There are different diagnostic techniques used to objectify the presence and severity of CoA.

Inspection and *patient history* might reveal some of the symptoms mentioned above. A telltale sign would be differential cyanosis, where the upper extremities are normally perfused and the lower extremities are hypoperfused.

On *palpitation* a weak or absent femoral pulse may be noted, which may have a prognostic value, especially in combination with a prominent brachial pulse [25]. Radio-femoral pulse delay and palpable collaterals on palpation are both pathognomonic for CoA. Of note is that an origin of the right subclavian artery distal to the coarctation might mask this difference, as it would also be decreased and therefore the carotid pulse should be palpated as well. In addition ventricular dysfunction may decrease pulses both in the upper and lower extremities which may have effect on the gradient.

A suprasternal thrill may be palpable, and, in isolated CoA, a vascular murmur (often systolic) at the back or a continuous vascular murmur can be heard.

An *electrocardiogram* may reveal signs of left ventricular hypertrophy with or without secondary ST-segment abnormalities.

On *chest X-ray* rib notching as a result of dilated intercostal arteries, a dilated ascending aorta, kinking or double contouring in the descending aorta, and a dilated left subclavian artery can be found. Also cardiomegaly in the infant can be a sign of a coarctation.

Echocardiography is of great value in estimating site, structure, and severity of the CoA. Especially in newborns this technique gives excellent opportunities as the entire aortic arch, isthmus, arterial duct, and descending aorta are imaged from the suprasternal notch and from the right and left infraclavicular windows. It can also provide information on the function and severity of left ventricular hypertrophy as well as associated cardiac abnormalities and vessel diameters. In adolescents and adults, echocardiography of the isthmus and descending aorta may become difficult as the distance from the transducer increases and the airways may form a more prominent barrier. High systolic velocities are generally found, but a diastolic runoff phenomenon in the descending or abdominal aorta is presumably the most reliable sign of significant coarctation. Doppler flow tracing can show a "serrated" pattern with a rapid acceleration and a high-velocity systolic peak, followed by a gradual deceleration throughout diastole [Fig. 16.2].

CMR and CCT are the preferred noninvasive imaging techniques because these allow assessment of the entire aorta. It allows for the precise location and collateral anatomy to be imaged. In addition, the diameter of the ascending aorta, in case of a bicuspid valve, and the presence of aneurysms can be detected. 3D (or even 4D) reconstructions can provide insightful visual aid to the surgeon when planning reconstruction [Fig. 16.3].

Angiography. Also cardiac catheterization and manometry or angiography are important diagnostic modalities. Especially when the severity of the coarctation and gradient are not clear, the invasive measurement will be helpful in deciding on the indication for treatment.

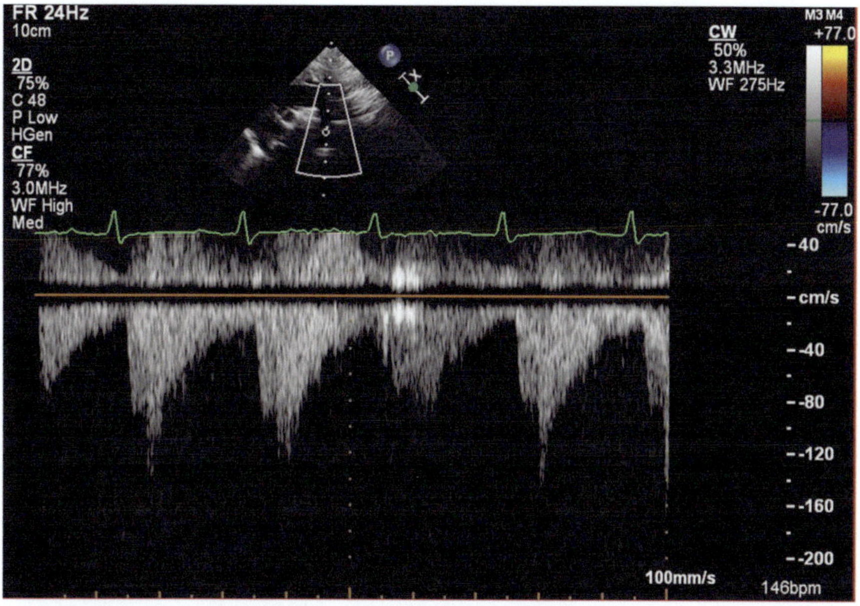

Fig. 16.2 Serrated diastolic runoff pattern in the aorta

16.3.4 Treatment

In case of severe coarctation, there is clear evidence that treatment of CoA will reduce left ventricular afterload and will improve the long-term outcome of the patient. There are however different treatment options with pros and cons for all techniques, and there is no clear superior technique.

16.3.4.1 Indication for Intervention

The decision to intervene should preferably be taken in a multidisciplinary setting where careful evaluation on the level of the individual patient is possible. According to the most recent guidelines, a pressure gradient between the upper and lower body extremities of >20 mmHg in combination with an upper body hypertension (>140/90 mmHg in adults), an abnormal blood pressure response during exercise, and a significant left ventricular hypertrophy are class I, level C indications for intervention [24]. When there is hypertension in combination with a 50 % narrowing of the aorta compared to the aortic diameter at the level of the diagram as measured on CT, MR, or invasive angiography, an intervention should be considered (class IIa, level C). And finally, in case of an anatomical narrowing (>50 %) in the absence of hypertension or a significant pressure gradient, an

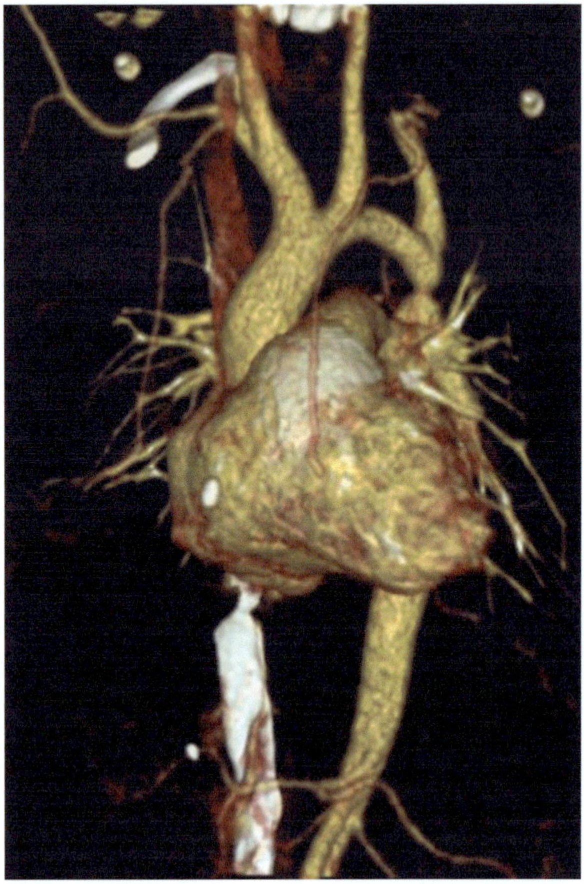

Fig. 16.3 3D reconstruction (CT) of aortic coarctation in a 6-month-old child. Very prominent *A. anonyma* and late branching a. subclavia sinistra

intervention may be considered (class IIb, level C). After intervention, endocarditis prophylaxis is advised for 6 months.

16.3.4.2 Choice of Intervention

There are two main therapies for the relief of CoA: surgical and percutaneous intervention. Surgery is the preferred treatment of infants with coarctation with an overall survival rate of 98 % at a median follow-up of 4.8 years of age. When considering surgery, there are several operative techniques to choose from: (extended) end-to-end anastomosis, patch aortoplasty, subclavian flap aortoplasty and resection with interposition of a graft, or others. All techniques have different advantages and disadvantages. With Dacron patch angioplasty, for example, there is a higher incidence of aneurysm formation, while in subclavian flap aortoplasty, a higher incidence of recoarctation has been found. The incidence of dissection is approximately equal among all modalities [26]. The (extended) end-to-end anastomosis is the most widely used technique and generally regarded as the safest and most effective method. However, this technique is not feasible in every situation.

The other option for gradient relief, percutaneous intervention, is used more often in full-grown children and adults. Catheter intervention is a safe and effective alternative to surgery, with good gradient relief for both native and recurrent coarctation. A balloon is used to disrupt the intimal and medial layers of the narrowed segment. Compared to surgery, balloon angioplasty is equally effective in reducing pressure gradient early after intervention; however, the risks of recoarctation and aneurysm formation are greater [27]. Generally a covered stent is deployed to prevent recoarctation and aneurysm formation. Stent placement after balloon angioplasty or surgery reduces the complications, improves luminal diameter, results in minimal residual gradient, and sustains hemodynamic benefit. Stent placement is not generally recommended in patients less than 25 kg due to the small aortic size and the potential injury to the femoral artery from the large sheath required for stent delivery. There is however little evidence regarding the long-term outcome of the effectiveness of the blood pressure reduction and late complications after stenting. No randomized trials have compared stenting to surgery [28], and it is therefore hard to objectively compare the two modalities.

16.3.4.3 Conservative Treatment

The acute medical treatment of CoA in the neonate is focused on maintaining patency of the ductus arteriosus. This is mainly done by administering a prostaglandin E1 inhibitor and diuretics can be given to alleviate symptoms of heart failure. In the adult patient, treatment is mainly focused on blood pressure control. This is normally achieved using beta-blockers, ACE inhibitors, and angiotensin-receptor blockers [29]. The use of ACE inhibitors has been associated with renal failure, especially when renal perfusion cannot be sustained [30].

In case of a less severe coarctation or increased intervention risk, the choice between intervention and conservative treatment is especially important. For example, in patients with Turner syndrome, more complications may be encountered after intervention than in the normal population, and the balance may shift toward a more conservative approach.

16.3.4.4 Long-Term Outcome

Patients with CoA historically have a reduced long-term survival, mainly influenced by early interventional and late hypertensive complications. Until the 1980s patients still only had an average life expectancy of 38 years [10], and patients often died before the age of 50 due to cardiovascular causes. Nowadays patients, who have been operated successfully, using the most recent techniques, have a good medium- to long-term survival with actuarial survival of 98 % at

40, 98 % at 50, and 89 % at 60 years of age [31]. Still atherosclerotic cardiovascular disease and cerebrovascular events contribute significantly to late morbidity and mortality. An important risk factor is late repair which is associated with hypertension, but even patients with repair at young age have a 30 % 10-year prevalence of hypertension [32]. Vigilant blood pressure control is therefore indicated, also in patients with good results after repair. Recoarctation requiring reintervention and descending aortic aneurysms occur in 34 % and 18 %, respectively. The lowest occurrence is found in patients treated with an end-to-end repair [31]. Higher rates of recoarctation tend to occur in smaller patient size, in younger age at repair, and in the presence of associated transverse arch hypoplasia. Indications for reintervention are similar to those for native coarctation. Aneurysms of the ascending aorta or in the region of the aortic isthmus are the most dangerous complications because they carry the risk of life-threatening rupture. Bicuspid aortic valve, aortic wall changes, and systemic hypertension may together be responsible for aneurysmal formation of the ascending aorta. Because the incidence of aneurysm formation after surgery or balloon angioplasty appears to increase with longer follow-up periods, all patients need careful periodic surveillance. Generally, aortic aneurysms are treated surgically. Alternatively, endovascular stent grafts have been used to repair aortic aneurysms successfully without major complications.

16.3.4.5 Pregnancy

Cardiac output increases by almost 50 % during pregnancy and rises even further during labor. There are cases of aortic dissection described during pregnancy in women with CoA [33, 34], but in general pregnancy is well tolerated. There might be a mildly elevated risk of miscarriage. Some studies show an increased rate of miscarriage [35], where others show a risk that is comparable to the general population [33]. Hypertensive disorders are more frequently found. In the normal population, these hypertensive disorders of pregnancy occur in approximately 8 % of all pregnancies, whereas in CoA patients, hypertension and (pre)eclampsia probabilities are estimated in some studies to be 0.183 (SE 0.285) and 0.061 (SE 0.211), respectively [35]. Women with CoA are in principal advised to deliver vaginally [36].

16.3.4.6 Quality of Life

No specific research on the psychological function of CoA patients has been published so far, but there are studies on other types of CHD. These studies show that although patients score significantly better on most scales of subjective health being compared to normative data [37, 38], patients do show signs of reduced sexual functioning. Sexuality has received not so much attention by physicians despite a clear need for information by patients. In addition, not much information is available on sports participation in these patients. Patients often grow up in a protective environment where sports participation is discouraged, while even for complex CHD patients, participating in sports can have a positive influence on exercise capacity and subjective physical function without a clear increased risk of sudden death or cardiac arrhythmias. Topics such as contraceptives, sexuality, pregnancy, and sports participation need more attention from medical specialists and caregivers.

16.4 Associations

In this paragraph we will discuss a number of syndromes and other congenital cardiovascular defects that are seen in combination with CoA.

There is no known single causal genetic defect for CoA, but it often occurs together with several other left-sided defects such as BAV. It is seldom associated with right-sided defects. There is a myriad of genetic syndromes which are known to have a relatively frequent occurrence of CoA and genetic abnormalities occur in 6.2 % of patients with a CoA. They have however different genetic origins and therefore a single genetic cause for CoA is improbable. Almost all syndromes described below have a frequent occurrence of several congenital heart defects and therefore it seems plausible that there is a common developmental pathway. A patent arterial duct is found in almost half (43 %) of CoA patients, and also septal defects are very common (39 % ventricular defects, 20 % atrial septal defects, and 4.4 % atrioventricular septal defects). We will discuss the aortic valve separately, but also the mitral, tricuspid, and pulmonary valves are found to be abnormal in, respectively, 4.9 %, 2.4 %, and 1 % of CoA patients.

16.4.1 Bicuspid Aortic Valve

The aortic valve is normally made up of three cusps; however, in 1–2 % of the general population, abnormal cusp formation during valvulogenesis leads adjacent cusps to fail to segregate and form one single cusp. BAV can cause significant morbidity as the valve is prone to leakage or stenosis and is often accompanied by ascending aortic dilatation. Histopathological changes of the aortic media such as loss of smooth muscle and medial layer elastic fibers can be seen in the ascending aorta of BAV patients, and it has been argued that BAV and CoA are part of the same aortopathy. BAV is, as CoA, more often seen in males than in females (2:1, male/female). In 50–75% of the patients with a coarctation, also BAV is present [39]. The prevalence of CoA in BAV patients is less well studied but is approximately 7 % [40]. Aortic dilatation seems more severe in patients with both BAV and CoA than in patients with an isolated CoA [41]. The dilatation varies from patient to patient, and clear associations with age and hypertension could not be proven. A current parameter in BAV research is the cusp anatomy; different valve types are discerned [42], based on their morphological cusp phenotype, of which the type with fusion of the left and right coronary cusp is associated with CoA [7].

16.4.2 Hypoplastic Left Heart Syndrome

Hypoplastic left heart syndrome (HLHS) occurs in 0.016–0.036 % of live births and occurs more often in males [43]. It is the clinical presentation in 11 % of CoA patients. It entails severe left-sided outflow obstruction due to an abnormal development of the left-sided cardiac structures, a predominant underdevelopment of the left ventricle and aorta, and sometimes also mitral atresia or stenosis. The degree of left ventricular outflow obstruction can vary from patient to patient [43], and the right heart may also be enlarged and hypertrophic. Coarctation of the aorta in juxta position is commonly present [44–46]. HLHS is a duct-dependent lesion, and it needs a series of univentricular surgical palliations to correct the situation or heart transplantation may be considered. The coarctation of patients with HLHS is histologically similar to isolated coarctation as ductal tissue has been found at the coarctation site [47].

16.4.3 Taussig-Bing Anomaly and Transposition Complexes

In 1949 Helen Taussig and Richard Bing described the first case of what is now known as the Taussig-Bing anomaly (TBA), an uncommon form of double outlet right ventricle (DORV) in which both the aorta and pulmonary artery arise from the right ventricle [48]. The pulmonary artery overrides a subpulmonary ventricular defect. It is associated with additional aortic arch obstruction in 39–52 % of patients, substantially complicating the surgical management [49, 50]. Approximately 6.7 % of coarctation patients have this anomaly. Also a complete transposition of the great arteries and transposition complexes are found to be associated with an aortic obstruction at subaortic level or in the aortic arch [51, 52].

16.4.4 Kabuki Syndrome

This syndrome with an estimated prevalence of 1 in 32,000 received its name from the supposed resemblance of its typical facial features to makeup worn by the artists in a traditional Japanese dance drama called "Kabuki." In Kabuki syndrome, 69–91 % of patients have a congenital heart defect; most of these lesions are left-sided obstructions of which 29 % an aortic coarctation [53, 54]. It is caused by a mutation of two genes located on the short arm (or p-arm) of the X chromosome KMT2D or KDM6A (or MLL2) and inherits in an autosomal dominant fashion. In a study describing the KMDA6A knocked-down zebrafish, prominent defects in heart development were found [55].

16.4.5 Shone's Syndrome

Shone's complex or Shone's syndrome, first described in eight cases in 1963, includes a supravalvular mitral valve membrane, a "parachute mitral valve," a subaortic stenosis, and a coarctation of the aorta (CoA) [56]. In addition BAV was also present in 30–83 % of these patients [56–58]. CoA is seen in approximately 96 % of patients; however, only 63 % patients exhibit all four symptoms. It is managed surgically, where the level of involvement of the mitral valve and presence of secondary pulmonary hypertension are the main determinant of clinical outcome in these patients.

16.4.6 Myhre Syndrome

Myhre syndrome is a very rare syndrome (prevalence <1/1.000.000), caused by a heterozygous mutation in the SMAD4 gene on chromosome 18q21 [59]. A study of 32 patients describes congenital heart defects in 17 patients, including patent ductus arteriosus, aortic coarctation (12.5 %), mild-to-moderate valvular aortic stenosis (12.5 %), and membranous ventricular septal defect (3.3 %).

16.4.7 Williams-Beuren Syndrome

Williams-Beuren syndrome is caused by a deletion on chromosome 7q11.23 and occurs in approximately 1 in 10,000 live births [60]. One of the deleted genes is the ELN gene which codes for the protein elastin [61]. The syndrome was first described by Williams et al. in 1961 in four patients and then in the following year also by Beuren et al. in an additional five patients. Congenital cardiovascular defects occur in about 80 % of all patients where some form of arterial stenosis is the predominant form occurring in 40–75 % of patients [62]. It differs however from the typical juxta-ductal CoA in that its preferred location is at the sinotubular junction (supravalvular aortic stenosis) and is also often seen as an elongated hypoplastic segment [61], of which the first is the most common, occurring in approximately 75 % of the children.

16.4.8 Noonan Syndrome

Noonan syndrome (NS) occurs in approximately 1/1000 to 1/2000 live births [63], and it is one of the most common syndromic causes of congenital heart disease second only to Down syndrome [64]. It inherited in an autosomal dominant manner, although many individuals have a de novo mutation. Mutations recognized to cause the syndrome include mutations in the *PTPN11*, *SOS1*, *RAF1*, *KRAS*, *NRAS*, and *BRAF* genes. The congenital heart disease occurs in between 50 and 80 % of patients, with pulmonary valve stenosis and hypertrophic cardiomyopathy being the most common (50–60 % and 20 % of patients, respectively). However, other structural defects such as atrial septal defect, patent ductus arteriosus, and tetralogy of Fallot have also been described [64]. The left-sided outflow obstructions can occur at the valvular or supravalvular level or as classic aortic coarctation [65, 66]. CoA itself is seen in approximately 8.8 % of patients [65] and is more often seen in patients with a PTPN11 mutation [64].

16.4.9 Alagille Syndrome

Alagille syndrome (AGS) is a multisystem disorder affecting the liver, heart, eyes, face, skeleton, and other systems occurring in 1 in 70,000 newborns. Up to 70 % of patients have a mutation in the Jagged1 gene, which fulfills a function in the Notch signaling pathway. The remaining 30 % is probably also caused by a mutation in this large gene, but not yet found due to testing limitations [67]. The cardiovascular defects are predominantly of the pulmonary arteries (67 %) [68]. In a study describing 268 individuals with AGS, aortic coarctation was only found in three cases (1.1 %), still substantially higher than in the normal population.

16.4.10 The 22q11.2 Deletion Syndrome

The 22q11.2 deletion syndrome is the most common microdeletion syndrome and is known for its wide variety of signs and symptoms. It has been described under many different names of which some well-known include the Shprintzen syndrome, the DiGeorge syndrome, and the velo-cardiofacial anomaly. Its incidence is approximately 1 in 3000 persons and 75 % of patients have a form of CHD. A common 3 Mb hemizygous deletion of 22q11.2 is detected in the majority of patients. Smaller deletions within this 3 Mb region together with rare deletions outside of the region account for the other 30 % [69]. This syndrome occurs in 0.9 % of patients with a CoA. Other CHDs are tetralogy of Fallot, pulmonary stenosis, pulmonary stenosis, and septal defects.

16.4.11 Turner Syndrome

Of the aforementioned syndromes, Turner syndrome (TS) is probably the most well-known, with a prevalence of approximately 1 in 2500 live-born girls [70]. It has a broad variety of features, among which short stature, infertility, and a webbed neck. Aortic pathology is seen quite frequently in TS. Aortic dilatation and especially aortic dissection are seen more often, probably associated with BAV and CoA [1, 70]. In up to 17 % of patients, a CoA is found. The presence of CoA in TS patients is often associated with BAV (RR, 4.6) [71, 72]. More recently Ho et al. found that in 50 % of Turner patients, aortic coarctation appeared to be associated with an elongated transverse aortic arch [1]. Supposedly other abnormalities such as an aberrant right subclavian artery (8 %) and common origin of the innominate and left carotid artery (8 %) belong to the same cardiovascular phenotype [70].

16.4.12 Miscellaneous

In addition to the syndromes and associations mentioned above, there are other associations with CoA; congenital rubella syndromes are known to cause cardiac and cardiovascular disease especially pulmonary artery stenosis and patent ductus arteriosus in 50 % of patients [73]. But also aortic coarctation has been reported in these children.

References

1. Ho VB, Bakalov VK, Cooley M, Van PL, Hood MN, Burklow TR, Bondy CA (2004) Major vascular anomalies in Turner syndrome: prevalence and magnetic resonance angiographic features. Circulation 110(12):1694–1700. doi:10.1161/01.CIR.0000142290.35842.B0
2. Campbell M (1970) Natural history of coarctation of the aorta. Br Heart J 32(5):633–640
3. Verheugt CL, Uiterwaal CS, Grobbee DE, Mulder BJ (2008) Long-term prognosis of congenital heart defects: a systematic review. Int J Cardiol 131 (1):25–32. doi:S0167-5273(08)00793-6 [pii] 10.1016/j.ijcard.2008.06.023
4. Morgagni G (1760) De sedibus et causis morborum. Epist XVIII. 1760:6, vol 6. Epist XVIII
5. Abbott ME (1928) Coarctation of the aorta of the adult type: II. A statistical study and historical retrospect of 200 recorded cases with autopsy, of stenosis or obliteration of the descending arch in subjects above the age of two years. Am Heart J 3:574
6. Vergales JE, Gangemi JJ, Rhueban KS, Lim DS (2013) Coarctation of the aorta – the current state of surgical and transcatheter therapies. Curr Cardiol Rev 9(3):211–219. doi:CCR-EPUB-04-54830 [pii]
7. Warnes CA (2003) Bicuspid aortic valve and coarctation: two villains part of a diffuse problem. Heart 89(9):965–966
8. van der Linde D, Konings EE, Slager MA, Witsenburg M, Helbing WA, Takkenberg JJ, Roos-Hesselink JW (2011) Birth prevalence of congenital heart disease worldwide: a systematic

review and meta-analysis. J Am Coll Cardiol 58 (21):2241–2247. doi:S0735-1097(11)03079-8 [pii] 10.1016/j.jacc.2011.08.025
9. Toro-Salazar OH, Steinberger J, Thomas W, Rocchini AP, Carpenter B, Moller JH (2002) Long-term follow-up of patients after coarctation of the aorta repair. Am J Cardiol 89 (5):541–547. doi:S0002914901022937 [pii]
10. Cohen M, Fuster V, Steele PM, Driscoll D, McGoon DC (1989) Coarctation of the aorta. Long-term follow-up and prediction of outcome after surgical correction. Circulation 80(4):840–845
11. Brown ML, Burkhart HM, Connolly HM, Dearani JA, Cetta F, Li Z, Oliver WC, Warnes CA, Schaff HV (2013) Coarctation of the aorta: lifelong surveillance is mandatory following surgical repair. J Am Coll Cardiol 62 (11):1020–1025. doi:S0735-1097(13)02530-8 [pii] 10.1016/j.jacc.2013.06.016
12. Campbell M, Polani PE (1961) The aetiology of coarctation of the aorta. Lancet 1 (7175):463–468
13. Talner CN (1998) Report of the New England regional infant cardiac program, by Donald C. Fyler, MD, Pediatrics, 1980;65(suppl):375–461. Pediatrics 102(1 Pt 2):258–259
14. Ho SY, Anderson RH (1979) Coarctation, tubular hypoplasia, and the ductus arteriosus. Histological study of 35 specimens. Br Heart J 41(3):268–274
15. Russell GA, Berry PJ, Watterson K, Dhasmana JP, Wisheart JD (1991) Patterns of ductal tissue in coarctation of the aorta in the first three months of life. J Thorac Cardiovasc Surg 102 (4):596–601
16. Keith LM, Persaud TVN (December 19, 2011) The developing human: clinically oriented embryology 9/e. Elsevier India, pp 327–329
17. Niwa K, Perloff JK, Bhuta SM, Laks H, Drinkwater DC, Child JS, Miner PD (2001) Structural abnormalities of great arterial walls in congenital heart disease: light and electron microscopic analyses. Circulation 103(3):393–400
18. Isner JM, Donaldson RF, Fulton D, Bhan I, Payne DD, Cleveland RJ (1987) Cystic medial necrosis in coarctation of the aorta: a potential factor contributing to adverse consequences observed after percutaneous balloon angioplasty of coarctation sites. Circulation 75 (4):689–695
19. Nistri S, Sorbo MD, Marin M, Palisi M, Scognamiglio R, Thiene G (1999) Aortic root dilatation in young men with normally functioning bicuspid aortic valves. Heart 82(1):19–22
20. Bauer M, Pasic M, Meyer R, Goetze N, Bauer U, Siniawski H, Hetzer R (2002) Morphometric analysis of aortic media in patients with bicuspid and tricuspid aortic valve. Ann Thorac Surg 74(1):58–62
21. Bonderman D, Gharehbaghi-Schnell E, Wollenek G, Maurer G, Baumgartner H, Lang IM (1999) Mechanisms underlying aortic dilatation in congenital aortic valve malformation. Circulation 99(16):2138–2143
22. Vogt M, Kuhn A, Baumgartner D, Baumgartner C, Busch R, Kostolny M, Hess J (2005) Impaired elastic properties of the ascending aorta in newborns before and early after successful coarctation repair – proof of a systemic vascular disease of the prestenotic arteries? Circulation 111(24):3269–3273. doi:10.1161/Circulationaha.104.529792
23. Oliver JM, Gallego P, Gonzalez A, Aroca A, Bret M, Mesa JM (2004) Risk factors for aortic complications in adults with coarctation of the aorta. J Am Coll Cardiol 44 (8):1641–1647. doi:S0735-1097(04)01536-0 [pii] 10.1016/j.jacc.2004.07.037
24. Baumgartner H, Bonhoeffer P, De Groot NM, de Haan F, Deanfield JE, Galie N, Gatzoulis MA, Gohlke-Baerwolf C, Kaemmerer H, Kilner P, Meijboom F, Mulder BJ, Oechslin E, Oliver JM, Serraf A, Szatmari A, Thaulow E, Vouhe PR, Walma E, Task Force on the Management of Grown-up Congenital Heart Disease of the European Society of C, Association for European Paediatric C, Guidelines ESCCfP (2010) ESC Guidelines for the management of grown-up congenital heart disease (new version 2010). Eur Heart J 31 (23):2915–2957. doi:ehq249 [pii] 10.1093/eurheartj/ehq249
25. Novitzky D, Sanchez HE, Human D, Barnard CN (1984) The significance of femoral pulses in coarctation of the aorta. S Afr Med J 65(19):755–757

26. Jurcut R, Daraban AM, Lorber A, Deleanu D, Amzulescu MS, Zara C, Popescu BA, Ginghina C (2011) Coarctation of the aorta in adults: what is the best treatment? Case report and literature review. J Med Life 4(2):189–195
27. Forbes TJ, Kim DW, Du W, Turner DR, Holzer R, Amin Z, Hijazi Z, Ghasemi A, Rome JJ, Nykanen D, Zahn E, Cowley C, Hoyer M, Waight D, Gruenstein D, Javois A, Foerster S, Kreutzer J, Sullivan N, Khan A, Owada C, Hagler D, Lim S, Canter J, Zellers T, Investigators C (2011) Comparison of surgical, stent, and balloon angioplasty treatment of native coarctation of the aorta: an observational study by the CCISC (Congenital Cardiovascular Interventional Study Consortium). J Am Coll Cardiol 58 (25):2664–2674. doi:S0735-1097(11)03440-1 [pii] 10.1016/j.jacc.2011.08.053
28. Padua LM, Garcia LC, Rubira CJ, de Oliveira Carvalho PE (2012) Stent placement versus surgery for coarctation of the thoracic aorta. Cochrane Database Syst Rev 5:CD008204. doi:10.1002/14651858.CD008204.pub2
29. Moltzer E, Mattace Raso FU, Karamermer Y, Boersma E, Webb GD, Simoons ML, Danser AH, van den Meiracker AH, Roos-Hesselink JW (2010) Comparison of Candesartan versus Metoprolol for treatment of systemic hypertension after repaired aortic coarctation. Am J Cardiol 105(2):217–222 . doi:10.1016/j.amjcard.2009.08.674S0002-9149(09)02327-3 [pii]
30. Schoolwerth AC, Sica DA, Ballermann BJ, Wilcox CS, Council on the Kidney in Cardiovascular D, the Council for High Blood Pressure Research of the American Heart A (2001) Renal considerations in angiotensin converting enzyme inhibitor therapy: a statement for healthcare professionals from the Council on the Kidney in Cardiovascular Disease and the Council for High Blood Pressure Research of the American Heart Association. Circulation 104 (16):1985–1991
31. Choudhary P, Canniffe C, Jackson DJ, Tanous D, Walsh K, Celermajer DS (2015) Late outcomes in adults with coarctation of the aorta. Heart 101 (15):1190–1195. doi:heartjnl-2014-307035 [pii] 10.1136/heartjnl-2014-307035
32. Bhatt AB, Defaria Yeh D (2015) Long-term outcomes in coarctation of the aorta: an evolving story of success and new challenges. Heart 101 (15):1173–1175. doi:heartjnl-2015-307641 [pii] 10.1136/heartjnl-2015-307641
33. Beauchesne LM, Connolly HM, Ammash NM, Warnes CA (2001) Coarctation of the aorta: outcome of pregnancy. J Am Coll Cardiol 38(6):1728–1733. doi:S0735-1097(01)01617-5 [pii]
34. Plunkett MD, Bond LM, Geiss DM (2000) Staged repair of acute type I aortic dissection and coarctation in pregnancy. Ann Thorac Surg 69(6):1945–1947. doi:S0003-4975(00)01278-9 [pii]
35. Vriend JW, Drenthen W, Pieper PG, Roos-Hesselink JW, Zwinderman AH, van Veldhuisen DJ, Mulder BJ (2005) Outcome of pregnancy in patients after repair of aortic coarctation. Eur Heart J 26 (20):2173–2178. doi:ehi338 [pii] 10.1093/eurheartj/ehi338
36. Krieger EV, Landzberg MJ, Economy KE, Webb GD, Opotowsky AR (2011) Comparison of risk of hypertensive complications of pregnancy among women with versus without coarctation of the aorta. Am J Cardiol 107 (10):1529–1534. doi:S0002-9149(11)00345-6 [pii] 10. 1016/j.amjcard.2011.01.033
37. Menting ME, Cuypers JA, Opic P, Utens EM, Witsenburg M, van den Bosch AE, van Domburg RT, Meijboom FJ, Boersma E, Bogers AJ, Roos-Hesselink JW (2015) The unnatural history of the ventricular septal defect: outcome up to 40 years after surgical closure. J Am Coll Cardiol 65 (18):1941–1951. doi:S0735-1097(15)00904-3 [pii] 10.1016/j.jacc.2015.02.055
38. Cuypers JA, Opic P, Menting ME, Utens EM, Witsenburg M, Helbing WA, van den Bosch AE, Ouhlous M, van Domburg RT, Meijboom FJ, Bogers AJ, Roos-Hesselink JW (2013) The unnatural history of an atrial septal defect: longitudinal 35 year follow up after surgical closure at young age. Heart 99 (18):1346–1352. doi:heartjnl-2013-304225 [pii] 10.1136/heartjnl-2013-304225
39. Roos-Hesselink JW, Scholzel BE, Heijdra RJ, Spitaels SE, Meijboom FJ, Boersma E, Bogers AJ, Simoons ML (2003) Aortic valve and aortic arch pathology after coarctation repair. Heart 89(9):1074–1077

40. Schaefer BM, Lewin MB, Stout KK, Gill E, Prueitt A, Byers PH, Otto CM (2008) The bicuspid aortic valve: an integrated phenotypic classification of leaflet morphology and aortic root shape. Heart 94 (12):1634–1638. doi:hrt.2007.132092 [pii] 10.1136/hrt.2007.132092
41. Oliver JM, Alonso-Gonzalez R, Gonzalez AE, Gallego P, Sanchez-Recalde A, Cuesta E, Aroca A, Lopez-Sendon JL (2009) Risk of aortic root or ascending aorta complications in patients with bicuspid aortic valve with and without coarctation of the aorta. Am J Cardiol 104 (7):1001–1006. doi:S0002-9149(09)01125-4 [pii] 10.1016/j.amjcard.2009.05.045
42. Sievers HH, Schmidtke C (2007) A classification system for the bicuspid aortic valve from 304 surgical specimens. J Thorac Cardiovasc Surg 133 (5):1226–1233. doi:S0022-5223(07) 00237-1 [pii] 10.1016/j.jtcvs.2007.01.039
43. Morris CD, Outcalt J, Menashe VD (1990) Hypoplastic left heart syndrome: natural history in a geographically defined population. Pediatrics 85(6):977–983
44. Brenner JI, Berg KA, Schneider DS, Clark EB, Boughman JA (1989) Cardiac malformations in relatives of infants with hypoplastic left-heart syndrome. Am J Dis Child 143 (12):1492–1494
45. Roberts WC, Morrow AG, Braunwald E (1962) Complete interruption of the aortic arch. Circulation 26:39–59
46. Hinton RB, Jr., Martin LJ, Tabangin ME, Mazwi ML, Cripe LH, Benson DW (2007) Hypoplastic left heart syndrome is heritable. J Am Coll Cardiol 50 (16):1590–1595. doi:S0735-1097 (07)02390-X [pii] 10.1016/j.jacc.2007.07.021
47. Machii M, Becker AE (1995) Nature of coarctation in hypoplastic left heart syndrome. Ann Thorac Surg 59(6):1491–1494. doi:000349759500154D [pii]
48. Taussig HB, Bing RJ (1949) Complete transposition of the aorta and a levoposition of the pulmonary artery; clinical, physiological, and pathological findings. Am Heart J 37 (4):551–559
49. Sadow SH, Synhorst DP, Pappas G (1985) Taussig-Bing anomaly and coarctation of the aorta in infancy: surgical options. Pediatr Cardiol 6(2):83–89. doi:10.1007/BF02282743
50. Konstantinov IE (2009) Taussig-Bing anomaly: from original description to the current era. Tex Heart Inst J 36(6):580–585
51. Tchervenkov CI, Korkola SJ (2001) Transposition complexes with systemic obstruction. Semin Thorac Cardiovasc Surg Pediatr Card Surg Annu 4:71–82. doi:S1092912601000060 [pii]
52. Vogel M, Freedom RM, Smallhorn JF, Williams WG, Trusler GA, Rowe RD (1984) Complete transposition of the great arteries and coarctation of the aorta. Am J Cardiol 53(11):1627–1632
53. Yuan SM (2013) Congenital heart defects in Kabuki syndrome. Cardiol J 20(2):121–124. doi: VM/OJS/J/33959 [pii] 10.5603/CJ.2013.0023
54. Yoon JK, Ahn KJ, Kwon BS, Kim GB, Bae EJ, Noh CI, Ko JM (2015) The strong association of left-side heart anomalies with Kabuki syndrome. Korean J Pediatr 58(7):256–262. doi:10.3345/kjp.2015.58.7.256
55. Van Laarhoven PM, Neitzel LR, Quintana AM, Geiger EA, Zackai EH, Clouthier DE, Artinger KB, Ming JE, Shaikh TH (2015) Kabuki syndrome genes KMT2D and KDM6A: functional analyses demonstrate critical roles in craniofacial, heart and brain development. Hum Mol Genet 24 (15):4443–4453. doi:ddv180 [pii] 10.1093/hmg/ddv180
56. Shone JD, Sellers RD, Anderson RC, Adams P Jr, Lillehei CW, Edwards JE (1963) The developmental complex of "parachute mitral valve," supravalvular ring of left atrium, subaortic stenosis, and coarctation of aorta. Am J Cardiol 11:714–725
57. Ma XJ, Huang GY, Liang XC, Liu XQ, Jia B (2011) Atypical Shone's complex diagnosed by echocardiography. Pediatr Cardiol 32(4):442–448. doi:10.1007/s00246-011-9886-y
58. Grimaldi A, Vermi AC, Maisano F, Sacco F, Castiglioni A, Zangrillo A, Alfieri O (2011) Echocardiographic patterns of incomplete Shone's syndrome in adults. J Heart Valve Dis 20 (5):552–556
59. Michot C, Le Goff C, Mahaut C, Afenjar A, Brooks AS, Campeau PM, Destree A, Di Rocco M, Donnai D, Hennekam R, Heron D, Jacquemont S, Kannu P, Lin AE, Manouvrier-

Hanu S, Mansour S, Marlin S, McGowan R, Murphy H, Raas-Rothschild A, Rio M, Simon M, Stolte-Dijkstra I, Stone JR, Sznajer Y, Tolmie J, Touraine R, van den Ende J, Van der Aa N, van Essen T, Verloes A, Munnich A, Cormier-Daire V (2014) Myhre and LAPS syndromes: clinical and molecular review of 32 patients. Eur J Hum Genet 22 (11):1272–1277. doi: ejhg2013288 [pii] 10.1038/ejhg.2013.288

60. Stromme P, Bjornstad PG, Ramstad K (2002) Prevalence estimation of Williams syndrome. J Child Neurol 17(4):269–271
61. Pober BR (2010) Williams-Beuren syndrome. N Engl J Med 362 (3):239–252. doi:362/3/239 [pii] 10.1056/NEJMra0903074
62. Collins RT, 2nd (2013) Cardiovascular disease in Williams syndrome. Circulation 127 (21):2125–2134. doi:127/21/2125 [pii] 10.1161/CIRCULATIONAHA.112.000064
63. Noonan JA (1968) Hypertelorism with Turner phenotype. A new syndrome with associated congenital heart disease. Am J Dis Child 116(4):373–380
64. Roberts AE, Allanson JE, Tartaglia M, Gelb BD (2013) Noonan syndrome. Lancet 381 (9863):333–342. doi:S0140-6736(12)61023-X [pii] 10.1016/S0140-6736(12)61023-X
65. Marino B, Digilio MC, Toscano A, Giannotti A, Dallapiccola B (1999) Congenital heart diseases in children with Noonan syndrome: an expanded cardiac spectrum with high prevalence of atrioventricular canal. J Pediatr 135(6):703–706. doi:S0022-3476(99)70088-0 [pii]
66. Burch M, Sharland M, Shinebourne E, Smith G, Patton M, McKenna W (1993) Cardiologic abnormalities in Noonan syndrome: phenotypic diagnosis and echocardiographic assessment of 118 patients. J Am Coll Cardiol 22 (4):1189–1192. doi:0735-1097(93)90436-5 [pii]
67. Kamath BM, Spinner NB, Emerick KM, Chudley AE, Booth C, Piccoli DA, Krantz ID (2004) Vascular anomalies in Alagille syndrome: a significant cause of morbidity and mortality. Circulation 109 (11):1354–1358. doi:10.1161/01.CIR.0000121361.01862.A4 01.CIR.0000121361.01862.A4 [pii]
68. Emerick KM, Rand EB, Goldmuntz E, Krantz ID, Spinner NB, Piccoli DA (1999) Features of Alagille syndrome in 92 patients: frequency and relation to prognosis. Hepatology 29 (3):822–829. doi:S0270913999001251 [pii] 10.1002/hep.510290331
69. Shaikh TH, Kurahashi H, Saitta SC, O'Hare AM, Hu P, Roe BA, Driscoll DA, McDonald-McGinn DM, Zackai EH, Budarf ML, Emanuel BS (2000) Chromosome 22-specific low copy repeats and the 22q11.2 deletion syndrome: genomic organization and deletion endpoint analysis. Hum Mol Genet 9(4):489–501. doi:ddd064 [pii]
70. Mortensen KH, Andersen NH, Gravholt CH (2012) Cardiovascular phenotype in Turner syndrome – integrating cardiology, genetics, and endocrinology. Endocr Rev 33 (5):677–714. doi:er.2011-1059 [pii] 10.1210/er.2011-1059
71. Sachdev V, Matura LA, Sidenko S, Ho VB, Arai AE, Rosing DR, Bondy CA (2008) Aortic valve disease in Turner syndrome. J Am Coll Cardiol 51 (19):1904–1909. doi:S0735-1097(08)00716-X [pii] 10.1016/j.jacc.2008.02.035
72. Mortensen KH, Hjerrild BE, Andersen NH, Sorensen KE, Horlyck A, Pedersen EM, Lundorf E, Christiansen JS, Gravholt CH (2010) Abnormalities of the major intrathoracic arteries in Turner syndrome as revealed by magnetic resonance imaging. Cardiol Young 20 (2):191–200. doi:S1047951110000041 [pii] 10.1017/S1047951110000041
73. Oster ME, Riehle-Colarusso T, Correa A (2010) An update on cardiovascular malformations in congenital rubella syndrome. Birth Defects Res A Clin Mol Teratol 88(1):1–8. doi:10.1002/bdra.20621

Chapter 17
Tetralogy of Fallot and Pulmonary Atresia with Ventricular Septal Defect

Koichiro Niwa

Abstract Aortic dilatation and regurgitation in unrepaired tetralogy of Fallot imposes volume overload on both ventricles. A significant subset of adults late after repair of tetralogy of Fallot exhibits progressive aortic root dilatation, which may lead to aortic regurgitation and predispose to dissection and rupture that can be fatal, and necessitating aortic valve and aortic root surgery. The aortic dilatation relates medial abnormalities coupled with previous long-standing volume overload of the ascending aorta. Risk factors for aortic dilatation and regurgitation in tetralogy of Fallot relate to specific hemodynamic abnormalities, such as pulmonary atresia, right aortic arch, and a history of an aortopulmonary shunt, and patient demographics such as male sex and the association of chromosome 22q11 deletion. There is no current consensus on beta-blocker or angiotensin II receptor blocker (ARB) administration for limiting progressive dilatation of the aortic root in patients with repaired tetralogy of Fallot. Aortic root surgery should be considered for these patients and address aortic regurgitation and/or prevent the risk of aortic dissection. Thus, in tetralogy of Fallot meticulous follow-up of the aortic root after repair is recommended.

Keywords Aortic dilatation • Tetralogy of Fallot • Pulmonary atresia with ventricular septal defect • Aortic dissection • Cystic medial necrosis • Aortic regurgitation

17.1 Introduction

Aortic root dilatation is known to be a feature of tetralogy of Fallot (TOF). Increased aortic flow attributable to right-to-left shunting prior to repair is thought to be the underlying pathogenic mechanism [1–3]. Aortic root dilatation is greater in patients with extreme TOF or in other words pulmonary atresia with ventricular septal defect particularly in those who have not undergone repair (Fig. 17.1)

K. Niwa, M.D., Ph.D., FACC, FAHA, FJCC (✉)
Cardiovascular Center, St Luke's International Hospital, 9-1 Akashi-cho, Tokyo 104-8560, Japan
e-mail: koniwa@luke.ac.jp; kniwa@aol.com

K. Niwa, H. Kaemmerer (eds.), *Aortopathy*, DOI 10.1007/978-4-431-56071-5_17

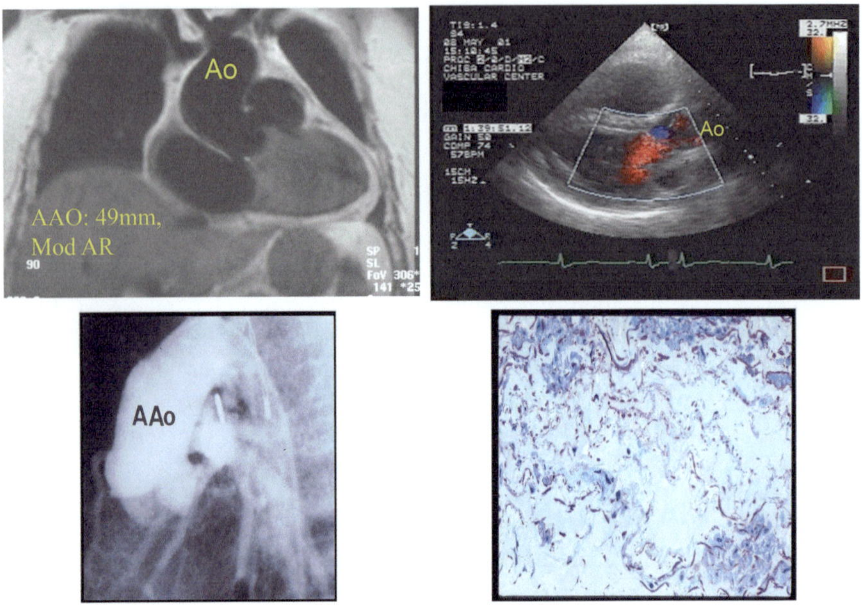

Fig. 17.1 *Upper panel*: 35-year-old male with repaired tetralogy of Fallot (MRI and Echo). *Lower Panel:* Infant (6 months old) with ventricular septal defect with pulmonary atresia angiography and necropsy specimen: grade 3 histologic grading scores

[1, 3]. Aortic root dilatation with high elasticity of aortic wall may lead to aortic regurgitation, which in turn may necessitate surgery. Aortic valve or aortic root replacement was required in a relatively small number of adult patients with repaired TOF in a single-center report [4]. In Japanese multicenter study of 4010 adults with repaired TOF, 24 patients (0.6 %) of them experienced aortic root surgery or valve replacement [5] (Fig. 17.2). Increased aortic flow and previous trauma to the aortic root, during initial TOF repair, as well as intrinsic medial abnormality of aortic wall are thought to be responsible for aortic regurgitation in this surgical series. Furthermore, aortic root dilatation may predispose to aortic dissection and rupture, even if the number of dissection of the aorta is still small (Fig. 17.3).

A subset of adult patients with TOF exhibits ongoing dilatation of the aortic root late after repair, which may lead to aortic regurgitation necessitating aortic valve and root surgery. This aortic root dilatation relates to previous long-standing volume overload of the aorta and possibly to intrinsic properties of the aortic root itself.

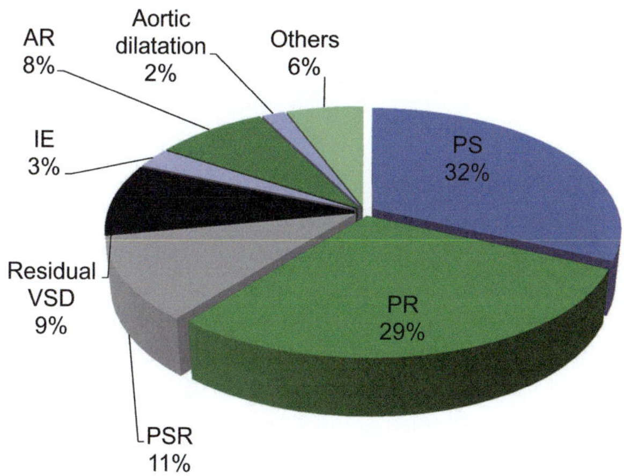

Fig. 17.2 Reason for reoperation in repaired TOF patients > 15 years. N = 236/4010 (5.9 %). *PS* pulmonary stenosis, *PR* pulmonary regurgitation, *PSR* both PS and PR, *VSD* ventricular septal defect, *IE* infective endocarditis, *AR* aortic regurgitation

	Sex Age (y)	Diagnosis	Ao Size (mm)	AR	Aorta	Journal
Kim WH	M,23	TOF	70	severe	Dissection	IJC 2005
Wijesekera VA	M, 60	TOF	55	severe	Dissection	IJC 2014
Rathi VK	M, 36	TOF	93x83	ND	Dissection	IJC 2005
Konstantinov IE	M, 18	TOF chr 22q11 del	60X70	mild	Dissection	JTCS 2010
Dearani JA	M, 26	VSD PA	ND	ND	Dissection	SEM TCSPCSA 2009

Fig. 17.3 Case reports of TOF (tetralogy of Fallot) and aortic dissection [5]. *Ao* aorta, *AR* aortic regurgitation, *ND* not done

17.2 Aortic Root Dilatation in Unrepaired Tetralogy of Fallot

Aortic root dilatation is a well-known feature of unrepaired TOF and is greatest in patients with pulmonary atresia with ventricular septal defect. A medial abnormality coupled with increased aortic flow attributable to the right-to-left shunting is thought to be the pathogenic mechanisms for this dilatation [6, 7]. Aortic regurgitation in TOF imposes volume overload on both ventricles, but more importantly on the right ventricle that also confronts systemic afterload [7]. Aortic root dilatation may lead to aortic regurgitation, which may necessitate surgery [7, 8].

17.3 Aortic Root Dilatation and Aortic Regurgitation, Ventricular Performance in Repaired Tetralogy of Fallot

Mild aortic regurgitation is reported in 15–18 % of the patients with repaired TOF [6]. Aortic valve or aortic root replacement is required in a small percentage of these patients [8]. However, remarkable aortic root dilatation was reported with the ratio of observed/expected aortic root size by standard nomogram N = 1.5 in 15 % of adults with repaired TOF (TOF with dilated aorta) (Fig. 17.4) [7]. These patients had special characteristics and manifestation compared with those with < 1.5 of observed/expected aortic root size (those without dilated aorta) (Figs. 17.5, 17.6, 17.7, and 17.8) [7], such as a longer shunt-to-repair interval with a higher incidence of pulmonary atresia, right aortic arch, moderate to severe aortic regurgitation, aortic valve replacement, and increased left ventricular end-diastolic dimensions. In repaired TOF with aortic dilatation study, approximately 15 % of adult patients with repaired TOF had dilated aortic root. Observed to expected aortic root size was 1.7 ± 0.2 in repaired TOF patients with dilated aorta and 1.2 ± 0.2 in those without

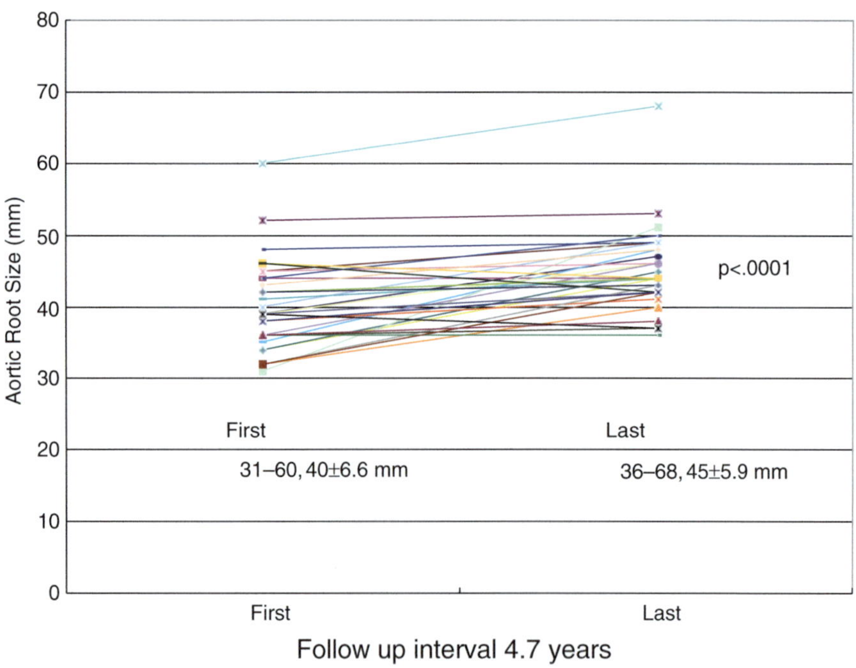

Fig. 17.4 Absolute aortic root size in 32 adult patients with repaired TOF and dilated aortic roots (dilators, 32/216 (15 %) patients with aortic root: > 40 mm). Range and mean value of aortic root size was 31–60 (40 ± 6.6) mm at the first and 36–68 (45 ± 5.9) mm at the last echo study, P < .0001. Mean time interval between the first and last echocardiogram was 4.9 ± 2.9 years

Fig. 17.5 Patient characteristics in repaired TOF with aortic dilatation (dilators vs. non-dilators)

	Dilators (n=32)	Non-Dilators (n=54)	p Value
Sex (Male : Female)	24 : 8	30 : 24	**.012**
Age (years)	36 ± 8.0 (23-52)	37 ± 9.1 (23-60)	.49
Pulmonary atresia	6 (19%)	0	< **.0001**
Right aortic arch	16 (50%)	14 (26%)	**.031**
Absent pulmonary valve	3 (9%)	0	**.011**
Blood pressure > 140/90	1 (3%)	0	.12
Cardiothoracic ratio (%)	59 ± 5.3 (48-69)	54 ± 5.9 (41-67)	**.024**

Fig. 17.6 Operative history of repaired TOF with aortic dilatation (dilators vs. non-dilators). *AVR* aortic valve replacement, *PA* pulmonary atresia, *VSD* ventricular septal defect

	Dilators (n=32)	Non-Dilators (n=54)	p Value
Age at repair (years)	14 ± 8.2 (5-37)	14 ± 9.2 (3-49)	.61
Follow after repair (years)	22 ± 7.1 (4-33)	24 ± 7.4 (4-36)	.58
Shunt-repair interval (years)	12 ± 8.3 (3-34)	8 ± 6.1 (2-28)	**.048**
AVR and arch repair	2 (6%)	0	**.023**
Aortopulmonary shunt	19	29	.48
Transannular patch	18 (56%)	26 (48%)	.88
Conduit repair (for PA)	6 (19%)	0	< **.0001**
Residual VSD	3 (9%)	2 (4%)	.13

Fig. 17.7 Aortic root size by echo in repaired TOF with aortic dilatation (dilators vs. non-dilators). *AoRo* aortic root

	Dilators (n=32)	Non-Dilators (n=54)	p Value
AoRo size (mm) last	45 ± 5.9 (36-68)	34 ± 4.6 (27-42)	< **.0001**
AoRo observed/expected size last	1.7 ± 0.2 (1.5-2.7)	1.2 ± 0.1 (1-1.4)	< **.0001**
Indexed AoRo size (cm/m^2) last	2.5 ± 0.5 (2.1-4.9)	1.8 ± 0.2 (1.3-2.0)	< **.0001**
AoRo rate of change (mm/year)	1.7 ± 3.8 (-2.0-10)	0.03 ± 1.6 (-2.0-3.5)	**.0011**
Indexed AoRo rate of change (mm/m^2/year)	0.08 ± 0.14 (-0.1-0.6)	0.01 ± 0.06 (-0.2-0.2)	< **.0001**

(Fig. 17.7). Aortic root size was larger than in healthy controls [9] even in those without dilated aorta. Aortic root size markedly increased late after TOF repair in those with a dilated aorta. This dramatic change was far beyond any change expected in healthy controls [9, 10] attributable to increased age. According to aortic dilatation report [7], the cardiothoracic ratio in the patients with dilated aorta was greater than those without. Enlarged left ventricular size was also observed by echocardiography in the patients with dilated aorta. Left ventricular enlargement in adult with repaired TOF is thought to be attributable to previous long-standing

Fig. 17.8 Cardiac function by echo in repaired TOF with aortic dilatation (dilators vs. non-dilators). *AR* aortic regurgitation, *LVEDD* left ventricular end-diastolic dimension, *LVEF* left ventricular ejection fraction, *TR* tricuspid regurgitation, *PR* pulmonary regurgitation, *RVP*/*LVP* ratio of right ventricular/left ventricular pressure

	Dilators (n=32)	Non-Dilators (n=54)	p Value
AR: moderate to severe	4 (13%)	0	**.0068**
LVEDD (mm)	49 ± 6.6 (34-61)	45 ± 5.0 (34-56)	**.0021**
LVEF (%)	54 ± 11 (35-76)	54 ± 12 (23-78)	.38
TR: moderate to severe	9 (28%)	12 (22%)	.52
PR: moderate to severe	11 (34%)	25 (46%)	.89
RV enlargement: moderate to severe	11 (34%)	18 (33%)	.69
RVP/LVP>0.5	4 (13%)	6 (11%)	.51

left-to-right shunts leading to volume overload. There was no significant difference in left ventricular ejection fraction between those with dilated aorta and those without (Fig. 17.8). Furthermore, there was no relationship between left ventricular size and severity of aortic regurgitation (AR) in patients with a dilated aortic root. It suggests that left ventricular enlargement in an adult cohort of patients with repaired TOF and, in part, a dilated aortic root may be attributable to previous long-standing left-to-right arterial shunts (aortopulmonary shunting) leading to volume overload and not attributable to a direct effect of AR [6].

17.4 Potential Factors Relating to Late Aortic Root Dilatation in TOF

Risk factors for aortic dilatation and AR in TOF have been analyzed by focusing on hemodynamic abnormalities and patient demographics. Severe cyanosis, severe right ventricular outflow tract obstruction, older age at repair, a larger aortic size at the time of repair, and a history of an aortopulmonary shunt parameters related to long-standing volume overload of the aortic root were the reported risk factors [7]. Right aortic arch, male sex, and the association of chromosome 22q11 deletion were also reported to be risk factors [7, 11]. Tetralogy patients with a right aortic arch tend to have a higher incidence of severe right ventricular outflow obstruction [12]. Males have a lower aortic wall compliance [13]. Currently, repair of TOF is routinely performed during the first year of life in most institutions, negating the need for palliative arterial shunts. Early repair dramatically reduces the period of volume overload of the aortic root and may have a beneficial long-term effect by limiting aortic root dilatation. There was a relation between male sex, pulmonary atresia, right aortic arch, longer time interval from palliation to repair, and progressive aortic root dilatation. In contrast, there was no difference in age at repair or length of follow-up from repair between TOF with dilated aorta and those without. Progressive right ventricular outflow tract obstruction in unrepaired TOF, with the extreme form being pulmonary atresia, increases right-to-left shunt through the ventricular septal defect and in turn the volume overload on the aortic root. In addition, left-to-right shunting attributable to palliative arterial shunts had a significant volume overload on the aortic root and the left ventricle [14], whereas left ventricular ejection fraction remained unchanged. Long-standing volume overload of the aortic root may contribute to aortic root dilatation [6, 15].

There is no gender predominance among patients with TOF [13]. In contrast, there was a clear male predominance among patients with dilated aortic root [7] even after indexing for body surface area and adapting for age [9]. Aortic root size in healthy men is significantly greater than that of healthy women [9, 10]. This was also the case in repaired TOF patients. Aortic elasticity and distensibility are known to decline with age; these changes occur earlier and are accelerated among men [13]. This may also be applicable to TOF patients and may explain in part the male predominance among those with dilated aorta.

Right aortic arch and/or absent pulmonary valve were more frequently observed among those with dilated aorta. Right aortic arch has been reported in 25 % of patients with TOF and is more common in patients with pulmonary atresia with ventricular septal defect [12]. Furthermore, right aortic arch, pulmonary atresia, or absent pulmonary valve syndrome are common morphologic features among TOF patients with 22q11 deletion [16, 17]. This high incidence of right aortic arch (50 %) and pulmonary atresia (19 %) (Fig. 17.5) in patients with marked aortic root dilatation and the relatively common coexistence of absent pulmonary valve syndrome may suggest a possible link between aortic root dilatation and chromosome 22 q11 deletion [18].

17.5 Aortic Dissection in Repaired Tetralogy of Fallot

Two cases of aortic root dissection in repaired TOF were reported initially from two institutions [19, 20]. The patients were male with an aortic root size of 70.5 mm and 93 × 83 mm, respectively. These are the first reports of aortic dissection in TOF and are important because aortic root dilatation and AR predispose to aortic dissection or rupture that can be fatal, even the number is small. Following these reports of dissection, there are three other reports of dissection in repaired TOF with the aortic root sizes of 55–70 mm [21–23], (Fig. 17.3). Including the other reports on dissection in TOF, minimal aortic root size in TOF patients with dissection was 55 mm (Fig. 17.3).

Because aortic valve or aortic root replacement is occasionally required in repaired TOF [5, 7, 8, 15], meticulous follow-up of the aortic root after repair and timely surgery in patients with aortic root dilatation are recommended.

17.6 Cause of Aortic Dilatation

Independent variables that alter the structure of ascending aortic media include Marfan syndrome, annuloaortic ectasia or Turner syndrome, systemic hypertension [24], aging [25], pregnancy [26], and others (Fig. 17.9). In patients with systemic hypertension, abnormalities of aortic medial elastin and collagen are prevalent [24]. With advancing age, layers of parallel aortic elastic fibers fragment, smooth muscle decreases especially in the thoracic aorta [25]. In pregnancy, gestational changes in ascending aortic media are characterized by elastic fiber fragmentation and hypertrophy/hyperplasia of smooth muscle cells [26]. Marfan syndrome is characterized by a defect in the chromosome 15 gene that codes for fibrillin-1 [27], in the absence of which elastin is more readily degraded by metalloproteinase [28]. Apoptosis reportedly plays a pathogenetic role in the medial abnormalities of abdominal aortic aneurysm [29, 30]. Deletion of transforming growth factor-β (TGF-β) receptor has a relation with aortic dilatation [31]. The genetic fault in Marfan syndrome apparently impairs aortic medial elastic fibers more extensively than impairment in CHD, and the incidence of ascending aortic dilatation, dissection, or rapture is higher, and the degree of aortic root medial lesions is greater in former than the latter [1]·

So-called cystic medial necrosis of the aortic root has commonly been found in Marfan syndrome, bicuspid aortic valve, and coarctation of the aorta [1]. Patients with a dilated aortic root in TOF share similar histological changes of the aortic root, suggestive of cystic medial necrosis indistinguishable from the aortic root in patients with Marfan syndrome [1]. Higher histologic grading scores in TOF patients are found even in infants, which suggests the intrinsic abnormality has crucial role for this dilatation [32]. Evidence for the role of aortic overflow over time in TOF includes the associations of higher age at operation, pulmonary atresia versus pulmonary stenosis, and longer presence of surgical aortopulmonary shunting with aortic dilation [7, 33]. There is a 12 % increase in mean aortic diameter after surgical aortopulmonary shunting [33].

Fig. 17.9 Variables alter structure of ascending aortic media. *TGF* transforming growth factor

1, Systemic hypertension.
2, Aging.
3, Pregnancy.
4, Chromosome: Marfan, Turner, Noonan, Chromosome 22q11.2 deletion.
5, Gene: Fibrillin-1 defect (15q21.1).
6, Deletion of TGF-β1 receptor, Defective ALK5 signaling in the neural crest.
7, Medial smooth muscle cell apoptosis.
8, Metallo-proteinase and elastin.
9, Hemodynamic abnormality (increased aortic flow).
10, Intrinsic abnormality of aortic wall in CHD (cystic medial necrosis).

Furthermore, whether aortic root dilatation is the result of long-standing volume overload of the aortic root or attributable to intrinsic aortic root abnormalities, or more likely both, needs to be additionally investigated.

17.7 Aortic Regurgitation

AR with a dilated aortic root is common in unrepaired or repaired pulmonary atresia with ventricular septal defect [15, 21, 34]. In TOF with pulmonary stenosis, however, when other causes of AR such as infective endocarditis [35], surgical damage of the valve [6, 21], and bicuspid aortic valve [1, 35] are excluded, significant AR is relatively uncommon [6, 36].

AR in unrepaired TOF patients may be due to annular dilation, weaker support of the right coronary cusp by the deficient outflow septum, and cusp prolapse [37]. Only in a very small number of patients can surgical trauma potentiate AR. Frequency and degree of AR can be higher in case of late TOF repair [33].

It has been reported that 15–18 % patients with repaired TOF had mild AR, and the cause of AR has been suggested to be aortic root dilatation [37]. Dodds et al. [8] reported 16 patients with repaired TOF, aortic root dilatation, and AR who underwent aortic valve replacement, including four patients with aortic root replacement. Eleven of these 16 patients developed progressive AR despite an uncomplicated repair and follow-up. Two of them had TOF with pulmonary stenosis, and the remainder had pulmonary atresia with ventricular septal defect. The authors speculated that AR might have been attributable to progressive dilatation of the aortic root after repair. In the aortic root study [7], mean aortic root size in the four patients with significant AR – all form those with dilated aorta – was significantly larger compared with 28 patients without dilated aorta. Of note, only one of these four patients had pulmonary atresia with ventricular septal defect, the remaining had TOF with pulmonary stenosis. In Japanese recent study, 20/236 reoperations (8 %) in repaired TOF were due to AR [5] (Fig. 17.1). Thus, possibly progressive aortic root dilatation is the major cause of AR after repair of TOF. Furthermore, AR secondary to aortic root dilatation can occur both in patients with repaired TOF and pulmonary stenosis or repaired pulmonary atresia with ventricular septal defect [37].

17.8 New Clinical Entity "Aortopathy" in TOF

Chong WY [38] found that in 67 children with 8.3 years after TOF repair, aortic dilation (z-score > 2) was observed in 88 %, 87 %, 61 %, and 63 % at the annulus, sinus of Valsalva, sinotubular junction, and ascending aorta, respectively. Significantly increased stiffness, reduced strain, and distensibility of the aorta are observed in those with dilated aorta.

Senzaki H [39] reported they observed an abnormal ventriculoarterial coupling (decreased aortic stiffness) in repaired TOF. They compared arterial function between 38 repaired TOF and 55 controls and found that the former had higher characteristic of impedance (158 vs. 105), pulse wave velocity (561 cm/s vs. 417 cm/s), arterial wave reflection (reflection coefficient: 0.21 (0.12) vs. 0.16 (0.06)), and lower total peripheral arterial compliance (0.93 vs. 1.24) and finally found the increase in aortic wall stiffness was closely associated with the increase in aortic root diameter. Therefore, central and peripheral arterial wall stiffness is increased after TOF repair. Abnormal arterial elastic properties have negative impact on the left ventricle and provoke aortic dilatation, and it may induce left ventricular hypertrophy and systolic and diastolic dysfunction of the left ventricle with age. Also in repaired TOF patients, other researchers found decreased aortic elasticity and increased augmentation index [40]. Possibly this specific abnormal arterial hemodynamics in repaired TOF negatively influences left ventricular after load and aortic dilatation, and it may induce systolic and diastolic dysfunction of LV which may sometimes influence the right ventricle with age.

We can recognize these pathophysiological abnormalities of the aorta and abnormal aortoventricular interaction, i.e., aortic dilation, AR, aortic pathophysiological abnormalities, and decreased coronary artery flow and left ventricular dysfunctions, as a new clinical entity “aortopathy” [41, 42].

17.9 Prevention of Aortic Root Dilatation in TOF

ß-blockers and/or angiotensin receptor blockers (ARB) are the drug of choice for prevention of progressive aortic root dilatation in Marfan syndrome [43]. Aortic root dissection has been thus far rarely reported in patients with repaired TOF; nevertheless, aortic root replacement was performed in two patients with dilated aortic root diameters of 47–68 mm [8] and 2 % of repaired TOF patients in Japanese study [5] (Fig. 17.2). There is no consensus at present on ß-blocker or ARB administration for prevention of progressive dilatation of the aortic root in repaired or unrepaired TOF. Aortic dissection was happened in repaired TOF with aortic root size equal or over 55 mm. Aortic root surgery may be considered for patients with TOF and aortic root dilatation exceeding 55 mm [44], particularly when the primary indication for surgery is pulmonary valve implantation. However, this is a general recommendation, and available data to date are very limited (Table 17.1, [45]).

Aortic root dilatation and rate of change were significantly greater in patients with dilated aortic roots. This subset of TOF patients showed a male predominance and shared common morphologic features [46], namely, pulmonary atresia and right aortic arch, which may help identify patients at risk of progressive aortic dilatation, AR, and possibly – with further follow-up – aortic dissection. In previous studies, patients underwent repair of TOF at a relatively older age (beyond the age of 10 years) [6, 8].

Table 17.1 Prevalence of repaired TOF with aortic root size 55 mm or >55 mm

Author name that reported	Repaired TOF with aortic root size > 55 mm/total repaired TOF	References
Dodds III GA	3/ 400	[8]
Ishizuka T	1/427	[36]
Mongeon FP	11/474 (> 50 mm)	[45]
Niwa K	2/216	[7]
Nagy CD	2/109	[47]

17.10 Conclusions

1. Medial abnormalities in the ascending aorta were prevalent in repaired TOF, encompassing a wide age range, and may predispose to dilatation, aneurysm, and rupture necessitating aortic valve and root surgery, and that is often accompanied with AR.
2. A subset of adult patients with TOF exhibits ongoing dilatation of the aortic root even late after repair, which may relate to previous long-standing volume overload of the aorta and possibly to intrinsic properties of the aortic root.
3. This aortic dilatation is often associated with decreased elasticity and increased stiffness of the aorta, and it may reduce coronary arterial flow and negative impact on left ventricle function.
4. Therefore, this association in repaired TOF – dilated aorta, aortic pathophysiological abnormalities (abnormal aortic medial abnormalities, reduced aortic elasticity), and left ventricular dysfunction – should be called as aortopathy.
5. This aortopathy possibly induces not just aortic dilatation, but that will accelerate cardiac failure with age; therefore, we can recognize this complex lesion as new concept – aortopathy.
6. There is no consensus at present on the timing and dose of ß-blockers and/or ARB administration for prevention of progressive dilatation of the aortic root in patients with repaired TOF.
7. Meticulous follow-up of the aortic root after repair of TOF is thus recommended.

References

1. Niwa K, Perloff JK, Bhuta SM et al (2001) Structural abnormalities of great arterial walls in congenital heart disease. Light and electron micro- scopic analyses. Circulation 103:393–400
2. Roberts CS, Roberts WC (1991) Dissection of the aorta associated with congenital malformation of the aortic valve. J Am Coll Cardiol 17:712–716
3. Mckusick VA (1972) Association of congenital bicuspid aortic valve and Erdheim's cystic medial necrosis. Lancet 299:1026–1027
4. Seki M, Kurishima C, Kawasaki H et al (2012) Aortic stiffness and aortic dilation in infants and children with tetralogy of Fallot before corrective surgery: evidence for intrinsically abnormal aortic mechanical property. Eur J Cardiothorac Surg 41:277–282

5. Mizuno A, Niwa K, Matsuo K et al (2013) Survey of reoperation indications in tetralogy of Fallot in Japan. Circ J 77:2942–2947
6. Capelli H, Ross D, Somerville J (1982) Aortic regurgitation in tetrad of Fallot and pulmonary atresia. Am J Cardiol 49:1979–1983
7. Niwa K, Siu S, Webb G et al (2002) Progressive aortic root dilatation in adults late after repair of tetralogy of Fallot. Circulation 106:1374–1378
8. Dodds GA III, Warnes CA, Danielson GK (1997) Aortic valve replacement after repair of pulmonary atresia and ventricular septal defect or tetralogy of Fallot. J Thorac Cardiovasc Surg 113:736–741
9. Roman MJ, Devereux RB, Kramer-Fox R et al (1989) Two-dimensional echocardiographic aortic root dimensions in normal children and adults. Am J Cardiol 64:507–512
10. Vasan RS, Larson MR, Levy D (1995) Determinations of echocardiographic aortic root size. The Framingham heart study. Circulation 91:734–740
11. Zecchel R, Ho SY, Davlouros PA et al (2001) Histology of the aorta, and aortic root dilatation in adults with tetralogy of Fallot. J Am Coll Cardiol 37:468A
12. Rao BNS, Anderson RC, Edwards JE (1971) Anatomic variations in the tetralogy of Fallot. Am Heart J 81:361–371
13. Sonesson B, Lanne T, Vesnersson E et al (1994) Sex difference in the mechanical properties of the abdominal aorta in human being. J Vasc Surg 20:959–965
14. Jarmakani JMM, Graham TP Jr, Cenent RV et al (1972) Left heart function in children with tetralogy of Fallot before and after palliative or corrective surgery. Circulation 46:478–490
15. Marelli AJ, Perloff JK, Child JS et al (1994) Pulmonary atresia with ventricular septal defect in adults. Circulation 89:243–251
16. Matsuoka R, Takao A, Kimura M et al (1994) Confirmation that the conotruncal anomaly face syndrome is associated with deletion within 22q11.2. Am J Med Genet 53:285–289
17. Johnson MC, Strauss AW, Dawton B et al (1995) Deletion within chromosome 22 is common in patients with absent pulmonary valve syndrome. Am J Cardiol 76:66–69
18. John AS, McDonald-McGinn DM, Zackai EH et al (2009) Aortic root dilatation in patients with 22q11.2 deletion syndrome. Am J Med Genet A149A:939–942
19. Kim WH, Seo JW, Kim SJ et al (2005) Aortic dissection late after repair of tetralogy of Fallot. Int J Cardiol 101:515–516
20. Rathi VK, Doyle M, Williams RB et al (2005) Massive aortic aneurysm and dissection in repaired tetralogy of Fallot; diagnosis by cardiovascular magnetic resonance imaging. Int J Cardiol 101:169–170
21. Wijesekera VA, Kiess MC, Grewal J et al (2014) Aortic dissection in a patient with a dilated aortic root following tetralogy of Fallot repair. Int J Cardiol 174:833–834
22. Konstantinov IE, Fricke TA, d'Udekem Y et al (2010) Aortic dissection and rupture in adolescents after tetralogy of Fallot repair. J Thorac Cardiovasc Surg 140:e71–e73
23. Dearani JA, Burkhart HM, Stulak JM et al (2009) Management of the aortic root in adult patients with conotruncal anomalies. Semin Thorac Cardiovasc Surg Pediatr Card Surg Annu 12:122–129. doi:10.1053/j.pcsu.2009.01.013
24. Carlson RG, Lillehei CW, Edwards JE (1970) Cystic medial necrosis of the ascending aorta in relation to age and hypertension. Am J Cardiol 25:411–415
25. Schlatmann TJ, Becker AE (1977) Histologic changes in the normal aging aorta: implications for dissecting aortic aneurysm. Am J Cardiol 39:13–20
26. Monalo-Estrell P, Barker AE (1967) Histopathologic findings in human aortic media associated with pregnancy. Arch Pathol 83:336–341
27. Dietz HC, Pyeritz RE (1995) Mutations in the human gene for fibrillin-1 (FBN1) in the Marfan syndrome and related disorders. Hum Mol Genet 4:1799–1809
28. Segura AM, Luna RE, Horiba K et al (1998) Immunohistochemistry of matrix metalloproteinases and their inhibitors in thoracic aortic aneurysms and aortic valves in patients with Marfan's syndrome. Circulation 98(Suppl II):II-331–II-338

29. Bonderman D, Gharehbaghi-Schnell E, Walleneck G et al (1999) Mechanisms underlying aortic dilatation in congenital aortic valve malformations. Circulation 99:2138–2143
30. Ihling C, Szombathy T, Nampoothiri K et al (1999) Cystic medial degeneration of the aorta is associated with p53 accumulation, Bax upregulation, apoptotic cell death, and cell proliferation. Heart 82:286–293
31. Wang J, Nagy A, Larsson J et al (2006) Defective ALK5 signaling in the neural crest leads to increased postmigratory neural crest cell apoptosis and severe outflow tract defects. BMC Dev Biol 6:51–64
32. Tan JL, Davlouros PA, McCarthy KP et al (2005) Intrinsic histological abnormalities of aortic root and ascending aorta in tetralogy of Fallot: evidence of causative mechanism for aortic dilatation and aortopathy. Circulation 112:961–968
33. Bhat AH, Smith CJ, Hawker RE (2004) Late aortic root dilatation in tetralogy of Fallot may be prevented by early repair in infancy. Pediatr Cardiol 25:654–659
34. Bull K, Somerville J, Ty E et al (1995) Presentation and attrition in complex pulmonary atresia. J Am Coll Cardiol 25:491–499
35. Abraham KA, Cherian G, Rao VD et al (1979) Tetralogy of Fallot in adults- A report on 147 patients. Am J Med 66:811–816
36. Ishizaka T, Ichikawa H, Sawa Y et al (2004) Prevalence and optimal management strategy for aortic regurgitation in tetralogy of Fallot. Eur J Cardiothorac Surg 26:1080–1086
37. Rieker RP, Berman MA, Stansel HC Jr (1975) Postoperative studies in patients with tetralogy of Fallot. Ann Thorac Surg 19:17–25
38. Chong WY, Wong WH, Chiu CS et al (2006) Aortic root dilation and aortic elastic properties in children after repair of tetralogy of Fallot. Am J Cardiol 97:905–909
39. Senzaki H, Iwamoto Y, Ishido H et al (2008) Arterial haemodynamics in patients after repair of tetralogy of Fallot: influence on left ventricular after load and aortic dilatation. Heart 94:70–74
40. Cheung YF, Ou X, Wong SJ (2006) Central and peripheral arterial stiffness in patients after surgical repair of tetralogy of Fallot: implications for aortic root dilatation. Heart 92:1827–1830
41. Niwa K (2013) Aortopathy in congenital heart disease in adults: aortic dilatation with decreased aortic elasticity that impacts negatively on left ventricular function. Korean Circ J 43:215–220
42. Zanjani KS, Niwa K (2013) Aortic dilatation and aortopathy in congenital heart diseases. J Cardiol 61:16–21
43. Shores J, Berger KR, Murphy EA et al (1994) Progression of aortic dilatation and the benefit of long-term β-adrenergic blockade in Marfan's syndrome. N Engl J Med 330:1335–1341
44. Warnes CA, Williams RG, Bashore TM et al. (2008) ACC/AHA 2008 guidelines for the management of adults with congenital heart disease: a report of the American College of Cardiology/American Heart Association Task Force on Practice Guidelines. J Am Coll Cardiol 52:e1–121, Circulation 118:e714–e833. http://circ.ahajournals.org/cgi/content/full/118/23/e714
45. Mongeon FP, Gurvitz MZ, Broberg CS et al (2013) Aortic root dilatation in adults with surgically repaired tetralogy of Fallot: a multicenter cross-sectional study. Circulation 127:172–179
46. Niwa K (2005) Aortic root dilatation in tetralogy of Fallot long-term after repair – histology of the aorta in tetralogy of Fallot: evidence of intrinsic aortopathy. Int J Cardiol 103:117–119
47. Nagy CD, Alejo DE, Corretti MC et al (2013) Tetralogy of Fallot and aortic root dilation: a long-term outlook. Pediatr Cardiol 34:809–816

Chapter 18
Hypoplastic Left Heart Syndrome

Ryo Inuzuka

Abstract With more patients with hypoplastic left heart syndrome (HLHS) palliated through surgical revision and surviving into adulthood, long-term performance of the right-sided structures in the systemic position has become a clinical concern. Aortopathy, progressive dilation of aortic root, is one of such problems. Aortopathy in patients with HLHS is becoming a legitimate issue as it is related to aortic regurgitation, aortic dissection, and potential ventricular dysfunction, which might require surgical re-intervention. Although pathophysiology of aortic root dilation in patients with HLHS is largely unknown, several aspects of HLHS are considered to be related to the pathogenesis, such as anatomical, genetic, and hemodynamic factors, which will be described in detail in this chapter. Further elucidation of risk factors for progressive aortic dilation in HLHS as well as its mechanisms is required to establish disease-specific and stratified approach, as no specific recommendations for the management of aortic dilation in HLHS are currently available.

Keywords TGF-β signaling • Bicuspid aortic valve • Heritability • Hypoplastic left heart syndrome

18.1 Neo-aortic Root Dilation in HLHS

Hypoplastic left heart syndrome (HLHS) is a congenital malformation that is characterized by severe underdevelopment of the structures in the left heart-aorta complex [1]. Therefore, newborns with HLHS lack crucial components of systemic circulation (aortic atresia or mitral atresia with hypoplastic left ventricle and aortic root), which can be temporarily compensated by blood flow from pulmonary artery through patent ductus arteriosus. The current strategy of treating HLHS involves right ventricular recruitment for systemic perfusion, aortic arch reconstruction, and accomplishment of Fontan circulation in which systemic venous return was directed to the pulmonary vasculature without the use of a ventricular pump

R. Inuzuka, M.D., Ph.D. (✉)
Department of Pediatrics, University of Tokyo, 7-3-1 Hongo, Bunkyo-ku, 113-0033 Tokyo, Japan
e-mail: inuzukar-tky@umin.ac.jp

K. Niwa, H. Kaemmerer (eds.), *Aortopathy*, DOI 10.1007/978-4-431-56071-5_18

[2, 3]. Owing to significant improvement in surgical results based on the management protocol, long-term durability of the right-sided structures in the systemic position has become a clinical concern [4, 5].

Cohen et al. reviewed 53 patients with HLHS who had undergone Fontan operation and found that the neo-aortic root progressively dilated out of proportion to body size over time, with 52 patients (98 %) having a Z-score > 2 during a median follow-up period of 9.2 years (Fig. 18.1) [5]. They showed that all of neo-aortic valve annulus, sinuses of Valsalva, and sinotubular junction were dilated (Fig. 18.2). Moreover, neo-aortic root dilation was related to neo-aortic regurgitation, which was present in 61 % of patients at the last follow-up, with deterioration over time in 26 patients (49 %). With more patients with HLHS palliated through surgical revision and surviving into adulthood, neo-aortic root dilation is becoming a legitimate issue. Surgical re-intervention for neo-aortic root dilation and neo-aortic regurgitation is increasingly reported [6–12]. Even a sudden cardiac death due to a ruptured dissection of aortic aneurysm is reported [13]. Furthermore, in other forms of congenital heart disease (CHD), dilated aorta was associated with increased stiffness of the aortic wall, which negatively influences the systemic ventricular systolic and diastolic functions due to increased afterload and ventricular hypertrophy [14, 15].

18.2 Pathophysiology

"Aortopathy" in HLHS refers to neo-aortic root dilation, which is derived from pulmonary arterial tissue. While pathophysiology of aortopathy in patients with HLHS is largely unknown, several aspects of HLHS were considered to be related to the pathogenesis of neo-aortic root dilation.

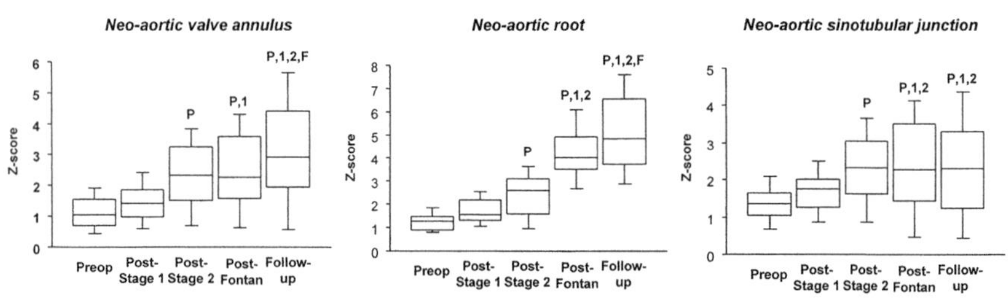

Fig. 18.1 Progressive neo-aortic dilation in patients with hypoplastic left heart syndrome. Box plots depicting the median value (*middle line of box*), the 25th and 75th percentiles (*upper and low boundaries of box*), and 10th and 90th percentiles (*upper and lower error bars*) for Z-scores of the neo-aortic valve annulus (*left*), root (*middle*), and sinotubular junction (*right*) in the study population. Significant differences ($p > 0.05$) by general factorial analysis of variance with the Bonferroni correction for multiple comparisons are indicated by the following symbols: P = differs significantly from the preoperative Z-score; 1 = differs significantly from the stage 1 Z-score; 2 = differs significantly from the bidirectional superior cavopulmonary anastomosis Z-score; F = differs significantly from the Fontan Z-score (Reproduced from Figure 3 of J Am Coll Cardiol. 2003;42:533–540 with permission of Elsevier Limited [5])

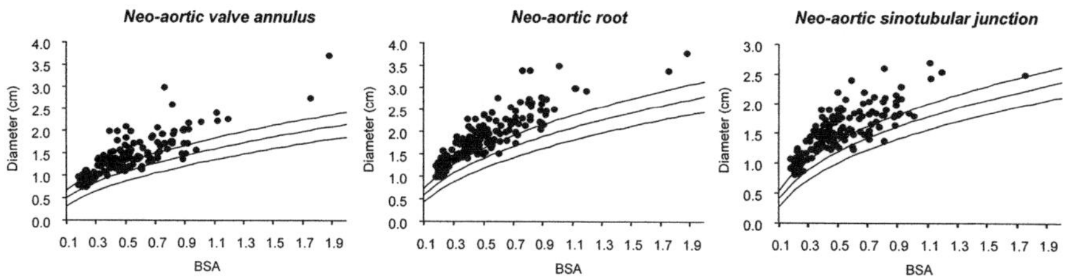

Fig. 18.2 Diameters of the neo-aortic valve annulus, root, and sinotubular junction. The diameters of the neo-aortic valve annulus (*left*), root (*middle*), and sinotubular junction (*right*) are plotted against body surface area (BSA) and compared with the normal distribution (mean with 95 % confidence intervals) (Reproduced from Figure 2 of J Am Coll Cardiol. 2003;42:533–540 with permission of Elsevier Limited [5])

18.2.1 Anatomical and Histological Factors

Patients after Norwood procedure for HLHS have native pulmonary valve in the systemic position. The presence of pulmonary autograft in the systemic position (under systemic pressure), as occurs in patients after the Ross procedure and arterial switch operation, is considered to be an independent risk factor for aortic dilatation [16–18]. A remodeling process of pulmonary autograft in systemic position has been studied in patients after Ross procedure by Rabkin-Aikawa et al. [19]. They found granulation tissue as an early sign of damaged arterial wall of the autograft, which progresses to accumulation of collagen and focal loss of normal muscle cells and elastin, which suggests scarring formation. These histological findings may explain progressive dilation of pulmonary autograft over time. Histopathological examinations of dilated aortic wall are also conducted in patients with HLHS, which showed cystic medial degenerative changes both in native and graft tissues, which is similar to aortopathy associated with bicuspid aortic valves and connective tissue disorders [7, 9]. Moreover, lack of supportive structure of semilunar valves may be related to neo-aortic root dilation. The normal aortic root annulus is wedged between the left and right atrioventricular valve annuli and thick left ventricular myocardium, whereas the pulmonary valve complex has only slight support from the thin right ventricular myocardium [5, 20].

18.2.2 Genetic Factors

While the genetic basis of HLHS remains largely unknown, several studies suggest that HLHS is heritable and is genetically related to bicuspid aortic valve which is known to be associated with aortopathy [21, 22]. HLHS has been shown to be predisposed to certain well-defined genetic disorders, such as Turner and Jacobsen syndromes [23, 24]. The widely accepted concept is that HLHS is a severe form of left-sided valve malformation secondary to embryonic alterations in blood flow, such as mitral or aortic stenosis [22]. In fact, in the embryonic chick, ligation of the left atrium resulted in left ventricular hypoplasia due to diminished flow through the left ventricle [25]. Observations of familial clustering of HLHS and bicuspid aortic valve prompted an investigation to determine the size of the genetic effect of HLHS by Hinton et al. [22, 26, 27]. They performed echocardiograms on family members of HLHS probands with aortic valve hypoplasia and dysplasia to assess the presence of cardiovascular malformations. Overall, 21 out of 38 (55 %) families had more than one affected individual, and 36 % of participants had cardiovascular malformations, including 11 % with bicuspid aortic valve. Maximum likelihood-based variance decomposition showed that the heritability of HLHS alone and with associated cardiovascular malformations were as high as 99 % and 74 % ($p > 0.00001$), respectively, suggesting that HLHS is determined largely by genetic effects. Similar analysis assuming an autosomal recessive trait reduced estimated heritability of HLHS, which questioned the assumption that HLHS is inherited as a simple Mendelian autosomal recessive condition and implicated HLHS as a complex trait. The sibling recurrence risk for HLHS was 8 % and 22 % for cardiovascular malformations. The genetic basis of HLHS and its relationship to bicuspid aortic valve was further investigated by the same group [21]. They performed family-based nonparametric genome-wide linkage analysis to identify disease loci for HLHS and bicuspid aortic valve. The recurrence risk ratio of BAV in HLHS families (8.05) was nearly identical to that in bicuspid aortic valve families (8.77). Linkage to multiple chromosomal regions, such as 10q22 and 6q23, was identified in HLHS kindreds, suggesting genetic heterogeneity of HLHS. Moreover, a shared chromosomal locus on 14q23 was identified for HLHS and bicuspid aortic valve, which provides the first direct evidence of a genetic relationship between HLHS and bicuspid aortic valve.

Recent studies have revealed that the transforming growth factor (TGF)-β signaling plays an important role in vascular remodeling. It has been theorized that fibrillin interacts with latent TGF-β binding protein to control TGF-β activity [28]. Thus, fibrilin-1 deficiency as in Marfan syndrome causes dysregulated TGF-β activation, which can result in matrix degradation and aortic dilation [29]. Correspondingly, suppression of TGF-β signaling by angiotensin II receptor antagonists has been shown to prevent vascular damage in Marfan syndrome [30, 31]. In fact, increased TGF-β signaling is shown to be universally present in aneurysms of various etiologies, which are not limited to the fibrillin-1 deficiency [29, 32]. While dysregulation of TGF-β activation has not been well substantiated in CHD-associated aortic dilation, TGF-β signaling have been shown to contribute to cardiac embryogenesis such as in cardiac neural crest cell migration and the formation of the cardiac outflow tracts [33]. Moreover, fibrillin-1 gene variants in individuals with tetralogy of Fallot are reported to be at an eight times greater risk of aortic dilatation [34]. A novel mutation of SMAD3, which encodes an intracellular member of the TGF-β signaling pathway, is reported in a patient with HLHS with significant aortic aneurysm, but the causal relationship remains to be elucidated.

18.2.3 Hemodynamic Factor

In patients with tetralogy of Fallot, factors associated with excessive flow through the aorta, such as higher age at operation, pulmonary atresia, and longer presence of surgically created aortopulmonary shunts, are associated with an aortic dilatation [16, 35–38]. Therefore, chronic aortic overflow has been attributed to aortic dilation. In patients with HLHS, a valuable study comparing long-term outcome between those with modified BT shunt and those with the right ventricular to pulmonary artery shunt as initial shunt for Norwood procedure has suggested a contribution of aortic overflow [39, 40]. Neo-aortic annular dimension Z-scores were significantly greater in the modified BT shunt group before stage II operation. However, the differences were no longer significant in the longer term at 14 months.

18.3 Management

No specific recommendations for the management of aortic dilation in HLHS are currently available. Surgical indications may be extrapolated from guidelines for bicuspid aortic valve or connective tissue disorders. Even with concomitant neo-aortic regurgitation, successful experiences with valve-sparing surgery have been reported [6, 7, 12]. Use of β-blockers or angiotensin receptor blockers, which have been reported to be beneficial in slowing aortic-root enlargement in Marfan syndrome, may be considered for those with marked aortic dilation [31]. Again, the actual effect of these medications for those with HLHS remains unclear.

18.4 Conclusions

With more patients with HLHS palliated through surgical revision and surviving into adulthood, aortopathy in HLHS becomes more widely recognized. While successful surgical re-interventions are reported, further elucidation of risk factors for progressive aortic dilation as well as its mechanisms is required to establish disease-specific and stratified approach to aortic dilation in this growing population.

References

1. Tchervenkov CI, Jacobs ML, Tahta SA (2000) Congenital heart surgery nomenclature and database project: hypoplastic left heart syndrome. Ann Thorac Surg 69:S170–S179
2. Feinstein JA, Benson DW, Dubin AM, Cohen MS, Maxey DM, Mahle WT, Pahl E, Villafañe J, Bhatt AB, Peng LF, Johnson BA, Marsden AL, Daniels CJ, Rudd NA, Caldarone CA, Mussatto KA, Morales DL, Ivy DD, Gaynor JW, Tweddell JS, Deal BJ, Furck AK, Rosenthal GL, Ohye RG, Ghanayem NS, Cheatham JP, Tworetzky W, Martin GR (2012) Hypoplastic left heart syndrome: current considerations and expectations. J Am Coll Cardiol 59:S1–S42
3. Rychik J (2014) Hypoplastic left heart syndrome: can we change the rules of the game? Circulation 130:629–631
4. Norwood WI, Lang P, Hansen DD (1983) Physiologic repair of aortic atresia-hypoplastic left heart syndrome. N Engl J Med 308:23–26
5. Cohen MS, Marino BS, McElhinney DB, Robbers-Visser D, van der Woerd W, Gaynor JW, Spray TL, Wernovsky G (2003) Neo-aortic root dilation and valve regurgitation up to 21 years after staged reconstruction for hypoplastic left heart syndrome. J Am Coll Cardiol 42:533–540
6. Erez E, Tam VK, Galliani C, Lashus A, Doublin NA, Peretti J (2012) Valve-sparing aortic root replacement for patients with a fontan circulation. J Heart Valve Dis 21:175–180
7. Pizarro C, Baffa JM, Derby CD, Krieger PA (2011) Valve-sparing neo-aortic root replacement after fontan completion for hypoplastic left heart syndrome. J Thorac Cardiovasc Surg 141:1083–1084
8. Herrmann JL, Lewis MJ, Fuller S, Mascio CE (2014) Aneurysm formation after the norwood procedure: case report and review of the literature. J Thorac Cardiovasc Surg 147:e55–e56
9. Shuhaiber JH, Patel V, Husayni T, El-Zein C, Barth MJ, Ilbawi MN (2006) Repair of symptomatic neoaortic aneurysm after third-stage palliation for hypoplastic left heart syndrome. J Thorac Cardiovasc Surg 131:478–479
10. Cameron D (2015) Surgery for congenital diseases of the aorta. J Thorac Cardiovasc Surg 149: S14–S17
11. Ehsan A, Singh H, Vargas SO, Sachweh J, Jonas RA (2005) Neoaortic aneurysm after stage i norwood reconstruction. Ann Thorac Surg 79:e23–e25
12. Kanzaki T, Yamagishi M, Miyazaki T, Maeda Y, Yaku H (2015) Valve-sparing neoaortic root replacement late after the norwood and fontan procedures. Ann Thorac Surg 99:309–312
13. Stolla M, Sweeney A, Alfieris GM, Metlay LA (2014) Aortic aneurysm with a ruptured dissection in a 15-year-old boy with hypoplastic left heart syndrome. J Thorac Cardiovasc Surg 147:e35–e36
14. Senzaki H, Iwamoto Y, Ishido H, Matsunaga T, Taketazu M, Kobayashi T, Asano H, Katogi T, Kyo S (2008) Arterial haemodynamics in patients after repair of tetralogy of fallot: influence on left ventricular after load and aortic dilatation. Heart 94:70–74
15. Inuzuka R, Seki M, Sugimoto M, Saiki H, Masutani S, Senzaki H (2013) Pulmonary arterial wall stiffness and its impact on right ventricular afterload in patients with repaired tetralogy of fallot. Ann Thorac Surg 96:1435–1441
16. May Khan A, Kim Y (2014) Aortic dilatation and aortopathies in congenital heart disease. Curr Opin Cardiol 29:91–96
17. Pasquali SK, Cohen MS, Shera D, Wernovsky G, Spray TL, Marino BS (2007) The relationship between neo-aortic root dilation, insufficiency, and reintervention following the ross procedure in infants, children, and young adults. J Am Coll Cardiol 49:1806–1812
18. Hourihan M, Colan SD, Wernovsky G, Maheswari U, Mayer JE, Sanders SP (1993) Growth of the aortic anastomosis, annulus, and root after the arterial switch procedure performed in infancy. Circulation 88:615–620
19. Rabkin-Aikawa E, Aikawa M, Farber M, Kratz JR, Garcia-Cardena G, Kouchoukos NT, Mitchell MB, Jonas RA, Schoen FJ (2004) Clinical pulmonary autograft valves: pathologic evidence of adaptive remodeling in the aortic site. J Thorac Cardiovasc Surg 128:552–561

20. Hokken RB, Bartelings MM, Bogers AJ, Gittenberger-de Groot AC (1997) Morphology of the pulmonary and aortic roots with regard to the pulmonary autograft procedure. J Thorac Cardiovasc Surg 113:453–461
21. Hinton RB, Martin LJ, Rame-Gowda S, Tabangin ME, Cripe LH, Benson DW (2009) Hypoplastic left heart syndrome links to chromosomes 10q and 6q and is genetically related to bicuspid aortic valve. J Am Coll Cardiol 53:1065–1071
22. Hinton RB, Martin LJ, Tabangin ME, Mazwi ML, Cripe LH, Benson DW (2007) Hypoplastic left heart syndrome is heritable. J Am Coll Cardiol 50:1590–1595
23. Natowicz M, Kelley RI (1987) Association of turner syndrome with hypoplastic left-heart syndrome. Am J Dis Child 141:218–220
24. Ye M, Coldren C, Liang X, Mattina T, Goldmuntz E, Benson DW, Ivy D, Perryman MB, Garrett-Sinha LA, Grossfeld P (2010) Deletion of ets-1, a gene in the jacobsen syndrome critical region, causes ventricular septal defects and abnormal ventricular morphology in mice. Hum Mol Genet 19:648–656
25. deAlmeida A, McQuinn T, Sedmera D (2007) Increased ventricular preload is compensated by myocyte proliferation in normal and hypoplastic fetal chick left ventricle. Circ Res 100:1363–1370
26. Ferencz C, Rubin JD, McCarter RJ, Brenner JI, Neill CA, Perry LW, Hepner SI, Downing JW (1985) Congenital heart disease: prevalence at livebirth. The baltimore-washington infant study. Am J Epidemiol 121:31–36
27. Brenner JI, Berg KA, Schneider DS, Clark EB, Boughman JA (1989) Cardiac malformations in relatives of infants with hypoplastic left-heart syndrome. Am J Dis Child 143:1492–1494
28. Habashi JP, Judge DP, Holm TM, Cohn RD, Loeys BL, Cooper TK, Myers L, Klein EC, Liu G, Calvi C, Podowski M, Neptune ER, Halushka MK, Bedja D, Gabrielson K, Rifkin DB, Carta L, Ramirez F, Huso DL, Dietz HC (2006) Losartan, an at1 antagonist, prevents aortic aneurysm in a mouse model of marfan syndrome. Science 312:117–121
29. Jones JA, Barbour JR, Stroud RE, Bouges S, Stephens SL, Spinale FG, Ikonomidis JS (2008) Altered transforming growth factor-beta signaling in a murine model of thoracic aortic aneurysm. J Vasc Res 45:457–468
30. Habashi JP, Doyle JJ, Holm TM, Aziz H, Schoenhoff F, Bedja D, Chen Y, Modiri AN, Judge DP, Dietz HC (2011) Angiotensin ii type 2 receptor signaling attenuates aortic aneurysm in mice through erk antagonism. Science 332:361–365
31. Lacro RV, Dietz HC, Sleeper LA, Yetman AT, Bradley TJ, Colan SD, Pearson GD, Selamet Tierney ES, Levine JC, Atz AM, Benson DW, Braverman AC, Chen S, De Backer J, Gelb BD, Grossfeld PD, Klein GL, Lai WW, Liou A, Loeys BL, Markham LW, Olson AK, Paridon SM, Pemberton VL, Pierpont ME, Pyeritz RE, Radojewski E, Roman MJ, Sharkey AM, Stylianou MP, Wechsler SB, Young LT, Mahony L, Investigators PHN (2014) Atenolol versus losartan in children and young adults with marfan's syndrome. N Engl J Med 371:2061–2071
32. Ruigrok YM, Rinkel GJ, van't Slot R, Wolfs M, Tang S, Wijmenga C (2006) Evidence in favor of the contribution of genes involved in the maintenance of the extracellular matrix of the arterial wall to the development of intracranial aneurysms. Hum Mol Genet 15:3361–3368
33. Wang J, Nagy A, Larsson J, Dudas M, Sucov HM, Kaartinen V (2006) Defective alk5 signaling in the neural crest leads to increased postmigratory neural crest cell apoptosis and severe outflow tract defects. BMC Dev Biol 6:51
34. Chowdhury UK, Mishra AK, Balakrishnan P, Sharma S, Kabra M, Ray R, Kalaivani M, Gupta R, Govindappa RM, Subramaniam GK (2008) Role of fibrillin-1 genetic mutations and polymorphism in aortic dilatation in patients undergoing intracardiac repair of tetralogy of fallot. J Thorac Cardiovasc Surg 136:757–766 , 766.e751–710
35. Zanjani KS, Niwa K (2013) Aortic dilatation and aortopathy in congenital heart diseases. J Cardiol 61:16–21
36. Chong WY, Wong WH, Chiu CS, Cheung YF (2006) Aortic root dilation and aortic elastic properties in children after repair of tetralogy of fallot. Am J Cardiol 97:905–909

37. Niwa K, Siu SC, Webb GD, Gatzoulis MA (2002) Progressive aortic root dilatation in adults late after repair of tetralogy of fallot. Circulation 106:1374–1378
38. Bhat AH, Smith CJ, Hawker RE (2004) Late aortic root dilatation in tetralogy of fallot may be prevented by early repair in infancy. Pediatr Cardiol 25:654–659
39. Ohye RG, Sleeper LA, Mahony L, Newburger JW, Pearson GD, Lu M, Goldberg CS, Tabbutt S, Frommelt PC, Ghanayem NS, Laussen PC, Rhodes JF, Lewis AB, Mital S, Ravishankar C, Williams IA, Dunbar-Masterson C, Atz AM, Colan S, Minich LL, Pizarro C, Kanter KR, Jaggers J, Jacobs JP, Krawczeski CD, Pike N, McCrindle BW, Virzi L, Gaynor JW, Investigators PHN (2010) Comparison of shunt types in the norwood procedure for single-ventricle lesions. N Engl J Med 362:1980–1992
40. Frommelt PC, Guey LT, Minich LL, Bhat M, Bradley TJ, Colan SD, Ensing G, Gorentz J, Heydarian H, John JB, Lai WW, Levine JC, Mahle WT, Miller SG, Ohye RG, Pearson GD, Shirali GS, Wong PC, Cohen MS, Investigators PHN (2012) Does initial shunt type for the norwood procedure affect echocardiographic measures of cardiac size and function during infancy?: the single vventricle reconstruction trial. Circulation 125:2630–2638

Chapter 19
Transposition of the Great Arteries After Arterial Switch Operation

Satoshi Masutani

Abstract The aorta in transposition of the great arteries (TGA) has unique anatomical and operative features; the pulmonary valve and root are used to form the neo-aortic valve and root, and the aortic root undergoes surgical insult with the arterial switch operation. Aortopathy, defined as aortic root dilatation caused by abnormalities in aortic pathophysiological function with low coronary artery flow and systemic ventricular dysfunction, is a clinically important sequel in TGA patients. Despite variation between individuals, aortopathy generally progresses with age; aortic root dilation is progressive, and aortic distensibility and freedom from significant aortic regurgitation (AR) decrease with age. Although aortopathy in TGA seems not as severe as that following the Ross operation, some patients with marked aortic root dilation or severe AR require repeat operations. Research on aortopathy in TGA is currently accumulating information on the nature of the aortopathy, individual risk and protective factors, and anatomical, histological, and functional characteristics. Because of the progressive nature of aortopathy, further longer serial follow-up data need to be accumulated to clarify life-span prognosis of aortopathy and develop effective therapeutic strategies to prevent/ameliorate aortopathy in TGA patients.

Keywords Transposition of great arteries • Aortopathy • Switch • Jatene • Aortic regurgitation

19.1 Introduction

Dilatation of the aortic root can be caused by abnormalities in aortic pathophysiological function, with low coronary artery flow and systemic ventricular dysfunction. This new clinical entity is called "aortopathy" [1]. Aortopathy is a clinically important entity that is associated with hypertension and atherosclerosis and with the need for surgery. Aortopathy is reported in various conditions, including

S. Masutani, M.D. (✉)
Pediatrics, Saitama Medical Center, Saitama Medical University, 1981 Kamoda, 350-8550 Kawagoe, Saitama, Japan
e-mail: masutani@saitama-med.ac.jp

K. Niwa, H. Kaemmerer (eds.), *Aortopathy*, DOI 10.1007/978-4-431-56071-5_19

systemic syndromes and specific congenital heart diseases [1]. Transposition of the great arteries (TGA) is one such underlying disease of aortopathy. This chapter will specifically focus on the aortopathy in TGA, which has unique anatomical aspects and surgical features.

19.2 TGA, Change of Surgeries, and Manipulation of Aorta

Transposition of the great arteries (TGA) is the second most common cyanotic congenital heart defect, with incidences estimated at 315 per million live births [2, 3]. Currently, most treated TGA patients live to adulthood, with a 20-year survival rate of nearly 90 % [4]. The arterial switch operation (ASO), the current mainstay therapeutic option for TGA patients, directly manipulates the aorta, using the original pulmonary valve and root as a neo-aortic valve and root. These points may be unique and important aspects of aortopathy in TGA patients. Thus, we summarize here the characteristics of TGA operations with particular focus on aortic manipulation.

TGA was classically treated with atrial switch operations such as the Senning and Mustard operations. These operations produce physiological correction of the abnormal circulation [5]. However, the atrial switch operation is linked to significant late morbidity and mortality, e.g., atrial arrhythmias, dysfunction of the morphologic right systemic ventricle, and heart failure [6]. Recently, the atrial switch operation has been largely replaced by the arterial switch operation (ASO), an anatomical repair, which was initiated by Jatene [7] with later modifications by Lecompte [8]. The early and midterm results of ASO are outstanding even in the presence of complex coronary artery patterns and associated cardiac defects [9].

Briefly, ASO involves the transection and reanastomosis of both great arteries above the sinuses of Valsalva and transplantation of the coronary arteries [10]. This procedure involves excision of the coronary artery from the aorta with a small cuff of the aortic wall attached (the "coronary button") [11]. The ascending aorta and the pulmonary trunk are transected and switched such that the new aorta is made up of the pulmonary root and valve and the rest is the aorta. The new pulmonary trunk consists of the aortic root and valve with pulmonary artery (PA) tissue. Before the transected vessels are anastomosed, the pulmonary trunk is relocated anterior to the aorta (the Lecompte maneuver); small holes are created in the neo-aorta, and the coronary artery buttons are reimplanted at these holes (coronary translocation) [11].

The original pulmonary valve and root are placed in the systemic circulation and serve as the systemic (neo-aortic) valve and root after ASO. These are unique aortic characteristics in TGA patients after ASO. Further, suture of the coronary button causes a scar in the coronary sinus. Previously, a significant proportion of patients undertook pulmonary arterial banding (PAB) [12] before ASO for LV training to avoid cardiopulmonary bypass during the early neonatal period, as part of a two-staged repair. In such patients, PAB can affect the tissue in the neo-aortic root and valve after ASO. Recently, one-stage ASO has overtaken PAB as the primary operation in most TGA patients. Based on the current understanding of aortic manipulation in the TGA operation, we review the aortopathy of TGA.

19.3 Time Course of Aortic Dilation and Regurgitation

Aortic dilation and regurgitation (AR) are key objective findings of aortopathy and are well-known complications after ASO in TGA [1]. Progressive dilation of the neo-aortic root is out of proportion to somatic growth, and the incidence of AR increases with follow-up [1]. Most reports have shown progression of aortic root dilation [13, 14] and increased occurrence of significant AR [14] over time [13, 15].

The Kaplan-Meier curve in Fig. 19.1 clearly shows that freedom from aortic root dilation (neo-aortic root z-score >=3.0) and from moderate/severe AR decreased over time in patients who underwent an ASO before 2000 [15]. Importantly, the dilation of the aorta is not proportional; it is most pronounced in the aortic root [5, 16], with the aortic annulus second, and less pronounced in the sinotubular junction, as shown in Fig. 19.2 [5].

Although aortic dilation shortly after ASO is a common finding, reports of the long-term fate of aortic dilation over 10 years have been quite inconsistent, with some reports showing further progression [5] and others no further progression [15, 16]. Detailed serial follow-up data showed rapid dilatation of the new aortic root z-score in the first year of life, followed by normalization of growth and no further progression of the aortic root until 20 years of age (Fig. 19.3) [17]. In

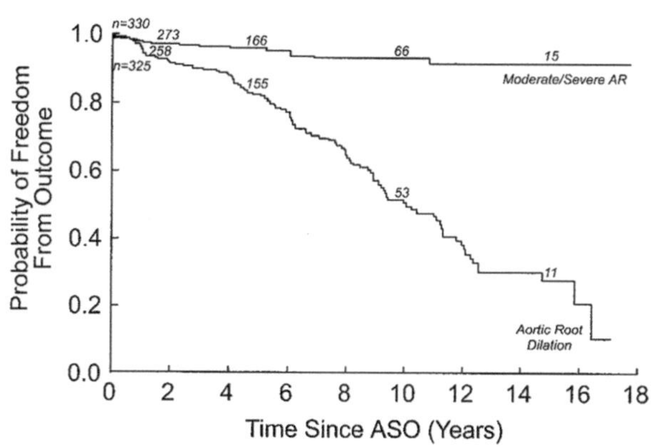

Fig. 19.1 Probability of freedom from neo-aortic root dilation (neo-aortic root z-score ≧ 3.0) and probability of freedom from moderate to more severe neo-aortic regurgitation, each independently over time since ASO. *AR* aortic regurgitation, *ASO* arterial switch operation (Reprinted with permission from Schwartz et al. [15])

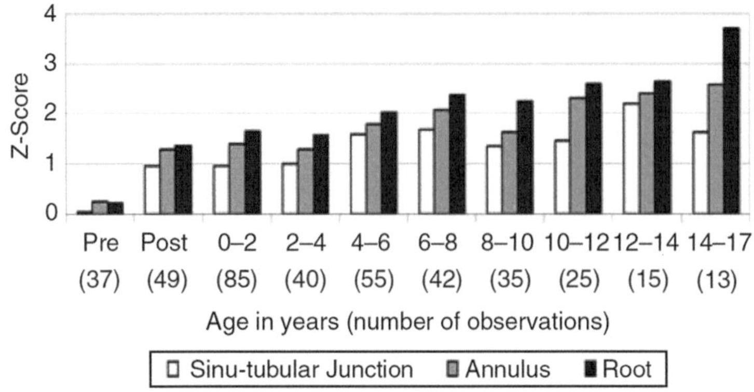

Fig. 19.2 Z-Score of the measurements at the basal and mid-sinusal levels and the sinotubular junction after the arterial switch operation. *Pre* preoperative measurement, *Post* postoperative measurement, *ASO* arterial switch operation (Reprinted with permission from Marino et al. [5])

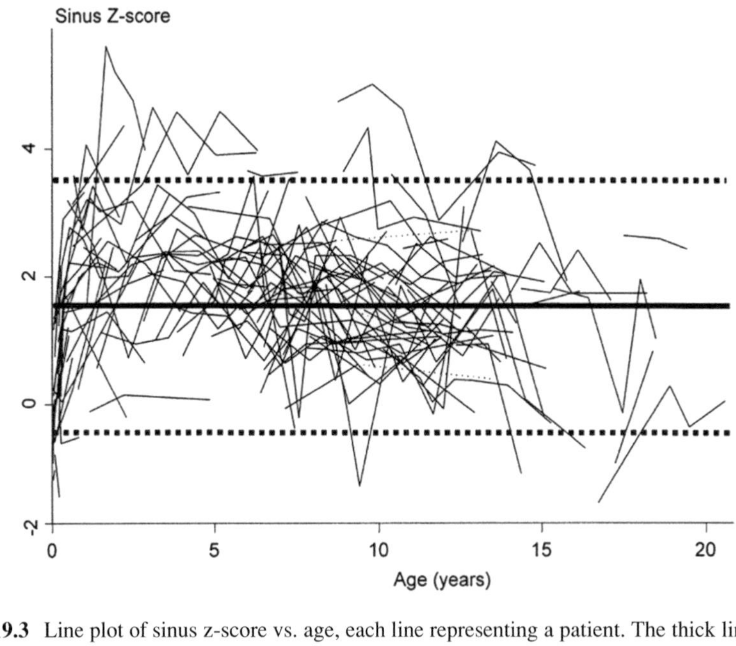

Fig. 19.3 Line plot of sinus z-score vs. age, each line representing a patient. The thick line is the overall trend of the patient lines, with 95 % prediction intervals. The sinus z-scores remain unchanged with age (Reprinted with permission from Hutter et al. [17])

contrast, recently published longer follow-up data from 17 to 30 years of age showed a progression of the aortic diameter during adulthood (Fig. 19.4) [13]. In this study, neo-aortic dilation >40 mm was present in 5 % of patients before reaching adulthood. As shown in Fig. 19.5, freedom from neo-aortic dilation was 56 % at 23 years of age and subsequently continued to decrease with age. During

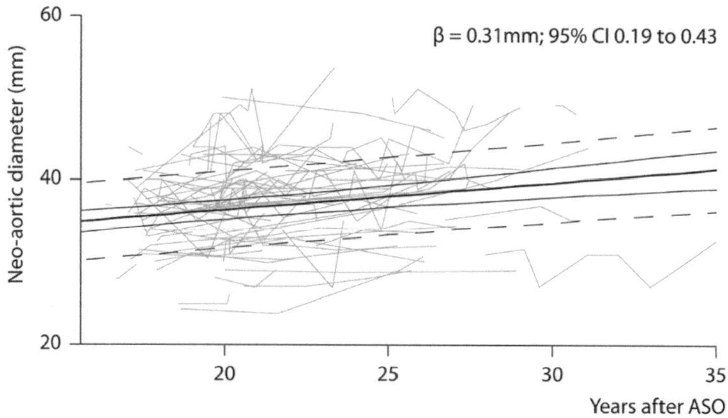

Fig. 19.4 Time trend for neo-aortic diameter in adult patients after arterial switch operation (ASO); (A) each line represents the individual mid-sinus-level neo-aortic measurements of one patient; *bold line*, mean neo-aortic growth; *plain lines*, 95 % CI of regression line; *dashed lines*, 95 % prediction interval (Reprinted with permission from van der Bom T et al. [13])

follow-up, a neo-aortic diameter wider than 45 mm was measured in 13 % of patients, and a neo-aortic diameter wider than 50 mm in 5 % of patients. Neo-aortic growth was on average linear and did not stabilize over time in early adulthood. Mean neo-aortic growth was 0.31 mm/year ($p < 0.001$ compared with normal value 0.08 mm/year) (Fig. 19.4) [13].

The characteristics of AR have been reported as follows: in 66 patients with trivial to mild neo-aortic insufficiency, 35 (53 %) had central insufficiency from lack of coaptation, 28 (42 %) had eccentric insufficiency, and 3 (4.5 %) had leaflet distortion due to unequal cusp size [5]. During childhood, 10 % of patients had moderate AR, and 4 % had received an artificial aortic valve for treatment of hemodynamically significant AR [13]. During a median follow-up of 7.2 years in adulthood, 4 % experienced neo-aortic complications. Neo-aortic root replacement (one root sparing, two Bentall procedures) was performed in three (4 %) patients with neo-aortic diameters of 53, 51, and 46 mm (the last had severe neo-aortic valve regurgitation) [13]. Aortic dissection or rupture in the TGA patients after ASO has also been reported recently [18–20].

Despite inconsistency in reports on late further progression or no progression, some patients progress to aortopathy after reaching adulthood. Great differences in diameters and serial changes between patients [13, 15, 17] have been consistently reported, as shown in the time trend plot for neo-aortic sinus diameter in adult patients after ASO (Fig. 19.4) [13]. This shows that individual factors may be important for progression of aortopathy in TGA patients.

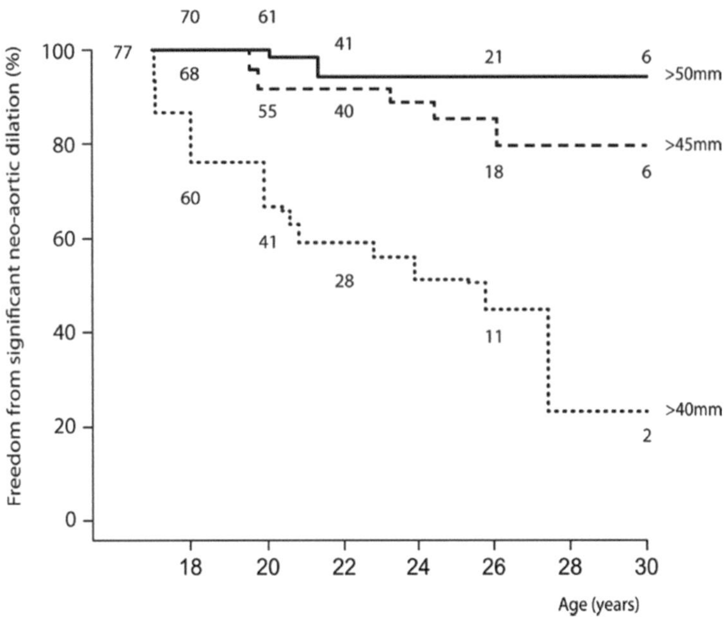

Fig. 19.5 Freedom from neo-aortic dilation. *Bold line*, first neo-aortic measurement >50 mm; *dashed line*, first neo-aortic measurement >45 mm; *dotted line*, first neo-aortic measurement >40 mm; patients with neo-aortic root dilation at baseline were included in the analysis and censored at the age of 17 years (Reprinted with permission from van der Bom T et al. [13])

19.4 Risk Factors for Aortic Dilation and Regurgitation

There are great differences in the baseline and serial changes in aortic diameters among TGA patients [13, 15, 17], and the risk factors for aortic dilation and regurgitation have been extensively analyzed to date. Previous PAB before ASO is a consistently reported risk factor for aortic dilation, while older age at the time of the ASO and the presence of VSD are other risk factors for AR [1].

In 1984, Sievers et al. reported dilation of the aorta and decreased distensibility after two-stage repair (ASO after PAB) in TGA patients [12]. After one-stage ASO became the standard strategy for TGA patients, the contribution of PAB could be analyzed to see if it contributes to the development of aortopathy. PAB has been consistently reported as a strong risk factor for aortic dilation [10, 15, 16, 21]. Existence of a ventricular septal defect (VSD) [15, 16, 21, 22] (hazard ratio (HR) = 2.49 [16]) and Taussig-Bing anomaly [16] have been also reported to be risk factors. By the Kaplan-Meier method, independent predictors of aortic dilation, defined as a neo-aortic root z-score of ≧3.0, were previous PAB (hazard ratio [HR] = 2.4) and ASO performed later (HR = 19.0). The main risk factor identified for at least moderate AR was age ≧1 year at ASO (HR = 5.8), which was closely related to

VSD repair at ASO and previous PAB [15]. Male patients were more prone to greater rates of dilation compared with females in both TOF and TGA [3].

Bicuspid aortic valve is a known underlying disease that causes aortopathy in patients with normal ventriculo-arterial connections. A case has been reported of aortic root dilation and aortic insufficiency due to bicuspid pulmonary (neo-aortic) valve late after the ASO, which required a Bentall procedure [23]. However, the prevalences of AR and aortic reoperation were not particularly high during childhood in the analysis of 40 TGA patients with bicuspid neo-aortic valve; 22 % had aortic root dilation with a bicuspid neo-aortic valve z-score of ≧3.0, and 13 % had significant (mild to moderate) AR at mean follow-up of 7.7 years in an analysis of the 40 patients with a bicuspid pulmonary valve with no significant left ventricular outflow tract obstruction out of 980 neonates who underwent ASO for TGA [9]. Although it seems that bicuspid pulmonary (neo-aortic) valve did not represent a high risk for AR in childhood, a definite conclusion needs to await longer follow-up data. Subaortic LVOTO surgery at the time of ASO was another significant factor for at least moderate AR and a predictor of a shorter time to neo-aortic valve or root surgery (HR 10.9) [15]. Discrepancies in sizes between the aorta and pulmonary artery [24], or between the aortic and pulmonary valves (OR 2.05) [25], have been also reported risk factors for AR. Individual surgeons who performed the ASO had lower risks for aortic root dilation [15], indicating that differences in surgical technique may influence future aortopathy.

There are difficulties in distinguishing true risk factors from confounding factors for the following reasons. First, as with other congenital heart disease, there are many anatomical variations. Second, surgical strategies and timing in TGA patients vary greatly. Third, given the progressive nature of aortopathy, the conclusion of each study may differ due to observational period differences. Only about three decades have passed since the current main strategy of treating ASO with the Lecompte modification [8] was introduced, and thus the current observational period is not enough to conclude lifelong prognosis. Future large-scale prospective accumulation of data using a database would further clarify the risk factors for aortopathy in TGA patients. Assessment of individual genetic backgrounds such as polymorphisms may further clarify detailed individual factors.

19.5 Histological Findings

Cystic medial necrosis is observed in patients undergoing arterial switch operations in both the aorta and pulmonary artery (20 %) in the neonate; therefore, histological aortic abnormalities in TGA are not only induced by surgical insult but are also an intrinsic feature of TGA arteries [1]. This is supported by observations that aortopathy also occurs in TGA patients after the atrial switch operation [26–28], which does not involve manipulating the aorta.

Histologic examination of patients with unrepaired TGA has demonstrated that the pulmonary artery (PA) in TGA shows a very clear trend in loss of actin-positive smooth muscle cells as the patient grows older, which was not observed in the normal PA or aorta or in the aorta in TGA [29]. These results indicate the intrinsic vascular abnormalities in the PA (neo-aorta) in TGA, which may be responsible for the histological characteristics in the neo-aortic root dilation seen in TGA patients after ASO.

19.6 Anatomical Features of TGA After ASO

Comparisons with the Ross operation, which also involves aortic root manipulation and coronary implantation, may be useful to assess the characteristics in TGA after ASO. Development of aortic dilation, AR, and aortic stiffening in TGA patients seems less severe than that seen after the Ross operation, despite the shorter time of pressure load to the pulmonary valve in the systemic circulation in the Ross patients [30]. In ASO, the valve stays in its previous position, and only the great arteries and coronary arteries are transposed. In the Ross procedure, especially with the widely used full-root replacement technique, the entire valve, with the adjacent root tissue, is harvested and translocated to the aortic position and the coronary arteries are reimplanted [30]. A significantly dilated aortic root with z-scores > 3 was observed in 52 % of the Ross patients and 31 % of those with TGA at a median age of 10–11 years [30].

However, the frequency of root aneurysms after ASO seems higher than that after the atrial switch operation in TGA patients [26]. What are the characteristics of the ASO that may affect the neo-aorta? First, the complicated shape of the suture lines, plus the transplanted coronary arteries, and even the Lecompte maneuver itself, can alter the geometry of the neo-aortic root and thus cause neo-aortic AR to develop [25]. Second, the direction of original pulmonary (neo-aortic) valve is toward the original pulmonary artery. After ASO, the original pulmonary (neo-aortic) root is reconnected to the aorta without changing the valve direction toward the original pulmonary artery. Third, the curvature of the aortic arch was significantly steeper in ASO patients; this is more triangular-shaped in TGA compared with the rounded normal arch [11, 31]. These operative and structural features should affect arterial stiffening and the development of aortopathy, as will be discussed in next section.

19.7 Effects of Aortopathy on Left Ventricular and Arterial Function

Aortic dilation, AR, and aortic stiffening [32, 33] develop in TGA patients after ASO. Dilation of the aorta correlates with impaired distensibility [31] and increased stiffness of the aorta. The impairment of arterial distensibility is a known risk factor for cardiovascular morbidity and mortality because of the development of systolic arterial hypertension, premature atherosclerosis, and aneurysm formation [31]. TGA patients (mean age of 14.8 years) showed a progressive decrease of aortic distensibility, reduced left atrial passive emptying fraction, and increased stiffness of the thoracic aorta, indicated by increased pulse wave velocity [31]. This result indicates the close relationship between aortic properties and LV diastolic function.

Distensibility of the aortic wall may cause impaired coronary perfusion or reserve. However, coronary supply-demand balance was preserved in the pediatric ASO patients (age 5–9 years) despite the aortic root dilation and decreased distensibility of the aortic root [34]. Because such assessment is more important in adult patients given the progressive nature of the aortopathy and the increasing risk of coronary disease, future assessment in adults is strongly warranted.

Results on LV function have been inconclusive, with some studies reporting it as normal and some showing impairments. LV performance assessed by tissue Doppler imaging and speckle tracking echocardiography recovers to control values within the first postoperative year [35]. However, at medium-term follow-up (mean age of 12.4 years), there was slightly decreased longitudinal shortening and decreased LV torsion in patients with TGAs, although standard measurements of global ventricular function such as ejection fraction were normal [36]. In contrast, Hui et al. reported impaired LV contractility at medium-term follow-up (mean age of 9.4 years) [37]. They showed not only reduced ejection fraction as measured by the Pombo method but also impaired contractility shown by the stress-velocity relationship [38] ($<$-2SD in 61 % of patients) at baseline [37]. Moreover, dobutamine stress echocardiography unmasked wall motion abnormalities in 74 % of patients. Exercise myocardial perfusion scan showed reversible myocardial perfusion defects in 17 out of 22 patients, which corresponded to segments of hypokinesia as detected by dobutamine stress echocardiography [37]. Although their control group ejection fraction (80 ± 6 %) seems too high and that in TGA (70 ± 6 %) is still within normal range, the stress-velocity relationship, dobutamine stress echocardiography, and exercise studies reliably indicate the suboptimal LV function at rest and reserve function.

How should these inconsistent reports be interpreted? There were considerable differences in the reports with regard to aforementioned background, anatomical characteristics of included patients, evaluation method, and timing of evaluation. Hui et al. identified factors associated with impaired LV contractility: an older age at operation ($p = 0.01$), longer cardiopulmonary bypass ($p = 0.01$), circulatory arrest times ($p = 0.045$), and an unusual coronary artery pattern ($p = 0.059$) [37]. This indicates that individual factors are particularly important in LV function after ASO. Currently, the whole picture of the aortic-LV systolic-diastolic- left atrial functional relationship remains to be further clarified. Future studies are warranted to elucidate the effects of aortopathy on load-insensitive measures of LV contractility, relaxation, stiffness, and LV-arterial coupling.

19.8 Treatment of Aortic Dilation and AR

A few cases of aortic dissection or rupture in TGA patients after ASO have been reported recently [18–20]. Many centers will empirically proceed to surgical intervention when the neo-aortic diameter exceeds a certain limit or when there is severe aortic insufficiency [13]. Neo-aortic root replacements such as root sparing or Bentall procedures were performed at neo-aortic diameters over 50 mm or when severe neo-aortic valve regurgitation was present at lower diameters in one cohort [13]. Serial follow-up is needed to monitor ventricular and arterial conditions.

In Marfan syndrome, losartan, an angiotensin-II receptor-1 blocker, may, according to some studies, be effective in reducing the aortic root dilatation rate [39]. In contrast, there has been no proven medical therapy to prevent or to ameliorate aortopathy in TGA patients. Future studies are warranted to establish effective medical therapies in TGA patients.

19.9 Future Directions

Because disproportionate neo-aortic dilation continues into adulthood [13] and average life expectancy is increasing, further serial follow-up data is needed to clarify the lifelong prognosis in TGA patients. Lifestyle affects arterial functions; the significance of lifestyle in progression of aortopathy should be assessed in future studies. Further refinement of surgical procedures and the establishment of medical therapies to ameliorate aortopathy in TGA patients are also warranted.

19.10 Summary

Aortopathy is a known important sequel in TGA. Generally, aortic dilation progresses, the occurrence of AR increases, and aortic distensibility decreases with age. There are many variances in aortic conditions among TGA patients; some risk factors for aortopathy, such as previous PAB, have been identified. The extent of aortopathy seems related to LV functional abnormalities at rest and during stress. Recently, rupture of the aorta has been reported in patients after ASO. Reoperation for severe aortic dilation and/or severe AR is still needed for a small proportion of patients. Currently, no effective medical therapy has been established to prevent or ameliorate aortopathy in TGA patients.

References

1. Niwa K (2013) Aortopathy in congenital heart disease in adults: aortic dilatation with decreased aortic elasticity that impacts negatively on left ventricular function. Korean Circ J 43(4):215–220. doi:10.4070/kcj.2013.43.4.215
2. Hoffman JI, Kaplan S (2002) The incidence of congenital heart disease. J Am Coll Cardiol 39(12):1890–1900
3. Trippel A, Pallivathukal S, Pfammatter JP, Hutter D, Kadner A, Pavlovic M (2014) Dimensions of the ascending aorta in conotruncal heart defects. Pediatr Cardiol 35(5):831–837. doi:10.1007/s00246-014-0862-1
4. Villafane J, Lantin-Hermoso MR, Bhatt AB, Tweddell JS, Geva T, Nathan M, Elliott MJ, Vetter VL, Paridon SM, Kochilas L, Jenkins KJ, Beekman RH 3rd, Wernovsky G, Towbin JA (2014) D-transposition of the great arteries: the current era of the arterial switch operation. J Am Coll Cardiol 64(5):498–511. doi:10.1016/j.jacc.2014.06.1150
5. Marino BS, Wernovsky G, McElhinney DB, Jawad A, Kreb DL, Mantel SF, van der Woerd WL, Robbers-Visser D, Novello R, Gaynor JW, Spray TL, Cohen MS (2006) Neo-aortic valvar function after the arterial switch. Cardiol Young 16(5):481–489. doi:10.1017/s1047951106000953
6. Yurasek GK, Gauvreau K, Powell AJ, Geva T, Brown DW (2014) Great vessel root and artery dimensions in transposition of the great arteries repaired with atrial switch operation. Pediatr Cardiol 35(3):457–462. doi:10.1007/s00246-013-0800-7
7. Jatene AD, Fontes VF, Paulista PP, Souza LC, Neger F, Galantier M, Sousa JE (1976) Anatomic correction of transposition of the great vessels. J Thorac Cardiovasc Surg 72(3): 364–370
8. Lecompte Y, Zannini L, Hazan E, Jarreau MM, Bex JP, Tu TV, Neveux JY (1981) Anatomic correction of transposition of the great arteries. J Thorac Cardiovasc Surg 82(4):629–631
9. Angeli E, Gerelli S, Beyler C, Lamerain M, Rochas B, Bonnet D, Vouhe P, Raisky O (2012) Bicuspid pulmonary valve in transposition of the great arteries: impact on outcome. Eur J Cardiothorac Surg 41(2):248–255. doi:10.1016/j.ejcts.2011.03.063
10. Hourihan M, Colan SD, Wernovsky G, Maheswari U, Mayer JE Jr, Sanders SP (1993) Growth of the aortic anastomosis, annulus, and root after the arterial switch procedure performed in infancy. Circulation 88(2):615–620
11. Ntsinjana HN, Capelli C, Biglino G, Cook AC, Tann O, Derrick G, Taylor AM, Schievano S (2014) 3D morphometric analysis of the arterial switch operation using in vivo MRI data. Clin Anat (New York, NY) 27(8):1212–1222. doi:10.1002/ca.22458
12. Sievers HH, Lange PE, Arensman FW, Radley-Smith R, Yacoub MH, Harms D, Heintzen PH, Bernhard A (1984) Influence of two-stage anatomic correction on size and distensibility of the anatomic pulmonary/functional aortic root in patients with simple transposition of the great arteries. Circulation 70(2):202–208
13. van der Bom T, van der Palen RL, Bouma BJ, van Veldhuisen SL, Vliegen HW, Konings TC, Zwinderman AH, Blom NA, Koolbergen DR, Hazekamp MG, Mulder BJ (2014) Persistent neo-aortic growth during adulthood in patients after an arterial switch operation. Heart 100 (17):1360–1365. doi:10.1136/heartjnl-2014-305702
14. Co-Vu JG, Ginde S, Bartz PJ, Frommelt PC, Tweddell JS, Earing MG (2013) Long-term outcomes of the neoaorta after arterial switch operation for transposition of the great arteries. Ann Thorac Surg 95(5):1654–1659. doi:10.1016/j.athoracsur.2012.10.081
15. Schwartz ML, Gauvreau K, del Nido P, Mayer JE, Colan SD (2004) Long-term predictors of aortic root dilation and aortic regurgitation after arterial switch operation. Circulation 110 (11 Suppl 1):II128–II132. doi:10.1161/01.CIR.0000138392.68841.d3
16. McMahon CJ, Ravekes WJ, Smith EO, Denfield SW, Pignatelli RH, Altman CA, Ayres NA (2004) Risk factors for neo-aortic root enlargement and aortic regurgitation following arterial switch operation. Pediatr Cardiol 25(4):329–335. doi:10.1007/s00246-003-0483-6

17. Hutter PA, Thomeer BJ, Jansen P, Hitchcock JF, Faber JA, Meijboom EJ, Bennink GB (2001) Fate of the aortic root after arterial switch operation. Eur J Cardiothorac Surg 20(1):82–88
18. Frischhertz BP, Shamszad P, Pedroza C, Milewicz DM, Morris SA (2015) Thoracic aortic dissection and rupture in conotruncal cardiac defects: a population-based study. Int J Cardiol 184:521–527. doi:10.1016/j.ijcard.2015.03.061
19. Sharma R, Cohen B, Peters P, Shah P (2013) Aortic valve-sparing in aortic dissection with transposition of great arteries. Asian Cardiovasc Thorac Ann 21(2):202–204. doi:10.1177/0218492312449753
20. Shamszad P, Barnes JN, Morris SA (2014) Aortic dissection in hospitalized children and young adults: a multiinstitutional study. Congenit Heart Dis 9(1):54–62. doi:10.1111/chd.12090
21. Delmo Walter EM, Huebler M, Alexi-Meshkishvili V, Sill B, Berger F, Hetzer R (2010) Fate of the aortic valve following the arterial switch operation. J Card Surg 25(6):730–736. doi:10.1111/j.1540-8191.2010.01144.x
22. Bove T, De Meulder F, Vandenplas G, De Groote K, Panzer J, Suys B, DeWolf D, Francois K (2008) Midterm assessment of the reconstructed arteries after the arterial switch operation. Ann Thorac Surg 85(3):823–830. doi:10.1016/j.athoracsur.2007.10.043
23. Bobylev D, Breymann T, Boethig D, Ono M (2013) Aortic root replacement in a patient with bicuspid pulmonary valve late after arterial switch operation. Thorac Cardiovasc Surg 61(4):316–319. doi:10.1055/s-0032-1328933
24. Lim HG, Kim WH, Lee JR, Kim YJ (2013) Long-term results of the arterial switch operation for ventriculo-arterial discordance. Eur J Cardiothorac Surg 43(2):325–334. doi:10.1093/ejcts/ezs264
25. Michalak KW, Moll JA, Moll M, Dryzek P, Moszura T, Kopala M, Mludzik K, Moll JJ (2013) The neoaortic root in children with transposition of the great arteries after an arterial switch operation. Eur J Cardiothorac Surg 43(6):1101–1108. doi:10.1093/ejcts/ezs709
26. Ono M, Goerler H, Boethig D, Westhoff-Bleck M, Hartung D, Breymann T (2007) Valve-sparing operation for aortic root aneurysm late after Mustard procedure. Ann Thorac Surg 83(6):2224–2226. doi:10.1016/j.athoracsur.2006.12.043
27. Rutz T, Max F, Wahl A, Wustmann K, Khattab K, Pfammatter JP, Kadner A, Schwerzmann M (2012) Distensibility and diameter of ascending aorta assessed by cardiac magnetic resonance imaging in adults with tetralogy of fallot or complete transposition. Am J Cardiol 110(1):103–108. doi:10.1016/j.amjcard.2012.02.055
28. Ladouceur M, Kachenoura N, Lefort M, Redheuil A, Bonnet D, Celermajer DS, Iserin L, Mousseaux E (2013) Structure and function of the ascending aorta in palliated transposition of the great arteries. Int J Cardiol 165(3):458–462. doi:10.1016/j.ijcard.2011.08.847
29. Lalezari S, Hazekamp MG, Bartelings MM, Schoof PH, Gittenberger-De Groot AC (2003) Pulmonary artery remodeling in transposition of the great arteries: relevance for neoaortic root dilatation. J Thorac Cardiovasc Surg 126(4):1053–1060. doi:10.1016/S0022
30. Pees C, Laufer G, Michel-Behnke I (2013) Similarities and differences of the aortic root after arterial switch and ross operation in children. Am J Cardiol 111(1):125–130. doi:10.1016/j.amjcard.2012.08.059
31. Voges I, Jerosch-Herold M, Hedderich J, Hart C, Petko C, Scheewe J, Andrade AC, Pham M, Gabbert D, Kramer HH, Rickers C (2013) Implications of early aortic stiffening in patients with transposition of the great arteries after arterial switch operation. Circ Cardiovasc Imaging 6(2):245–253. doi:10.1161/circimaging.112.000131
32. Murakami T, Nakazawa M, Momma K, Imai Y (2000) Impaired distensibility of neoaorta after arterial switch procedure. Ann Thorac Surg 70(6):1907–1910
33. Chen RH, Wong SJ, Wong WH, Cheung YF (2014) Arterial mechanics at rest and during exercise in adolescents and young adults after arterial switch operation for complete transposition of the great arteries. Am J Cardiol 113(4):713–718. doi:10.1016/j.amjcard.2013.10.050

34. Murakami T, Takei K, Ueno M, Takeda A, Yakuwa S, Nakazawa M (2008) Aortic reservoir function after arterial switch operation in elementary school-aged children. Circ J 72(8): 1291–1295
35. Klitsie LM, Roest AA, Kuipers IM, Hazekamp MG, Blom NA, Ten Harkel AD (2014) Left and right ventricular performance after arterial switch operation. J Thorac Cardiovasc Surg 147(5): 1561–1567. doi:10.1016/j.jtcvs.2013.07.048
36. Pettersen E, Fredriksen PM, Urheim S, Thaulow E, Smith HJ, Smevik B, Smiseth O, Andersen K (2009) Ventricular function in patients with transposition of the great arteries operated with arterial switch. Am J Cardiol 104(4):583–589. doi:10.1016/j.amjcard.2009.04.029
37. Hui L, Chau AK, Leung MP, Chiu CS, Cheung YF (2005) Assessment of left ventricular function long term after arterial switch operation for transposition of the great arteries by dobutamine stress echocardiography. Heart 91(1):68–72. doi:10.1136/hrt.2003.027524
38. Colan SD, Borow KM, Neumann A (1984) Left ventricular end-systolic wall stress-velocity of fiber shortening relation: a load-independent index of myocardial contractility. J Am Coll Cardiol 4(4):715–724
39. Groenink M, den Hartog AW, Franken R, Radonic T, de Waard V, Timmermans J, Scholte AJ, van den Berg MP, Spijkerboer AM, Marquering HA, Zwinderman AH, Mulder BJ (2013) Losartan reduces aortic dilatation rate in adults with Marfan syndrome: a randomized controlled trial. Eur Heart J 34(45):3491–3500. doi:10.1093/eurheartj/eht334

Chapter 20
The Fontan Operation

Hideo Ohuchi

Abstract Aortopathy has been recognized as one of the major pathophysiologic features in patients with congenital heart disease (CHD) that includes dilatation and/or increased stiffness of the aorta. A body of evidence of "aortopathy" has been also reported in patients after the Fontan operation and most of studies had focused on the dilated stiffened ascending aorta (aAO). In general, Fontan patients have dilated aAO with smaller descending aorta (dAO) and the other peripheral arteries, including carotid artery, indicating vascular remodeling. However, these features of aAO and dAO may be different from those in Fontan patients with hypoplastic left heart syndrome (HLHS) who have dilated dAO. In non-HLHS Fontan patients, stiffened aAO itself is considered as one of the causes for progressive dilatation of the aorta. In addition to aging, body size, and late first Fontan operation, impaired glucose tolerance, diminished nitric oxide bioavailability, and inflammation are also thought to be additional risk factors for the stiffened aorta, and most of those factors are determinants of endothelial function. An increased pulse pressure due to the stiffened aorta leads to ventricular pressure overload as well as low perfusion for the coronary circulation and ultimately may result in systemic ventricular dysfunction, especially in Fontan patients with the non-left ventricular morphologic ventricle as a systemic ventricle. Furthermore, the dilated stiffened aorta is detrimental to cardiovascular response and exercise capacity in these patients. Thus, prospective study to establish therapeutic strategy for "aortopathy" may be needed to improve long-term outcome of these vulnerable patients.

Keywords Fontan • Aortopathy • Arterial stiffness • Pulse wave velocity • Augmentation index

---

H. Ohuchi (✉)
Departments of Pediatric Cardiology and Adult Congenital Heart Disease, National Cerebral and Cardiovascular Center, 5-7-1 Fujishirodai, Suita, Osaka 565-8565, Japan
e-mail: hohuchi@ncvc.go.jp

K. Niwa, H. Kaemmerer (eds.), *Aortopathy*, DOI 10.1007/978-4-431-56071-5_20

20.1 Introduction

Elastic property of the great arteries, such as ascending aorta (aAO), is important for cardiovascular system [1, 2] and deteriorates as human ages [3, 4]. Stiff great arteries are also demonstrated in a variety of patients, including those with cardiovascular and pulmonary diseases [5–7] as well as those with impaired glucose tolerance [8]. In addition to intrinsic histological changes, inflammation [9, 10] and diminished availability of nitric oxide [11, 12] are believed to be involved in the aortic stiffness. Along with adverse influence on coronary flow [1], stiff aorta has adverse impact on exercise capacity and renal function [13, 14] and has prognostic power in some cardiac patients [15].

Dilated aAO and its progression over time have been also recognized as one of characteristics in CHD patients, especially those with tetralogy of Fallot [16–18]. Progression of aortic valve regurgitation and aortic dissection during pregnancy are additional concerns in adult CHD patients. In addition, dilated aAO has decreased distensibility, and the increased stiffness itself may be responsible for the progressive dilatation. The aortic pathophysiology is now widely recognized as "aortopathy" in patients with CHD.

According to these backgrounds, there have been growing evidences of "aortopathy" in patients after the Fontan operation. However, most of them have focused on "aortopathy" in patients with hypoplastic left heart syndrome (HLHS) [19–21] that is one of specific subtypes of Fontan circulation where arch reconstruction is frequently required that might modify the aortopathy, while there have been, so far, a few studies of aortopathy in the other majority of Fontan patients [22–27]. Because long survivors of the Fontan operation have unsatisfied clinical complications with time [28], clinical researchers have drawn attention to the aortopathy as one of the causes for the late complications, and recent studies have established an evidence of the dilated and stiffened aAO in Fontan patients although the detailed pathophysiology of aortopathy is still scarce.

This chapter reviews growing evidences of aortopathy in a majority of Fontan patients without HLHS (see chapter of aortopathy in HLHS).

20.2 Previous Reports

Studies addressing aortopathy in Fontan patients, mainly focusing on non-HLHS patients, are summarized in Tables 20.1 and 20.2.

Table 20.1 Studies of aortopathy in patients after Fontan operation

References	First author	Journal	Year	Design	n	Age	BMI	Male (%)	Diagnosis	APC/ TCPC	NYHA	Peak VO2	ACEI/ ARB	ß	Diuretics
[24]	Myers KA	JASE	2013	Fontan	22	14.9 (7.6–18.7)	19.5 (15.0–25.7)	–	TA(8), PA/IVS(4), CAVC(6), UVH(4)	NA	NA	–	64 %	18 %	5 %
				Control	23	15.2 (7.6–18.3)	18.9 (13.0–36.6)	–	Healthy	–	–	–	–	–	–
[23]	Lambert E	Int J Cardiol	2013	Fontan	18	25±1	25±1	44	TA(4), DILV(8), CAVC(2), MA(1), other(2)	9/9	NA	–	94 %	39 %	11 %
				Control	23	23±1	24±1	35	Healthy	–	–	–	–	–	–
[22]	Sarkola T	Heart & Vessel	2013	Fontan	28	14.8±1.3	20.4±3.1	54	SV(12), PA(11), HLHS(5)	0/28	NA	67±14(%)	50 %	13 %	NA
				Control	54	14.8±1.6	21.3±3.8	63	Healthy	–	–		–	–	–
[25]	Tomkiewicz-Pajak L	CV Ultrasound	2014	Fontan	25	24.7±6.2	21.7±2	56	TA(12), PA/IVS/TGA(8), DILV(3), DORV(2)	2/23	15/18/2	–	12 %	–	NA
				Control	25	26.9±3.4	22.6±3	60	Healthy	–	–	–	–	–	–
[30]	Kojima T, et al.	Circ J	2014	Dilated	6/31	3.5±0.7	–	58	UVH(21), PA/IVS(6), DORV (3), TA(1)	0/6	NA	–	32 %	33 %	–
				Non-dilated	6/25	4.5±0.7	–	58	UVH(15), PA/IVS(5), DORV (3), TA(2)	0/6	NA	–	7 %	26 %	–
[35]	Saiki H	Ann Thrasic Surg	2014	Fontan	34	11.5±8.6	–	47	NA	NA	NA	–	NA	NA	NA
				Control	20	13.4±6.0	–	60	PVC/IM/ASD/VSD	–	–	–	NA	NA	NA
[26]	Muller J	Int J Cardiol	2015	Fontan	87	23.9±10.5	21.9±5.0	57	NA	NA	NA	71.2±18.4 (%)	34 %	10 %	NA
				Control	322	29.4±18.4	23.0±4.4	49	Healthy	–	–	–	8 %	20 %	NA
[27]	Bhat DP	Pediatr Cardiol	2015	Fontan	22	13.1±4.2	22.4±6.6	50	LV-SV(12), HLHS(10)	0/22	NA	–	41 %	NA	NA
				Control	22	13.8±2.6	21.6±4.3	68	Healthy	–	–	–	–	–	–
[29]	Ohuchi H	Int Heart J	2017	Fontan	130	18±8	19±4	61	UVH(40), TA(31), DORV (23), MA(14), others	10/120	78/42/10	54±11(%)	33 %	28 %	65 %
				Control	36	16±6	20±3	50	VSD(29), PDA(7)	–	–	–	–	–	–

ACEI angiotensin-converting enzyme inhibitor, *ARB* angiotensin receptor blocker, *APC* atriopulmonary connection, *ASD* atrial septal defect, *BMI* body mass index, *ß* beta-blocker, *CAVC* common atrioventricular cannel, *DILV* double inlet left ventricle, *DORV* double outlet right ventricle, *HLHS* hypoplastic left heart syndrome, *IM* innocent murmur, *LV-SV* left ventricular-type systemic ventricle, *MA* mitral atresia, *NA* not available, *NYHA* New York Heart Association, *PA/IVS* pulmonary atresia with intact ventricular septum, *PDA* patent ductus arteriosus, *PVC* premature ventricular contraction, *SV* systemic ventricle, *TA* tricuspid atresia, *TCPC* total cavopulmonary connection, *TGA* transposition of the great arteries, *UVH* univentricular heart, VO_2 oxygen uptake, *VSD* ventricular septal defect

Table 20.2 Aortopathy-associated variables in patients after Fontan operation

	Cardiovascular variables				Aortic dimensions				Aortopathy variables							
References	HR	SBP	DBP	PP	aAO	CCA	dAO	aAO/dAO	PWV	AI	aAO SI ß	CCA SI ß	dAO SI ß	aAO/dAO SI ß	TAC	CCA compliance
[24]	74(49–96)	105 (82–140)	66(45–80)	38.5 (29–68)	–	–	–	–	4.88 (3.58–9.94) ***	–	4.15 (1.79–14.4) *	–	–	–	1.29 (0.70–3.33)	–
	72 (55–114)	107 (93–135)	64(41–74)	45 (30–73)	–	–	–	–	3.64 (2.68–4.85)	–	3.04 (1.56–5.68)	–	–	–	1.32 (0.74–4.25)	–
[23]	63±2	109±2	67±2	–	–	–	–	–	6.01±0.23	4.93±2.4†***	–	–	–	–	–	–
	70±3*	117±2*	65±2	–	–	–	–	–	5.82±0.46	–9.81±2.27†	–	–	–	–	–	–
[22]	–	101±10*	53±9	–	–	5.02±0.51**	11.2±2.7	–	5.2±1.1 (7.4±1.7)**	–	–	3.85±0.95	3.58±2.23	–	–	–
	–	107±9	53±6	–	–	5.36±0.44	11.9±2.2	–	5.0±1.0 (6.3±1.0)	–	–	4.29±1.12	3.18±1.05	–	–	–
[25]	64.8±12.6	127.2±13.9	79.4±7.3	–	–	–	–	–	7.81±1.0	17.01±3.3***	–	–	–	–	–	–
	68.9±16.2	124±10.6	77.7±5.2	–	–	–	–	–	7.91±0.8	6.05±11	–	–	–	–	–	–
[30]		92.6±2.7	56.7±2.7	–	171±3(%)	–	–	–	4.84±0.1**	–	–	–	–	–	–	–
		87.2±2.7	58.0±3.4	–	126±3(%)	–	–	–	3.94±0.1	–	–	–	–	–	–	–
[35]	81±19*	101±10**	57±10	–	–	–	–	–	3.90±0.08*	–	–	–	–	–	–	1.25±0.07*
	71±13	109±13	59±8	–	–	–	–	–	3.56±0.10	–	–	–	–	–	–	1.51±0.09
[26]	–	123.5±11.8	70.6±11.3	–	–	–	–	–	–	16.2±8.6**	–	–	–	–	–	–
	–	125±13.2	67.3±11.1	–	–	–	–	–	–	14.2±10.6	–	–	–	–	–	–
[27]	–	88±28**	74±12**	–	–	–	–	–	–	16(5.2–20.8) †***	–	–	–	–	–	–
	–	114±8	64±5	–	–	–	–	–	–	–1.5 (–67.6–3.3)†	–	–	–	–	–	–
[29]	82±15	106±8	66±9***	37±9*	17.4±4.5**	–	8.5±1.3**	1.9±0.3***	–	–	3.2±0.7***	–	2.7±0.6***	1.2±0.3***	–	–
	–	106±13	74±8	32±7	15.1±2.1	–	9.9±1.2	1.5±0.2	–	–	2.2±0.3	–	2.2±0.3	1.0±0.1	–	–

aAO ascending aorta, *AI* augmentation index, *CCA* common carotid artery, *dAO* descending aorta, *aAO/dAO* ratio of aAO to dAO, *DSP* diastolic blood pressure, *HR* heart rate, *PP* pulse pressure, *PWV* pulse wave velocity, *SBP* systolic blood pressure, *SI* stiffness index (ß), *TAC* total aortic compliance, *2DE* two-dimensional echocardiography, † indicates AI normalized for a HR of 75

*, **, and *** indicate $p < 0.05$, <0.01, and <0.001, vs. control group, respectively

20.2.1 Aortic Size

Prevalence of abnormally dilated aAO is unknown although the pathophysiology may be clinically relevant. In our recent consecutive 130 patients, prevalence of the dilated aAO (standardized by body surface area) with $\geq$ 1SD and $\geq$ 2SD was 46.9 % (n = 61) and 26.2 % (n = 34), respectively. Standardized aAO tended to be larger in Fontan with non-left ventricular morphology as a systemic ventricle than those with left ventricle as a systemic ventricle (106 $\pm$ 18 % vs. 113 $\pm$ 24 %, p = 0.051). There have been no data on the determinants of dilated aAO in these patients. In our series, age, body mass index, and cardiac index were closely associated with standardized diameters of the aAO [29].

20.2.2 Aortic Geometry

Clinical relevance of aortic arch geometry has been studied in patients after repair of coarctation of the aorta in terms of the association with systemic hypertension, especially during exercise [30], and there have been few studies addressing impact of aAO shape abnormality on exercise physiology in the other type of CHD. In our 130 patients, greater difference in aortic size between aAO and descending aorta (dAO), i.e., aAO/dAO ratio, was greater in the Fontan patients and was predictive of impaired response of systolic blood pressure during exercise (Fig. 20.1, [29]). In addition, diameter of the dAO was significantly smaller than that of the aAO and was correlated with the cardiac output.

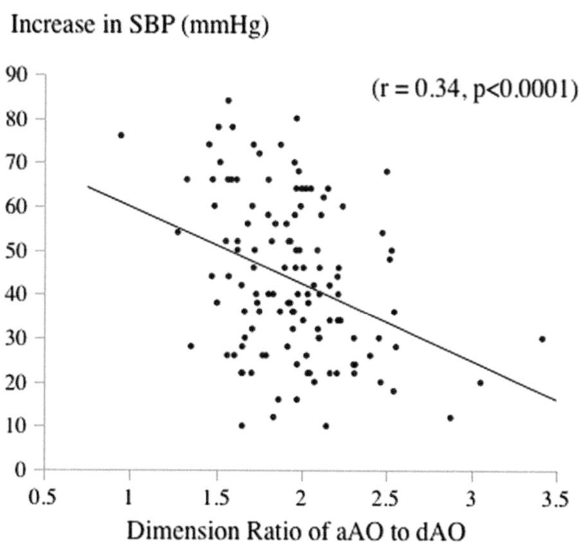

Fig. 20.1 Impact of aortic size ratio of ascending aorta (aAO) to descending aorta (dAO) on increase in systolic blood pressure (SBP) from rest to peak exercise

Morphology and even function of small arteries and veins can be evaluated by high-resolution ultrasound owing to recent advances of medical modalities. According to studies using very high-resolution ultrasound, adventitial thickness of the common carotid, brachial, radial, ulnar, femoral, and dorsal tibial arteries was thinner, and intima-media thickness of the cubital and tibial veins was also thinner in 28 Fontan patients (age, 14.8 ± 1.3) than in 54 age-matched controls, demonstrating vascular remodeling in Fontan patients [22]. Given that significant small dAO in our patients, low perfusion flow-associated vascular remodeling may exist in most parts of systemic arteries, except for dilated aAO, in the majority of non-HLHS Fontan patients.

20.2.3 Aortic Stiffness and Its Determinants

Several studies demonstrated stiffened aAO in Fontan patients. Kojima et al. demonstrated that pulse wave velocity (PWV) in the aorta was faster in patients with single ventricle with abnormally dilated aAO than in those without dilatation although the study included non-Fontan patients, and they speculated that the increased stiffness of the aAO was one of the determinants of the dilatation [31]. On the other hand, in adult Fontan patients, the augmentation index (AI), normalized by heart rate of the central and digital aorta, was greater in the Fontan patients than in the controls [23], although there was no difference in PWV between Fontan patients (n=18) and healthy controls. Myers et al. demonstrated that PWV and stiffness index were higher in 22 children and adolescent with Fontan circulation than in healthy controls although there was no difference in the total aortic compliance [24]. Tomkiewicz-Pajak et al. also demonstrated significantly higher AI in young adult Fontan patients (n=25) than in controls [25]. According to the study, hypoxia was an independent predictor of PWV although, again, no difference in PWV between the Fontan patients and controls was observed, indicating that hypoxia as well as arterial volume overload during the pre-Fontan period has an adverse impact on aortic distensibility. Furthermore, Muller et al. showed that Fontan circulation (n=87) itself was an independent predictor of high AI, i.e., stiffened aorta, in a large cohort of adolescent and young adult CHD (n=1125) [26]. This study also showed the other determinants of high AI that included older age, low body height, low heart rate, low exercise capacity, and no use of angiotensin-converting enzyme inhibitors. On the other hand, Bhat et al. showed high AI in 22 Fontan patients; however, history of arch repair, use of angiotensin-converting enzyme inhibitors, or systemic ventricular morphology had no impact on AI although the study included HLHS patients [27].

When compared with control subjects, stiffness index was higher in both aAO and dAO and stiffness was significantly higher in the aAO than in the dAO [29]. Interestingly, in addition to late age at Fontan operation, aAO stiffness was closely associated with plasma levels of brain natriuretic peptide, asymmetric dimethylarginine (naturally occurring amino acid that inhibits forms of nitric oxide synthase), and fasting glucose (Fig. 20.2, [29]). As for adverse impact of

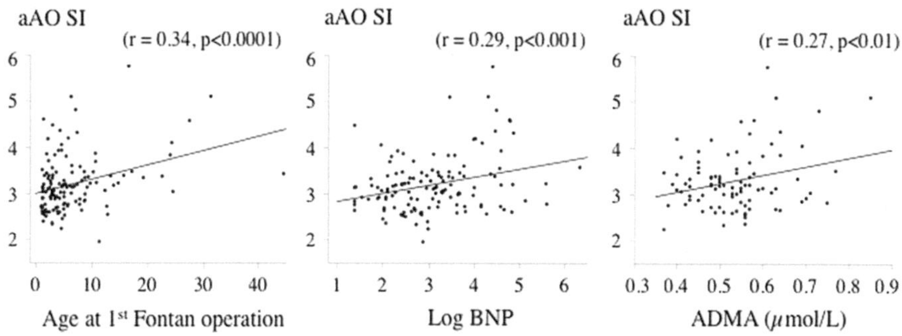

Fig. 20.2 Correlations between age at first Fontan operation, plasma levels of brain natriuretic peptide (BNP) and asymmetric dimethylarginine (ADMA), and stiffness index of the ascending AO (aAO SI)

late Fontan operation on aortic distensibility, as described in the study of Tomkiewicz-Pajak et al. [25], long-standing hypoxia and arterial volume overload may be responsible for the stiffened aorta probably, in part, due to endothelial dysfunction [32] because of independent association of aAO stiffness index with plasma levels of asymmetric dimethylarginine [29], implying diminished nitric oxide bioavailability. Furthermore, impaired glucose tolerance may also have negative impact on aortic distensibility in Fontan patients [29] as demonstrated in general population and non-CHD adults with cardiovascular disease [8].

Plasma levels of high sensitive C-reactive protein (hs-CRP) are associated with reduced aortic distensibility in the general population and in those with metabolic syndrome [9, 33], and acute inflammation actually decreases aortic distensibility [10]. Chronic inflammation may be also associated with reduced aortic distensibility in Fontan patients [29]. Plasma levels of hs-CRP and cytokines, such as interleukin-6, are increased in patients with heart failure [34] that is shared with Fontan pathophysiology with elevated sympathetic activity [23].

20.3 Clinical Relevance of Aortic Distensibility

20.3.1 Systemic Ventricular Function

PWV increases as the aorta stiffens so that aortic reflection waves can quickly return and reach the systemic ventricle even during systole, resulting in augmentation of the systolic pressure with lower diastolic pressure, i.e., increased pulse pressure [1, 2]. Thus, additional pressure load to the systemic ventricle may lead to ventricular dysfunction, especially if the morphologic right ventricle performs as a systemic ventricle. At the same time, low diastolic pressure of the aAO reduces the coronary flow [1]. Significant association of a high aAO stiffness index with high plasma levels of brain natriuretic peptide may support this concept [29].

20.3.2 *Exercise Physiology*

There have been several studies addressing impact of stiffened aorta on exercise capacity [9, 10], and the same story may hold true in Fontan patients, as demonstrated by Müller et al. and ours [26, 29]. Müller et al. demonstrated that higher AI was associated with lower peak oxygen uptake (VO_2), and our data showed that increased stiffness index of the aAO and dAO predicted lower peak VO_2 (Fig. 20.3). Possible mechanisms of the adverse impact of stiffened aorta on exercise capacity are, in part, due to pressure load to the systemic ventricle and reduced coronary flow during exercise. In addition, aortic shape, i.e., dilated aAO with small dAO, may be also detrimental to organ perfusion during exercise because of the impaired increase in blood pressure [29]. Thus, stiffened dilated aAO may be associated with low perfusion of multiple organs, ultimately resulting in progressive deterioration of multi-organ functions in the long-term postoperative period.

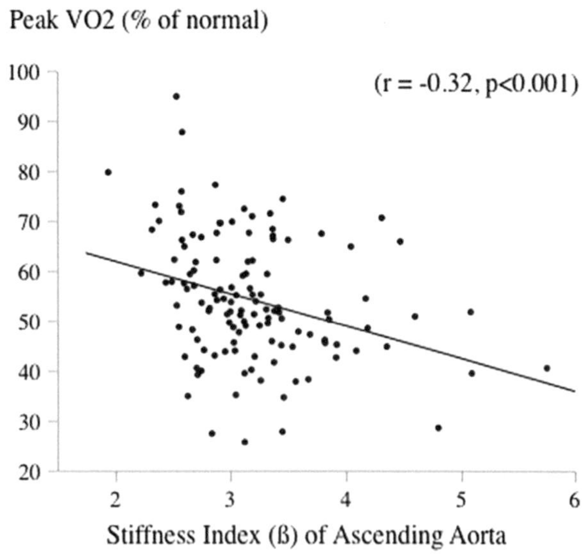

Fig. 20.3 Impact of ascending aortic stiffness on % predicted peak oxygen uptake (VO2) in patients after the Fontan operation

20.3.3 Renal Function

Stiffened aorta, especially the dAO, is closely associated with renal function [29]. The association with body mass index and hs-CRP implies that acquired pathological alternations, such as metabolic syndrome and heart failure, along with the intrinsic histological changes, may play a significant role for the progression of aortopathy and the related organ dysfunction, including renal dysfunction.

20.3.4 Aortic Dissection

Aortic dissection was reported in HLHS Fontan patient with extremely dilated aortic root (78 mm in diameter) and severe aortic valve regurgitation [35].

20.3.5 Cerebral Circulation

Carotid artery is also stiffer in children with Fontan circulation than in controls. Together with high central venous pressure, the stiffened carotid artery may be responsible for impaired cerebral perfusion in these patients [36], and this pathophysiology may be associated with a negative neurodevelopmental outcome.

20.4 Future Perspectives

Robust evidences of the dilated and stiffened aorta are emerging in patients after the Fontan operation. Some of these etiologies are intrinsic in nature; however, traditional risk factors, such as heart failure and metabolic factors, are now being recognized as significant additional contributors to Fontan "aortopathy." Thus, there is significant room for potential therapeutic strategies to improve long-term outcome of these patients. Prospective studies aiming at modifying risk factors, such as obesity, impaired glucose intolerance, and chronic inflammation, are required in the near future.

References

1. Nichols WW, O'Rourke MF (1998) Vascular impedance. In: McDonald's blood flow in arteries: theoretical, experimental and clinical principles, 4th ed. Edward Arnold, London, pp 54–97, 243–283, 347–395

2. Safar ME, Toto-Moukouo JJ, Bouthier JA, Asmar RE, Levenson JA, Simon AC et al (1987) Arterial dynamics, cardiac hypertrophy, and antihypertensive treatment. Circulation 75:1156–1161
3. Senzaki H, Akagi M, Hishi T, Ishizawa A, Yanagisawa M, Masutani S et al (2002) Age-associated changes in arterial elastic properties in children. Eur J Pediatr 161:547–551
4. Lakatta EG, Levy D (2003) Arterial and cardiac aging: major shareholders in cardiovascular disease enterprises: part I: aging arteries: a "set up" for vascular disease. Circulation 107:139–146
5. Blacher J, Guerin AP, Pannier B, Marchais SJ, Safar ME, London GM (1999) Impact of aortic stiffness on survival in end-stage renal disease. Circulation 99:2434–2439
6. Schillaci G, Pirro M, Mannarino MR, Pucci G, Savarese G, Franklin SS et al (2006) Relation between renal function within the normal range and central and peripheral arterial stiffness in hypertension. Hypertension 48:616–621
7. Sabit R, Bolton CE, Edwards PH, Pettit RJ, Evans WD, McEniery CM et al (2007) Arterial stiffness and osteoporosis in chronic obstructive pulmonary disease. Am J Respir Crit Care Med 175:1259–1265
8. Henry RMA, Kostense PJ, Spijkerman AMW, Decker JM, Nijpels G, Heine RJ et al (2003) Arterial stiffness increases with deteriorating glucose tolerance status: the Hoorn Study. Circulation 107:2089–2095
9. Yasmin Y, CM ME, Wallace S, IS M, JR C, IB W (2004) C-reactive protein is associated with arterial stiffness in apparently healthy individuals. Arterioscler Thromb Vasc Biol 24:969–974
10. Vlachopoulos C, Dima I, Aznaouridis K, Vasiliadou C, Ioakeimidis N, Aggeli C et al (2005) Acute systemic inflammation increases arterial stiffness and decreases wave reflections in healthy individuals. Circulation 112:2193–2200
11. Ramsey MW, Goodfellow J, Jones CJ, Luddington LA, Lewis MJ, Henderson AH (1995) Endothelial control of arterial distensibility is impaired in chronic heart failure. Circulation 92:3212–3219
12. Wilkinson IB, Qasem A, McEniery CM, Webb DJ, Avolio AP, Cockcroft JR (2002) Nitric oxide regulates local arterial distensibility in vivo. Circulation 105:213–217
13. Vaitkevicius PV, Fleg JL, Engel JH, O'Connor FC, Wright JG, Lakatta LE et al (1993) Effects of age and aerobic capacity on arterial stiffness in healthy adults. Circulation 88(part 1):1456–1462
14. Bonapace S, Rossi A, Cicoira M, Franceschini L, Golia G, Zanolla L et al (2003) Aortic distensibility independently affects exercise tolerance in patients with dilated cardiomyopathy. Circulation 107:1603–1608
15. Laurent S, Boutouyrie P, Asmar R, Gautier I, Laloux B, Guize L et al (2001) Aortic stiffness is an independent predictor of all-cause and cardiovascular mortality in hypertensive patients. Hypertension 37:1236–1241
16. Niwa K, Perloff JK, Bhuta SM, Laks H, Drinkwater DC, Child JS et al (2001) Structural abnormalities of great arterial walls in congenital heart disease: light and electron microscopic analyses. Circulation 103:393–400
17. Chong WY, Wong WH, Chiu CS, Cheung YF (2006) Aortic root dilation and aortic elastic properties in children after repair of tetralogy of Fallot. Am J Cardiol 97:905–909
18. Yetman AT, Graham T (2009) The dilated aorta in patients with congenital cardiac defects. J Am Coll Cardiol 53:461–467
19. Cardis BM, Fyfe DA, Mahle WT (2006) Elastic properties of the reconstructed aorta in hypoplastic left heart syndrome. Ann Thorac Surg 81:988–991
20. Schlangen J, Fischer G, Petko C, Hansen JH, Voges I, Rickers C, Kramer HH, Uebing A (2013) Arterial elastance and its impact on intrinsic right ventricular function in palliated hypoplastic left heart syndrome. Int J Cardiol 168:5385–5389
21. Voges I, Jerosch-Herold M, Wegner P, Hart C, Gabbert D, Al Bulushi A, Fischer G, Andrade AC, Pham HM, Kristo I, Kramer HH, Rickers C (2015) Frequent dilatation of the descending

aorta in children with hypoplastic left heart syndrome relates to decreased aortic arch elasticity. J Am Heart Assoc 4:e002107. doi:10.1161/JAHA.115.002107
22. Sarkola T, Jaeggi E, Slorach C, Hui W, Bradley T, Redington AN (2013) Assessment of vascular remodeling after the Fontan procedure using a novel very high resolution ultrasound method: arterial wall thinning and venous thickening in late follow-up. Heart Vessel 28:66–75
23. Lambert E, d'Udekem Y, Cheung M, Sari CI, Inman J, Ahimastos A, Eikelis N, Pathak A, King I, Grigg L, Schlaich M, Lambert G (2013) Sympathetic and vascular dysfunction in adult patients with Fontan circulation. Int J Cardiol 167:1333–1338
24. Myers KA, Leung MT, Terri Potts M, Potts JE, Sandor GG (2013) Noninvasive assessment of vascular function and hydraulic power and efficiency in pediatric Fontan patients. J Am Soc Echocardiogr 26:1221–1227
25. Tomkiewicz-Pajak L, Dziedzic-Oleksy H, Pajak J, Olszowska M, Kolcz J, Komar M, Podolec P (2014) Arterial stiffness in adult patients after Fontan procedure. Cardiovasc Ultrasound 12:15. doi:10.1186/1476-7120-12-15
26. Müller J, Ewert P, Hager A (2015) Increased aortic blood pressure augmentation in patients with congenital heart defects - A cross-sectional study in 1125 patients and 322 controls. Int J Cardiol 184:225–229
27. Bhat DP, Gupta P, Aggarwal S (2015) Elevated aortic augmentation index in children following Fontan palliation: evidence of stiffer arteries? Pediatr Cardiol 36:1232–1238
28. Khairy P, Fernandes SM, Mayer JE Jr, Triedman JK, Walsh EP, Lock JE et al (2008) Long-term survival, modes of death, and predictors of mortality in patients with Fontan surgery. Circulation 117:85–92
29. Ohuchi H, Hayama Y, Negishi J, Noritake K, Miyazaki A, Yamada O, Shiraishi I (in press) Impact of abnormal aortic size and stiffness on exercise physiology in patients after the Fontan operation. Int Heart J (in press)
30. Ntsinjana HN, Biglino G, Capelli C, Tann O, Giardini A, Derrick G, Schievano S, Taylor AM (2013) Aortic arch shape is not associated with hypertensive response to exercise in patients with repaired congenital heart diseases. J Cardiovasc Magn Reson 15:101
31. Kojima T, Kuwata S, Kurishima C, Iwamoto Y, Saiki H, Ishido H, Masutani S, Senzaki H (2014) Aortic root dilatation and aortic stiffness in patients with single ventricular circulation. Circ J 78:2507–2511
32. Jin SM, Noh CI, Bae EJ, Choi JY, Yun YS (2007) Impaired vascular function in patients with Fontan circulation. Int J Cardiol 120:221–226
33. Ferreira I, Boreham CA, Twisk JW, Gallagher AM, Young IS, Murray LJ et al (2007) Clustering of metabolic syndrome risk factors and arterial stiffness in young adults: the Northern Ireland Young Hearts Project. J Hypertens 25:1009–1020
34. Vasan RS, Sullivan LM, Roubenoff R, Dinarello CA, Harris T, Benjamin EJ et al (2003) Inflammatory markers and risk of heart failure in elderly subjects without prior myocardial infarction: the Framingham Heart Study. Circulation 107:1486–1491
35. Egan M, Phillips A, Cook SC (2009) Aortic dissection in the adult Fontan with aortic root enlargement. Pediatr Cardiol 30:562–563
36. Saiki H, Kurishima C, Masutani S, Senzaki H (2014) Cerebral circulation in patients with Fontan circulation: assessment by carotid arterial wave intensity and stiffness. Ann Thorac Surg 97:1394–1399

Chapter 21
Future Research Projects on Aortopathy in Congenital Heart Anomalies

Masaru Miura

Abstract Several issues need to be resolved by future clinical research in aortopathy in the context of congenital heart diseases. Epidemiological issues include the incidence not only of aortic dilatation but also of cardiac events such as aortic dissection, heart failure, ischemic heart diseases, and death in the long term. Determining the etiology of congenital aortopathy requires clarification of pathologic, hemodynamic, and genetic factors related to aortic dilatation, as well as the interactions of these factors resulting in decreased elasticity and increased stiffness. Diagnostic issues include the definition of aortic diameter for dilatation and the evaluation of cardiovascular function using echocardiography and magnetic resonance angiography. Issues in therapy which need to be addressed include the use of randomized controlled trials to determine which medications are effective and safe for suppressing the progression of aortic dilatation and establishment of indications for surgical intervention to prevent cardiac events. These issues are ongoing concerns in clinical research and are garnering increasing interest as burgeoning topics still in need of reliable evidence and adequate research protocols. As an actual example of an ongoing prospective study, I introduce here a prospective cohort study design of aortopathy in adults with tetralogy of Fallot after corrective surgery.

Keywords Clinical research • Evidence • Prospective study

21.1 Introduction

Aortopathy occurs in several congenital heart diseases such as tetralogy of Fallot (TOF), transposition of the great arteries, coarctation of the aorta, persistent truncus arteriosus, single ventricle, hypoplastic left heart syndrome, and bicuspid aortic valve disease [1]. These diseases exhibit ongoing dilatation of the aortic root associated with reduced aortic elasticity, resulting in aortic regurgitation, left

M. Miura, M.D., Ph.D. (✉)
Division of Cardiology, Tokyo Metropolitan Children's Medical Center, 2-8-29 Musashidai, Fuchu, Tokyo 183-8561, Japan
e-mail: masaru_miura@tmhp.jp

K. Niwa, H. Kaemmerer (eds.), *Aortopathy*, DOI 10.1007/978-4-431-56071-5_21

ventricular failure, and, in rare cases, rupture of the aortic aneurysm and aortic dissection.

There is still a paucity of evidence pertaining to aortopathy in congenital heart diseases based on prospective clinical studies. Aortopathy is a recent recognized clinical entity, and its study is still in its infancy. Further, the number of patients with congenital heart diseases is small compared with those with acquired cardiac diseases, and the anatomical structure and hemodynamic status are various, resulting in difficulty in collecting sufficient numbers of homogeneous subjects. Finally, there are at present relatively modest numbers of cardiac events such as reoperation, aortic dissection, and death, although their occurrence is bound to increase in future years with the progressive aging of the population. Herein, I introduce an ongoing prospective cohort study of aortopathy in adults with TOF following corrective surgery.

21.2 Research Project in Aortopathy in Adults with TOF

21.2.1 Background

As described in previous sections, tetralogy of Fallot (TOF) is representative for congenital heart diseases causing aortopathy. According to studies in North America and Europe [2–5], the prevalence of aortic dilatation ranges widely from 7 to 51 % and is approximately 15 % in adolescents and adults with TOF. The prevalence of moderate to severe aortic regurgitation is reportedly 4–13 %. However, there is an absence of information for Asian countries. Further, because most of these reports are retrospective cross-sectional studies, time-dependent changes in aortic dilatation and the incidence of cardiac events in the long term are yet unknown.

Proposed mechanisms of aortic dilatation in TOF are complex and involve pathological [6, 7], hemodynamic [2, 8, 9], and genetic factors [10–12]. Thereby, reduced aortic elasticity and increased aortic rigidity lead to aortopathy [13–15]. Because of similarities to Marfan syndrome, beta-blockers are sometimes administered to patients with aortic dilatation. Angiotensin-converting enzyme (ACE) inhibitors and angiotensin II receptor blockers (ARB) are also used; however, it is also unclear if any medical treatments can suppress progressive aortic dilatation in patients with TOF.

21.2.2 Preliminary Questionnaire and Objective of the Prospective Cohort Study

In 2013, we performed a survey in institutions affiliated with the Japanese Society for Adult Congenital Heart Disease to investigate the current status of aortic dilatation in adults with TOF following corrective surgery. Additionally, we asked about the testing equipment used, willingness to participate in a prospective study, and the possible number of recruits. The number of patients indicated by the responses obtained from 45 institutions was 2197. Aortic dilatation was present in 134 (6.1 %) and moderate to severe aortic regurgitation in 141 (6.4 %).

On the basis of these results, we planned a new study entitled "The Prospective Cohort Research in Aortic Root Dilatation and Non-elasticity after Surgical Repair in Adults with TOF (TRANSIT)," registered with the University Hospital Medical Information Network clinical trial registry as number UMIN000017555. TRANSIT is an ongoing multicenter prospective observational cohort study, the first longitudinal examination of aortic dilatation in patients with TOF. The primary objective is to clarify time-dependent changes in aortic root diameters, and the secondary objective is to determine the incidence of aortic dilatation at the start and end of study, evaluate aortic stiffness, and determine the effects of medication.

21.2.3 Methods

Inclusion criteria for TRANSIT were an age of 20 years or older at registration, the presence of TOF including pulmonary atresia, and a history of corrective surgery before 10 years of age. Exclusion criteria were the presence of a double outlet right ventricle and the presence of other diseases causing aortic dilatation such as bicuspid aortic valve, coarctation of aorta, and Marfan syndrome. The registration period is from March 2015 to February 2018, with the following information collected at registration: birth month, gender, basic diagnosis, the presence of a residual ventricular septal defect, the presence of a left or right aortic arch, any chromosomal anomaly, the timing and type of operation undergone including reoperation, the presence and number of cardiac catheterizations, NYHA classification, medication, and history of pregnancy and delivery for women. The target sample size was 100 patients based on the preliminary survey and feasibility.

The time schedule is shown in Fig. 21.1. Physical measurements and medical tests including echocardiography are performed within 1 year of registration. In the first and the second year after commencement of the study, only clinical information was collected. In the third year, medical tests including echocardiography are performed again. The ankle-brachial index and pulse wave velocity test are performed when available. For echocardiographic assessments, moving images of the left ventricle from the long-axis view are anonymously recorded on disks and then sent to the data center for analysis to determine aortic root diameter, the main

Fig. 21.1 The time schedule for "TRANSIT" study

1 yr. Allowable period ±12 wk.

	Entry	Start	Yr. 1	Yr. 2	Yr. 3
Clinical information	●		●	●	●
Physical measurements		●			●
Echocardiography		●			●
Chest radiography		●			●
Electrocardiography		●			●
Blood test		●			●
ABI / PWV*		○			○

* For institutions where ankle brachial index (ABI) and pulse wave velocity (PWV) testing is available

target of measurement. Aortic diameter is measured using the leading-edge technique, and dilatation is defined when the actual value is 40 mm or larger or the ratio of the actual to expected value is over 1.5 times at the sinus of Valsalva and the sino-tubular junction. Left ventricular dimensions and wall thickness, trans-mitral flow pattern, mitral annulus velocity, aortic regurgitation, pulmonary stenosis, and pulmonary regurgitation are measured at each institution.

21.2.4 Outcome and Clinical Significance

The primary outcome is the time-dependent change in aortic root diameter, specifically, the enlargement rate per year in the diameter of the sinus of Valsalva and the sino-tubular junction. Secondary outcomes are the incidence of aortic dilatation at the start and end of the study and the risk factors, the evaluation of aortic stiffness based on pulse wave velocity, and the effect of medications, especially beta-blockers, ACE inhibitor, and ARB.

The clinical significance of the study is to clarify the incidence of, and changes in, aortic dilatation in adults with TOF. Incidentally to the main aims of this study, we may be able to clarify better the factors associated with aortic dilatation, such as aortic stiffness and the effects of medication. We hope to promote collaboration between pediatric cardiologists and internal cardiologists and thereby promote multicenter studies of adult congenital heart disease.

21.3 Future Themes of Research in Aortopathy

21.3.1 Epidemiological Issues

Several issues pertaining to aortopathy among patients with congenital heart diseases need to be resolved by clinical research (Table 21.1). The incidence and time-dependent changes in aortopathy, especially with regard to the triggered cardiac events including aortic regurgitation, heart failure, ischemic heart diseases, operation, aortic dissection, and death, are not accurately known. Most previous studies [2–5, 16–18] were retrospectively performed in a single institution, leading to distortion of data due to selection and information biases; *accordingly multi-institutional prospective studies should be performed.* The natural course of aortopathy accompanied by cardiac events, for example, aortic dissection [19], over a patient's lifetime remains a significant theme in research.

21.3.2 Etiological Issues

The etiology of aortopathy is complex, probably due to the involvement of multiple related factors and their interactions; hence the process of determining the etiology comprises multiple steps. At first, light microscopic examinations with various stains showed histological abnormalities including fibrosis, cystic medial necrosis, and elastic fragmentation in the aortic wall [6, 7]. To date few studies have used immunohistochemical or molecular-genetic pathological methods; thus, these methods may be encouraging for new studies. When patients undergo reoperation,

Table 21.1 Themes in clinical research on aortopathy

Epidemiology
Incidence of aortic dilatation
Occurrence of cardiac events: aortic dissection, heart
failure, ischemic heart disease, and death
Etiology
Pathology
Hemodynamics and cardiovascular function
Genetics
Surgical procedure
Diagnosis
Echocardiography
Magnetic resonance angiography
Treatment
Medication such as beta-blockers, angiotensin converting
Enzyme inhibitors and angiotensin receptor blockers
Surgical intervention

the biopsied tissue of the aorta can be collected intraoperatively and subjected to detailed pathological examination. Second, hemodynamic factors and cardiovascular function should be investigated, because volume overload [2, 8, 9] and decreased elasticity with increased stiffness [13–15] are associated with aortopathy. Third, although mutations and polymorphisms of *fibrillin-1* and *matrix metalloproteinase-3 and matrix metalloproteinase-9* [10, 11] were demonstrated in patients with aortopathy, genetic research in this domain remains insufficient. Comprehensive genetic analysis and epigenetic studies taking into account environmental factors such as smoking, diet, and stress provide vistas for further productive research. *Fourth, the relation of surgical methods to aortopathy is an attractive research theme, for example, pulmonary artery banding before arterial switch operation [20] and the procedure of Ross operation [21].*

21.3.3 Diagnostic Issues

Echocardiography is essential for research in aortopathy, because aortic dilatation is usually diagnosed on the basis of its findings. The diameter of the sinus of Valsalva and the sino-tubular junction may be measured using the inner edge-to-inner edge technique at mid-systole [22], but in most previous reports [2–5], these measurements were taken using the leading-edge technique at end-diastole [23, 24]. Although the definition of aortic dilatation varies from study to study, the optimal measurement site is the sinus of Valsalva or the sino-tubular junction, with the diameter being the actual diameter adjusted for the body surface area or z-score. A common agreement on a definition of aortopathy is desirable, inter alia, for the purpose of comparing studies.

As aortopathy induces left ventricular hypertrophy and dysfunction, research using techniques such as the speckle tracking method and three-dimensional echocardiography will doubtless prove helpful. Magnetic resonance angiography also plays an important role in clinical practice as well as in research for the assessment not only of aortic dilatation but also of aortic regurgitation, ventricular hypertrophy, and cardiac dysfunction.

21.3.4 Therapeutic Issues

The research on medical treatment is clinically important to *establish the administration criteria and* means of suppressing the progression of aortic dilatation. *The administration criteria should be decided on the basis of analysis of risk factors for aortopathy in each disease.* As beta-blockers, ACE inhibitors, ARB, and other medications have been experimentally used without evidence, their effectiveness and safety should be confirmed by clinical trials. In particular, ARB is thought to inhibit the activity of transforming growth factor (TGF)-beta related to aortic degeneration and dilatation, holding out the possibility of an effective drug intervention for aortopathy.

Indications for surgical intervention including aortic valve replacement, aortoplasty, and ascending aorta replacement for TOF are described as aortic root enlargement of at least 55 mm in diameter, significant aortic regurgitation associated with symptoms, and progressive left ventricular systolic dysfunction [25]; however, the evidence has not been established. *Further studies on reoperation for aortopathy are required* to prevent aortic dissection and cardiac death in the long term. Transcatheter aortic valve implantation may be indicated for aortic regurgitation without significant aortic dilatation.

21.3.5 Design and Protocol of Clinical Research

Previous retrospective studies have addressed the actual situation of aortopathy in adults with congenital heart disease but not suitable lifelong management based on evidence. Thus, long-term prospective cohort studies need to be conducted to resolve this issue. Randomized controlled trials to test the efficacy of drugs, especially for conditions like Marfan syndrome, need to be conducted. Clinical researchers need to recognize that the greatest contributing factors to aortopathy in previous reports were surrogate endpoints and the occurrence of cardiac events such as reoperation, aortic dissection, heart failure, ischemic heart disease, and death is the true endpoints.

Because the number of adults with congenital heart disease is limited, multi-institutional collaborative research is desirable to collect the requisite number of subjects. Besides the collection of subjects, the system can eliminate selection, information, and even ethnic bias, if performed nationwide. Such high-quality research projects require a clinical research center allowing the collaboration of clinical research coordinators, data managers, system engineers, and biostatisticians. It is also important to transit children and adolescents from pediatric units to internal medicine units for long-term follow-up.

In sum, clinical research on aortopathy in the context of congenital heart diseases is a burgeoning area of study where much work remains to establish the evidence and protocols for future clinical research.

References

1. Niwa K. (2013) Aortopathy in congenital heart disease in adults: aortic dilatation with decreased aortic elasticity that impacts negatively on left ventricular function. Korean Circ J 43:215–220
2. Niwa K, Siu SC, Webb GD et al (2002) Progressive aortic root dilatation in adults late after repair of tetralogy of Fallot. Circulation 106:1374–1378

3. Nagy CD, Alejo DE, Corretti MC et al (2013) Tetralogy of Fallot and aortic root dilation: a long-term outlook. Pediatr Cardiol 34:809–816
4. Mongeon FP, Gurvitz MZ, Broberg CS et al (2013) Aortic root dilatation in adults with surgically repaired tetralogy of Fallot: a multicenter cross-sectional study. Circulation 127:172–179
5. Cruz C, Pinhoa T, Lebreiroa A et al (2013) Echocardiographic assessment of aortic root dilatation in adult patients after tetralogy of Fallot repair. Rev Port Cardiol 32:477–482
6. Niwa K, Perloff JK, Bhuta SM et al (2001) Structural abnormalities of great arterial walls in congenital heart disease: light and electron microscopic analyses. Circulation 103:393–400
7. Tan JL, Davlouros PA, McCarthy KP et al (2005) Intrinsic histological abnormalities of aortic root and ascending aorta in tetralogy of Fallot: evidence of causative mechanism for aortic dilatation and aortopathy. Circulation 112:961–968
8. François K, Creytens D, De Groote K et al (2014) Analysis of the aortic root in patients with tetralogy of Fallot undergoing early repair: form follows function. J Thorac Cardiovasc Surg 148:1555–1559
9. Seki M, Kurishima C, Kawasaki H et al (2012) Aortic stiffness and aortic dilation in infants and children with tetralogy of Fallot before corrective surgery: evidence for intrinsically abnormal aortic mechanical property. Eur J Cardiothorac Surg 41:277–282
10. Chowdhury UK, Mishra AK, Balakrishnan P et al (2008) Role of fibrillin-1 genetic mutations and polymorphism in aortic dilatation in patients undergoing intracardiac repair of tetralogy of Fallot. J Thorac Cardiovasc Surg 136:757–766
11. Cheung YF, Hong WJ, Chan KW et al (2011) Modulating effects of matrix metalloproteinase-3 and -9 polymorphisms on aortic stiffness and aortic root dilation in patients after tetralogy of Fallot repair. Int J Cardiol 151:214–217
12. John AS, Rychik J, Khan M et al (2014) 22q11.2 deletion syndrome as a risk factor for aortic root dilation in tetralogy of Fallot. Cardiol Young 24:303–310
13. Senzaki H, Iwamoto Y, Ishido H et al (2008) Arterial haemodynamics in patients after repair of tetralogy of Fallot: influence on left ventricular after load and aortic dilatation. Heart 94:70–74
14. Chong WY, Wong WH, Chiu CS et al (2006) Aortic root dilation and aortic elastic properties in children after repair of tetralogy of Fallot. Am J Cardiol 97:905–909
15. Christensen JT, Lu JC, Donohue J et al (2014) Relation of aortic stiffness and strain by cardiovascular magnetic resonance imaging to age in repaired tetralogy of Fallot. Am J Cardiol 113:1031–1035
16. van der Bom T, van der Palen RL, Bouma BJ et al (2014) Persistent neo-aortic growth during adulthood in patients after an arterial switch operation. Heart 100:1360–1365
17. Schwartz ML, Gauvreau K, del Nido P, et al. (2004) Long-term predictors of aortic root dilation and aortic regurgitation after arterial switch operation. Circulation 110 (11 Suppl 1):II 128–32
18. Cohen MS, Marino BS, McElhinney DB et al (2003) Neo-aortic root dilation and valve regurgitation up to 21 years after stage reconstruction for hypoplastic left heart syndrome. J Am Coll Cardiol 42:533–540
19. Shamszad P, Barnes JN, Morris SA (2014) Aortic dissection in hospitalized children and young adults: a multiinstitutional study. Congenit Heart Dis 9:54–62
20. McMahon CJ, Ravekes WJ, Smith EO et al (2004) Risk factors for neo-aortic root enlargement and aortic regurgitation following arterial switch operation. Pediatr Cardiol 25:329–335
21. Skillington PD, Mokhles MM, Takkenberg JJ et al (2015) The Ross procedure using autologous support of the pulmonary autograft: techniques and late results. J Thorac Cardiovasc Surg 149(2 Suppl):S46–S52
22. Lopez L, Colan SD, Frommelt PC et al (2010) Recommendations for quantification methods during the performance of a pediatric echocardiogram: a report from the Pediatric Measurements Writing Group of the American Society of Echocardiography Pediatric and Congenital Heart Disease Council. J Am Soc Echocardiogr 23:465–495

23. Roman MJ, Devereux RB, Kramer Fox R et al (1989) Two-dimensional echocardiographic aortic root dimensions in normal children and adults. Am J Cardiol 64:507–512
24. Devereux RB, de Simone G, Arnett DK et al (2012) Normal limits in relation to age, body size and gender of two-dimensional echocardiographic aortic root dimensions in persons $\geq$15 years of age. Am J Cardiol 110:1189–1194
25. Silversides CK, Kiess M, Beauchesne L et al (2010) Canadian Cardiovascular Society 2009 Consensus Conference on the management of adults with congenital heart disease: outflow tract obstruction, coarctation of the aorta, tetralogy of Fallot, Ebstein anomaly and Marfan's syndrome. Can J Cardiol 26:e80–e97

MIX
Papier aus verantwortungsvollen Quellen
Paper from responsible sources
FSC® C105338

If you have any concerns about our products,
you can contact us on
ProductSafety@springernature.com

In case Publisher is established outside the EU,
the EU authorized representative is:
Springer Nature Customer Service Center GmbH
Europaplatz 3, 69115 Heidelberg, Germany

Printed by Libri Plureos GmbH
in Hamburg, Germany